CLINICAL GUIDE TO CARE PLANNING
Data ⇒ Diagnosis

Leslie D. Atkinson, R.N., M.S.N.
Nursing Program
Normandale Community College
Bloomington, Minnesota

Mary Ellen Murray, Ph.D., R.N.
Adjunct Assistant Research Scientist
Center for Nursing Research
School of Nursing
University of Michigan
Ann Arbor, Michigan

D1211144

McGRAW-HILL, INC.
Health Professions Division
New York   St. Louis   San Francisco
Auckland   Bogotá   Caracas   Lisbon   London
Madrid   Mexico City   Milan   Montreal   New Delhi
San Juan   Singapore   Sydney   Tokyo   Toronto

To Peter
To Craig
To our friendship

CLINICAL GUIDE TO CARE PLANNING
DATA ⇒ DIAGNOSIS

The clinical pathway examples, pages 460–481, are reproduced with the kind permission of the Battle Creek Health System, Battle Creek, Michigan.

1 2 3 4 5 6 7 8 9 0   DOCDOC   98765

ISBN 0-07-105466-9

This book was set in Times Roman by Keyword Publishing Services, Ltd.
The editors were Gail Gavert and Lester A. Sheinis;
the production supervisor was Clara B. Stanley;
the text and cover designer was Karen Quigley.
R. R. Donnelley & Sons Company was printer and binder.

This book is printed on acid-free paper.

Library of Congress Cataloging-in-Publication Data

Atkinson, Leslie D.
    Clinical guide to care planning: data ⇒ diagnosis/Leslie D. Atkinson,
    Mary Ellen Murray.
        p.   cm.
    Includes bibliographical references and index.
    ISBN 0-07-105466-9
    1. Nursing assessment. 2. Nursing care plans. 3. Nursing diagnosis.
I. Murray, Mary Ellen. II. Title.
    [DNLM: 1. Nursing Assessment. 2. Patient Care Planning. WY 100
A876c 1995]
RT46.A89   1995
610.73—dc20
DNLM/DLC
for Library of Congress   94–34820

Contents

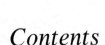

Preface

Clinical Guide to Care Planning: Data ⇒ Diagnosis is a "user-friendly text" that assists students in making accurate nursing diagnoses and planning client care. While we realize that many excellent books have been published on this subject, it has been our experience that students continue to have difficulty using them. Most texts seem to skip the key step that experienced nurses take without even being aware of it: They continuously match client data to data in their experience base of nursing diagnoses. This allows them to make nursing diagnoses rapidly and accurately. Lacking this experience base, the student struggles to match the data to the nursing diagnosis. This is why we developed our unique tool, the Data ⇒ Diagnosis Matching Guide. The guide condenses all related NANDA diagnoses and defining characteristics in a problem area into one or two pages. The student can then scan all data associated with several similar diagnoses to find the best data match.

The text provides 22 Focused Assessment Guides for problem areas. No general nursing assessment is included because most health care facilities or schools of nursing prefer students to use their own forms for a general nursing assessment. Each Focused Assessment Guide in this text was developed from the defining characteristics of the NANDA nursing diagnoses grouped by the authors into a problem area. Each Data ⇒ Diagnosis Matching Guide corresponds to a Focused Assessment Guide. This helps the student collect data to differentiate between related NANDA nursing diagnoses.

The other unique features of this text include:

■ specific examples of nursing diagnostic statements in two formats, general client outcomes with specific examples, general and specific nursing interventions, and examples of evaluative statements for each of the 109 NANDA approved nursing diagnoses

- an example of care planning for three nursing diagnoses from data collection through outcome evaluation, including an abbreviated nursing care plan
- a practice exercise to teach the diagnostic process and use of the Data ⇒ Diagnosis Matching Guide
- information and normal findings for physical problem areas to assist students in recognizing abnormal client data
- list of key terms associated with the nursing diagnosis to help students find additional interventions and rationales in their nursing fundamentals and/or medical-surgical nursing texts
- three case management examples using fourteen nursing diagnoses

We wish to thank Virginia E. Keck, Ph.D., R.N. (former Vice President, Nursing) and the care managers of the Battle Creek Health System, Kathleen Allen, B.S.N., R.N., Harriett DeRose, M.P.A., R.N., Rosalind Proos, M.S., R.N., and Deborah Buford, B.S.N., R.N., for their progressive work in development of the clinical pathways reproduced in the Appendix of this text.

As always, we continue to learn and grow in our understanding of nursing and the nursing process from the struggles of our students. We welcome comments, questions, and suggestions from students and educators using this text. Tell us what works—and what doesn't! Please write to

L. D. Atkinson
Nursing Program
Normandale Community College
9700 France Avenue South
Bloomington, Minnesota 55431

Acknowledgment: Nursing diagnoses, defining characteristics, or related factors are used with permission: North American Nursing Diagnosis Association (1992). *NANDA Nursing Diagnoses: Definitions and Classifications, 1992–1993.* Philadelphia: NANDA.

CLINICAL GUIDE TO CARE PLANNING

TO CARE PLANNING

Data ⇒ Diagnosis

Introduction to the Nursing Process and Care Planning

It is a no good, very bad week! As a student in nursing, life is tough. Tuition goes up each year, along with your weight, and your check book has taught you how to work with negative numbers. But those clinical experiences are real headbangers. Talk about stress! Your instructor gives you some patient's name, age, sex, and medical diagnosis and the rest is up to you. You are then expected to go into the room and be therapeutic with this stranger. By the way, the care plan detailing your therapeutic interventions is due tomorrow. Where do you begin? What are you supposed to be doing?

Not to worry! Help is on the way and you are holding it in your hand. Yes, that's right. A book on nursing diagnoses and care planning is going to get you through this and it should even help you to help the patient. Of course if you choose not to finish reading this introduction you will probably do fine on your own. NOT!

This is the bare bones of what is involved in making nursing diagnoses and care planning:

NURSING

First there is nursing:

Nursing is the diagnosis and treatment of human responses to actual or potential health problems (American Nurses Association; ANA 1980, 9).

1

This means nurses do not treat diseases such as cancer but they do treat the response clients have to the cancer and its treatment, such as nausea, inadequate nutrition, pain, anxiety, anticipatory grieving, and body image disturbances. Areas for nursing care involve (ANA 1991, 1):

___ disease or injury prevention
___ health promotion
___ health restoration
___ health maintenance

THE NURSING PROCESS

Then there is the Nursing Process: this is a problem-solving *process* applied to nursing and client care. It is the way you think as a nurse. The client has health care problems that nursing can prevent, lessen, or remedy. The nurse uses the nursing process to

___ identify client's health-related problems
___ select outcomes demonstrating improved health and functioning
___ plan what to do to achieve those outcomes
___ assist the client to carry out the plan
___ evaluate whether outcomes were achieved

| Nursing process | = | Assess Client | + | Diagnose Problems | + | Identify Outcomes | + | Plan and Implement Interventions | + | Evaluate Outcomes |

The nursing process results in a *product* called a nursing care plan. This is a guide for providing care to an individual client and it usually includes nursing diagnoses, expected client outcomes, and nursing interventions and treatments.

The first step in the nursing process is **assessment** of the client. The nurse collects data indicating the presence of current problems or the risk of problems developing. The client, the family, the chart, the client's nurse and other health care professionals are sources for this information. Clients are the major source of data, which are obtained by talking with them, observation, and examination.

Assessment (data collection	=	Observation of client	+	Interview of client, family, nurses	+	Examination of client	+	Chart Review

The next step in the nursing process is **diagnosing**. This is the process of analyzing data from the client and deciding if it represents a health problem appropriate for nursing intervention. The stated client problem is a **nursing diagnosis**.

Diagnosing (a process)	=	Analysis of client data	+	Problem Identification (broad area)	+	Formulation of the Nursing Diagnosis: 1. Select NANDA dx label 2. Individualize by including related factors

NURSING DIAGNOSES

A nursing diagnosis is

... a clinical judgement about the client's response to actual or potential health conditions or needs. Diagnoses provide the basis for determination of a plan of care to achieve expected outcomes (ANA 1991, 7).

... a clinical judgement about individual, family, or community responses to actual and potential health problems/life processes. Nursing diagnoses provide the basis for selection of nursing interventions to achieve outcomes for which the nurse is accountable (NANDA 1992, 83).

In 1973 a group of nurses first met to begin to identify, develop, and classify nursing diagnoses. This was the beginning of the North American Nursing Diagnosis Association (NANDA). Each NANDA diagnosis usually has a *definition, defining characteristics,* which are the clinical cues, signs and symptoms of the problem, and *related factors,*

factors that have some consistent relationship to the diagnosis. Related factors may precede the problem, contribute to the development and/or maintenance of the problem, or directly cause the problem (etiology). There are three types of defining characteristics (NANDA 1992, 10):

Critical: these signs/symptoms *must* be present in the client to make this diagnosis

Major: these signs/symptoms are present in 80–100% of clients with this diagnosis

Minor: these supporting signs/symptoms are present in 50–79% of clients with this diagnosis and provide supporting evidence for the diagnosis but may not be present

Diagnosing is a process of matching the client's data to the definition, defining characteristics, and related factors listed for NANDA nursing diagnoses. There are currently 109 NANDA approved nursing diagnoses. Since you cannot compare a client's data to each of the 109 NANDA diagnoses, you must narrow your search. Client data is first analyzed for deviations from normal or expected results which might indicate a problem or risk of a problem developing. This is *data analysis.*

This abnormal or high risk data is then grouped into separate, broad problem areas, such as problems with bowel function, pain problems, or nutrition problems. This is *problem identification.*

After problem identification, the nurse *formulates a nursing diagnosis.* This involves two activities. First the client data is matched to the NANDA diagnoses and the diagnosis with the best match is selected. Second, the NANDA diagnosis selected is individualized by adding the related factors, signs, and symptoms from the client's data base.

To select a NANDA diagnosis, the client data grouped under a broad problem area are compared to the definitions, defining characteristics, and related factors of the NANDA diagnoses associated with that problem area. For example, client data may indicate a problem in the broad area of urinary functioning: unrelieved sensation of a full bladder and urge to void, palpable bladder distension, voiding every hour or less in amounts of 50–100 mL. These data would be compared to the definitions and defining characteristics of the seven NANDA diagnoses associated with urine function: Altered Urinary Elimination, Stress Incontinence, Reflex Incontinence, Urge Incontinence, Functional Incontinence, Total Incontinence, and Urinary Retention. The NANDA diagnosis with the best match to the client's data is selected. The example of urinary data above best matches the definition and defining characteristics of Urinary Retention.

After matching the client data to a NANDA diagnosis, the diagnostic label is individualized by including the related factors for this client. In a three-part nursing diagnostic statement, the defining characteristics being experienced by this client are also included for additional individualization. For example, the NANDA diagnostic label, Urinary Retention, could be individualized into the nursing diagnosis, urinary retention related to effects of spinal anesthesia and swelling around urinary meatus as evidenced by distended bladder, small frequent voidings, and constant urge to void.

The two-part format for writing the nursing diagnosis includes the NANDA diagnostic label and the related factors (etiology) for a specific client.

Individualized nursing diagnosis	=	Client problem (NANDA diagnostic label)	+	Causes if known/ etiology ("related to …")

The PES format is a three-part format that includes the NANDA diagnostic label, the related factors for a specific client, and the defining characteristics presented by that client and used to make the nursing diagnosis.

Individualized nursing diagnosis	=	P Client Problem (NANDA dx label) +	+	E Cause/Etiology (related to …) +	+	S Signs/Symptoms (as evidenced by)

Often clients do not have actual, existing problems but they are likely to develop problems because of the presence of risk factors.

HIGH RISK NURSING DIAGNOSES

Risk factors are

> ... environmental, physiological, psychological, genetic, or chemical elements that increase the vulnerability of an individual, family or community to an unhealthy event (NANDA 1992, 84).

High risk nursing diagnoses are made when risk factors are identified in a client's data base. Nursing interventions are then selected to reduce or eliminate the risk factors and prevent the problem from occurring. These high risk nursing diagnoses are written in a two-part form using the NANDA diagnostic label and the client's risk factors. For example, High Risk for Activity Intolerance related to 2 weeks on bed rest, poor nutrition, and general muscle weakness.

| High risk nursing diagnosis | = | Potential client problem (NANDA dx label) "high risk for ..." | + | Client's risk factors + "related to ..." |

There are also nursing diagnoses in the NANDA list that do not seem like problems. These are wellness nursing diagnoses.

WELLNESS NURSING DIAGNOSES

A wellness nursing diagnosis describes ... human responses to levels of wellness in an individual, family, or community that have a potential for enhancement to a higher state (NANDA 1992, 84).

The NANDA wellness diagnoses include Health-seeking Behaviors, Family Coping: Potential for Growth, and Effective Breast-feeding. The related factors in a wellness nursing diagnostic statement identify factors indicating a client's readiness to move toward health promotion and/or factors that make success likely. For example, a wellness diagnostic statement for Effective Breast-feeding could be individualized and written as Effective breast-feeding related to prenatal and postpartum learning about breast-feeding, normal breast structure, full-term healthy newborn, strong family support system for breast-feeding.

After assessing and diagnosing, **identifying client outcomes** is the next step in the nursing process.

CLIENT OUTCOMES

Client outcomes are

> ... the desired result of nursing care; that which you hope to achieve with your client and which shows evidence that the problem identified in the nursing diagnosis has been prevented, remedied, or lessened (Murray, Atkinson, 1994, 66)

> ... measurable, expected, client-focused goals (ANA 1991, 7).

If the nursing diagnosis is pain, the outcome shows a reduction, elimination or prevention of pain; if the diagnosis is altered mobility, the outcome shows an improvement in mobility. An outcome statement includes several components:

$$\frac{\text{Client}}{\text{Outcome}} = \frac{\text{Client}}{\text{Behavior}} + \frac{\text{Criterion}}{\text{of Performance}} + \frac{\text{Time}}{\text{Frame}} + \frac{\text{Conditions}}{\text{(if needed)}}$$

Example:

Diagnosis: Hypothermia related to newborn delivery in cool room, evaporation from wet skin surfaces.

Outcome: Newborn's temperature to rise to 98°F (37°C) rectally or above within 1 hour of placement under overhead warmer.

The *client behavior* is an observable activity or measurement the client will demonstrate/achieve at some future time, e.g., drink, walk, report, achievement of specific vital signs/lab values. The behavior/measurement shows improvement in the problem identified in the nursing diagnosis. When developing outcomes, review the client's signs and symptoms associated with the diagnosis. Choose outcome behaviors that show reduction or elimination of these problematic signs and symptoms. In the example above, the behavior is the newborn's rise in temperature.

The *criterion of performance* is a stated level or value for the behavior selected in the outcome. It clarifies how well the behavior must be done to achieve the outcome, e.g., 1500 mL of fluids, less than 230 lb, one block, BP less than 150/100, temperature 97°F (36°C). In the example above, the criterion of performance is a rectal temperature of 98°F (37°C) or higher.

The *time frame* is a realistic estimate of how long the client should need to achieve the outcome behavior at the level specified, e.g., by 12:00 midnight, in two weeks, by discharge, within 30 minutes, in 4 hours. From the example above, the time frame is 1 hour.

The *condition* is added to the outcome statement if it is essential for achievement of the outcome. If it is not essential it is left out. In the example above, the condition under which this behavior, the temperature rise, will occur is under the overhead warmer.

PLANNING NURSING INTERVENTIONS

Planning nursing interventions is the next step in the nursing process. It involves selecting activities to perform with and for the client to achieve the identified outcomes. By achieving the intended outcomes, the client can prevent, reduce, or eliminate the diagnosed problems. The nurse tries to select realistic interventions based on the client's abilities and resources. The interventions are chosen to

___ achieve the outcomes at the level and time specified
___ reduce, eliminate, or cope with the client's problematic signs and symptoms
___ reduce, eliminate, treat or compensate for the client's causative, "related to," factors in the diagnostic statement

EVALUATION

Evaluation is the final step in the nursing process. It is

... the process of determining both the client's progress toward the attainment of expected outcomes and the effectiveness of nursing care (ANA 1991, 7).

Evaluation occurs continuously as the nurse identifies the client's response to interventions. The nurse and client decide whether the outcomes were achieved and what further interventions and treatments are needed to prevent, reduce, or eliminate the diagnosed problem. The nurse reviews the entire plan of care as the client's condition changes to make sure all diagnoses, outcomes, and interventions are still appropriate. New diagnoses are made as needed and resolved diagnoses are eliminated from the plan of care. When evaluating an outcome the nurse documents two parts in the client's chart.

Outcome Evaluation	=	Outcome met, Partially met, or Not met	+	Actual Client Behavior as Evidence

Examples:

Outcome met: Newborn's temperature is 98.4°F (36.9°C) rectally after 1 hour under the warmer.
Outcome not met: Newborn's temperature is 97.2°F (36.2°C) rectally after 1 hour under the warmer.

CASE MANAGEMENT

Case management is an expanded version of the nursing process that coordinates the efforts of physicians, nurses, physical therapists, dieticians, social service professionals, and others to treat client health problems. Case management is a health care delivery system organized using medical diagnostic groups (DRGs). This system is designed to provide quality client care in a cost-effective manner. It focuses on achievement of clinical outcomes. The nurse often assumes the case manager function, assuring coordination of a client's care by an interdisciplinary team.

A *case management plan* is developed for common DRGs to minimize delays, avoid omissions, and provide clinical practice guidelines for interventions and treatments. The case management plan has been called a second generation nursing care plan. Case management plans outline clinical guidelines for managing approximately 75% of clients with the same DRG, such as total joint replacement, mastectomy, or congestive heart failure. The plans are developed by physicians, nurses, and other care providers working together and sharing their professional expertise in treating and caring for clients in specific DRGs. The resulting plans are based on data, treatments, and responses from many clients with the same DRG rather than on data from an individual client. A case management plan includes

___ *admitting medical diagnosis (DRG)*
___ *nursing diagnoses (NANDA diagnostic labels)* experienced by a majority of clients with this medical diagnosis
___ *general client outcomes* for each nursing diagnosis on a daily time frame
___ *nursing interventions* specific to each nursing diagnosis (clinical/critical pathways most likely to achieve outcomes)
___ *interventions required of other health care professionals* on a daily time frame to achieve the outcomes and a timely discharge
___ *areas for individualizing the plan* for a specific client; blank area for additional nursing diagnoses

Examples of case management plans are in the Appendix.

HOW TO USE THIS BOOK

EVEN REAL NURSES NEED DIRECTIONS

Please read this section before using this text—it is guaranteed to save you time and grief. First complete the general nursing assessment form used by your school of nursing or health care facility. This will help you identify possible health-related nursing problems in broad areas such as bowel functioning, mobility, comfort/pain, and self-esteem. Now begin using this text. It has several sections which can be used sequentially or separately.

1. **Focused Assessment Guides:** specific questions to ask the client and family to clarify problems identified from the general nursing assessment

2. **Information and Normal Findings:** general information, normal values, and findings for physical problem areas/groups
3. **Data ⇒ Diagnosis Matching Guides:** a list of all NANDA diagonses dealing with a problem area is shown on one or two pages to help match data from the client to the definition and defining characteristics for a NANDA diagnosis
4. **General Outcomes and Interventions:** these apply to all or most of the nursing diagnoses listed in the Data ⇒ Diagnosis Matching Guide for a problem area such as pain, bowel, communication, or coping/adjustment
5. **Nursing Diagnosis Care Planning Guides:** individual care planning guides for each of the 109 NANDA nursing diagnoses; most guides include
___ Definition of diagnosis
___ Defining Characteristics (signs and symptoms)
___ Related Factors (cause/contributing factors/etiology)
___ Examples of individualized nursing diagnoses, client outcomes, interventions, and outcome evaluations for the NANDA diagnosis
___ Key index words to use in medical-surgical and fundamental nursing textbooks to locate other interventions and rationale for their use

6. **Case Management Plans:** plans for three example DRGs are located in the Appendix.

STEPS IN USING THIS BOOK

Step 1: In preparation for using this book, a general nursing assessment will need to be completed. Use the one provided by your school of nursing or health care facility. The general nursing assessment gives you examples of questions to ask and observations to make to rule problems in or out in broad physical and psychosocial areas. Avoid medical terminology which may not be understood by all clients. Forms vary greatly, but they usually ask about

___ client's normal pattern or behavior
___ effect of medical problem/treatment on functioning or behavior
___ coping strategies, compensation techniques, and outcomes

After completing the general nursing assessment for a problem area, such as respiratory/breathing function, you make a decision.

___ Yes, there is abnormal or unexpected data indicating a problem may be present in this area.

___ No, the data is all normal or expected and no problem is present.

If a problem is suggested by the data, you may proceed in one of two ways. Either ask the client the questions in this book's Focused Assessment Guide for that problem area then complete the general assessment, or do a complete general nursing assessment. Then turn to the Focused Assessment Guides for areas identified as possible problems.

Step 2: Use the Focused Assessment Guides to help you collect the data needed to clarify the problem. This additional data will enable you to differentiate between several related NANDA nursing diagnoses and provide direction for nursing interventions. The focused assessments in this book are more detailed than general nursing assessments and are compiled from the defining characteristics of NANDA nursing diagnoses grouped within problem areas. Use a Focused Assessment Guide only when a general nursing assessment gives you data suggesting a possible problem in an area. For example, if the client reports pain during the general nursing assessment, use the Pain Focused Assessment Guide to collect additional data. These data will help to differentiate between the nursing diagnoses: Acute Pain, Chronic Non-Malignant Pain, and Chronic Malignant Pain. There are Focused Assessment Guides for the following problem areas/groupings:

Physical Problem Areas
- Bowel
- Circulation
- Fluids/hydration
- Infant feeding/breast-feeding
- Mobility/activity
- Nutrition/eating

Psychosocial Problem Areas
- Communication/thinking/knowledge
- Coping/adjustment
- Family and growth/development
- Health management
- Roles/relationship

Physical Problem Areas
- Pain
- Physical safety/protection
- Respiratory/breathing
- Rest/sleep
- Self-care problems
- Sex/sexuality
- Skin/mucous membrane
- Temperature
- Urinary/voiding

Psychosocial Problem Areas
- Self-esteem
- Violence

The normals and information sections for the physical problem areas present information from physiology texts, medical-surgical textbooks, and fundamental nursing textbooks. Use this information to help identify abnormal or unexpected client data and to understand rationale for interventions.

Step 3: After completing the general nursing assessment and the appropriate focused assessments, turn to the Data⇒ Diagnosis Matching Guide for a problem area. This book contains 22 Data ⇒ Diagnosis Matching Guides, one for each problem area listed above. These will help you make an accurate diagnosis. On one or two pages you will find all the related NANDA diagnoses, abbreviated definitions, and essential data needed to make the most appropriate diagnosis. Take the client data obtained from the focused assessment and match it to the data found in the definition and defining characteristics for the NANDA diagnoses in the guide. Select the diagnosis with the best match.

Step 4: Turn to the page listed after the nursing diagnosis you selected from the Data ⇒ Diagnosis Matching Guide to find more complete information in the Nursing Diagnosis Care Planning Guide. These guides are presented for each of the 109 NANDA diagnoses. Each one contains the complete definition, all defining characteristics, and the factors related to that diagnosis. Compare your client's data to the more complete description to assure that you have made an accurate diagnosis. Now write an individualized nursing diagnosis for the client following the nursing diagnoses examples.

Step 5: Develop a plan of care for the client using the

Nursing Diagnosis Care Planning Guide for the NANDA diagnosis selected.

1. Review the General Outcomes and Interventions section which follows the Data ⇒ Diagnosis Matching Guide. These outcomes and interventions are appropriate for most diagnoses in this problem area. Consider individualizing them for the client and including them in the plan of care.
2. Review the Examples of Specific Outcomes section for the diagnosis; develop individualized outcomes appropriate for the client using the examples as a guide.
3. Review the Examples of Specific Interventions section for the diagnosis and select appropriate interventions for the client. Individualize them as needed.
4. Use the Key Index Words to locate additional interventions in medical-surgical and fundamental nursing textbooks.
5. If a Case Management Example is listed for this NANDA diagnosis, turn to the page reference to see how this diagnosis is integrated into an interdisciplinary plan of care. Exact NANDA terminology may not be used in these actual examples from health care facilities. This reflects the evolving nature of both case management plans and of NANDA terminology. Review the outcomes and critical/clinical pathways (nursing interventions on a time schedule) for inclusion in the individualized plan of care.

Step 6: Review the Examples of Specific Outcome Evaluations section for this diagnosis. After implementing your plan of care, evaluate the outcomes selected for the client. Update your nursing care plan based on outcome evaluation and new information obtained while giving care.

USING THIS BOOK: AN EXAMPLE

The following example for a respiratory/breathing problem will take you through the various sections of this text to show you how to make an accurate nursing diagnosis and develop a plan of care.

ASSESSING

Step 1: Start with a general assessment guide provided by your health care facility or school of nursing. Collect the client data indicated on the form. Examples of respiratory/breathing questions and observations from one general nursing assessment form are given below.

Questions and example client responses

___ "Do you feel short of breath or have any trouble breathing at rest?"
"No."

___ "Do you have any trouble or pain with coughing or taking deep breaths?"
"Yes, I hurt all the time but it gets really bad if I take any deep breath or cough."

___ "Do you have a productive cough?"
"I try not to cough because it hurts."

___ "Has your colostomy surgery [current health problem] affected your breathing?"
"I don't think so."

___ "Are you doing any breathing exercises to help your lungs clear?"
"No, my cancer is in my bowel not my lungs; besides it hurts."

Examples of observations

___ color pink, pale

___ respirations 26 per minute at rest, faster with minimal activity

___ no cough

___ lung sounds have moist crackles (rales) in both lower lobes

After completing each area of a general nursing assessment, there is a *decision point*. Does the data in this section indicate a possible problem? Refer to the Normals and Information section of this text for each problem area to help you decide if data is abnormal or unexpected and may indicate a problem. For the example data listed above, the decision is

___ Yes: respirations elevated, moist breath sounds, prefers not to cough or breathe deeply because of pain—*possible respiratory problem*

___ Yes: second problem of *pain* has also been identified

Step 2: Move to the Focused Assessment Guide if a problem is suggested by the data and collect more specific data. Alternatively you may first complete the general nursing assessment then use the Focused Assessment Guides for any problem areas it suggests. Since two problem areas have been suggested in this example, turn to the Respiratory/Breathing Focused Assessment on page 174 and the Pain Focused Assessment on page 127. Clarify both problems by further assessment.

Example of additional data from focused assessments
— Temperature (T) 99.8°F (37.7°C), Pulse (P) 98, Respirations (R) 26; Blood pressure (BP) 148/78 mmHg
— Hemoglobin 12.6 g/dL
— not using inspirometer although client claims to know how to use it
— diminished chest movements during ventilations; shallow breathing
— bowel surgery with general anesthesia two days ago to create a temporary colostomy as part of treatment for bowel cancer
— in bed most of the time; turns/repositions "as little as possible"
— pain is continuous; located through abdomen
— pain is rated 6 without activity and 10 with movement, coughing
— less pain after analgesic given for about 2 hours
— Demerol 75 mg IM every 4 hours prn ordered; 4–5 hours between doses on medication record

After completing the focused assessments for respiration/breathing and for pain in this example you would return to the general nursing assessment and complete it. If any more decision points indicate possible problems, clarify the problem by using the Focused Assessment Guide for that problem area.

DIAGNOSING

Step 3: Turn to the Respiratory/Breathing Data ⇒ Diagnosis Matching Guide page 177. Compare the definitions and data presented for the five NANDA diagnoses related to respiratory problems to the data obtained from the client. Select the diagnosis with the best match. Do the same for the pain data using the Pain Data ⇒ Diagnosis Matching Guide on page 129.

In the Respiratory/Breathing Data ⇒ Diagnosis Matching Guide, two NANDA diagnoses seem to match the data.

Ineffective Airway Clearance page 196
Ineffective Breathing Pattern page 199

In the Pain Data ⇒ Diagnosis Matching Guide, the diagnosis of Acute Pain, page 133, seems to be the best match to this client's data.

Step 4: Now turn to the pages listed after each diagnosis you have chosen from the Data ⇒ Diagnosis Matching Guide. This is the Care Planning Guide section of this text and it provides more complete information on these three diagnoses. Continue to evaluate the match between the client data and the definition, defining characteristics, and related factors listed for each diagnosis. All three diagnoses are a good match in this example and are chosen as the most accurate diagnoses for this client. Write the complete, individualized nursing diagnosis using the two- or three-part format.

Two-part format: NANDA dx label + client's related factors
__ Ineffective airway clearance related to reluctance to cough and deep breathe because of resulting pain.
__ Ineffective breathing pattern related to pain secondary to abdominal surgery.
__ Acute pain related to surgery, movement, coughing, and inadequate analgesic coverage.

Three-part format: NANDA dx label + client's related
factors + S&S
__ Ineffective airway clearance related to reluctance to cough and deep breathe because of resulting pain as evidenced by moist rales/crackles in lower lobes, shallow respirations, and elevated rate; reported effort by client to suppress cough.
__ Ineffective breathing pattern related to pain secondary to abdominal surgery as evidenced by rate of 26 per

minute, shallow breathing, reduced chest movement, reluctance to cough, deep breathe, or use inspirometer.
—— Acute pain related to surgery, movement, coughing, inadequate analgesic coverage as evidenced by client's report of continuous pain rated as a 6 and pain with movement and coughing rated as 10.

PLANNING NURSING CARE

Step 5a (Client Outcomes): Write client outcomes for each diagnosis by choosing client behaviors/measurements showing a reduction or elimination of the client's signs and symptoms associated with that diagnosis. Use the Care Planning Guide section for each diagnosis to help you.

Broader, longer-term outcomes or discharge outcomes are written to show maximum resolution or elimination of the problem. Review the Pain General Outcomes section page 130 and the Respiration/Breathing General Outcomes page 179. These examples will be broader, longer-term outcomes. Write longer-term, maximal outcomes for individual clients based on their unique data base.

Specific, shorter-term client outcomes are written to show smaller-step achievements, often on a daily basis, leading to achievement of broader, long-term outcomes. Use the Examples of Specific Outcomes section for each diagnosis as guide for short-term outcomes. See page 197 for Ineffective Airway Clearance, page 200 for Ineffective Breathing Pattern and page 135 for Acute Pain. The outcomes listed in this section are only examples. You need to formulate your own specific outcomes based on client's data.

Examples of outcomes

Nursing diagnosis	Ineffective airway clearance ...
Long-term outcome	Clear airway by discharge.
Short-term outcomes	Client coughing effectively within 2 hours.
	Clear breath sounds in 24 hours.

Nursing diagnosis	Ineffective breathing pattern ...
Long-term outcome	Effective breathing pattern by discharge.
Short-term outcome	Client's respiratory rate is 20 breaths per minute and of normal depth within 4 hours. Client does deep breathing, sustained maximal inspirations and/or inspirometers 3–4 times every hour while awake for the next 8 hours.
Nursing diagnosis	Acute pain ...
Long-term outcome	Pain free or minimal pain by discharge.
Short-term outcome	Client pain rating is 3 or less at rest within 1 hour Client states pain is 5 or less with movement, coughing, or deep breathing for the next 8 hours.

For example outcomes of pain (altered comfort) and altered respiratory function, look at the case management plans for total hip replacement and pneumonia in the appendixes.

Step 5b (Nursing Interventions): Select nursing interventions to help the client meet the outcomes. Choose interventions that treat both the problematic signs and symptoms (defining characteristics) that this client is experiencing *and* interventions to reduce, eliminate, or compensate for the related factors identified for this client.

___ Use the General Nursing Interventions section for respiratory/breathing problems, page 179, and for pain, page 131, for suggestions. Individualize them to the client as needed.

___ Use the Examples of Specific Nursing Interventions section for each of the three diagnoses for more specific actions: Acute Pain, page 135, Ineffective Breathing pattern, page 200, Ineffective Airway Clearance, page 197.

___ Look up key index words for each diagnosis in your fundamentals and medical-surgical textbooks to locate more interventions.

___ Look up the case management plan examples for total hip replacement and pneumonia in the appendixes.

See the nursing care plan at the end of this section for specific interventions for the three example nursing diagnoses.

EVALUATING

Step 6: Evaluate each of the outcomes selected for the client after giving nursing care. Use the Specific Examples of Outcome Evaluations section as a guide. The following nursing care plan shows outcome evaluations for the example outcomes.

NURSING CARE PLAN

Nursing Diagnoses	*Client Outcomes*
Ineffective airway clearance, r/t reluctance to cough, deep breaths due to pain	Clear airway by discharge. ___ Coughing effectively in 2 hours ___ Clear breath sounds in 24 hours
Ineffective breathing pattern related to pain is secondary to abdominal surgery	Effective Breathing Pattern by discharge. ___ R 20 per minute and of normal depth within 4 hours ___ Deep breathing, inspirometer or sustained maximal inspirations × 3 every hour while awake for next 8 hours
Acute pain related to surgery, movement, coughing, inadequate analgesics	Pain free/minimal pain by discharge. ___ Rates pain at 3 or less at rest within 1 hour. ___ Rates pain with movement, coughing, deep breathing as 5 or less during next 8 hours

Respiratory Interventions

Explain relationship between shallow breathing, collection of secretions in lower lobes, pain, reluctance to cough, and deep breathe

Manage pain (see Pain Interventions)

Assess knowledge of breathing exercises/use of inspirometer

Teach as needed deep breathing, SMIs, use of inspirometer, splinting while coughing

Encourage cough/deep breaths × 5 every hour followed by SMIs × 3

Assess lung sounds before and after chest physiotherapy; assess vital signs every 4 hours

Encourage good nutrition and fluids to 2000 mL/day; record I&O

Promote rest and sleep

Assist to turn and reposition every 2 hours

Out of bed as soon as possible

Ambulate qid as soon as possible

Outcome Evaluation

Outcome met: good coughing during last 2 hours

Outcome met: clear breath sounds after 24 hours of coughing and deep breathing

Outcome met: coughing, deep breathing and SMIs × 3 every hour for last 8 hours

Outcome met: R 18–20 per minute after 4 hours of deep breathing/coughing, turning; normal depth on inspiration

Outcomes met: clear airway and effective breathing pattern at discharge

Pain Interventions

Discuss pain management outcomes

Discuss inadequate pain management with physician and resulting respiratory problems; request alternate opioid analgesics and possible NSAID*

Outcome Evaluation

Outcome met: pain rated as 1–2 one hour after receiving 10 mg morphine IM

Outcome met: pain rated as 4–5 during coughing, turning, and deep breathing during last 8 hours

*Nonsteroid antiinflammatory drug (aspirin, acetaminophen, ibuprofen).

Pain Interventions

Administer maximum ordered dose of new opioid analgesic initially; as pain is controlled, titrate dose down to achieve good pain relief

Administer on around-the-clock schedule vs prn
Administer NSAID* and opioid if ordered by physician
Teach slow rhythmic breathing
Encourage distractions; music
Administer higher opioid dose 30 minutes before painful treatments, therapy
Support body in good alignment
Reposition every 2 hours
Assess for any side effects of analgesics and prevent/treat as needed: constipation, N&V, sedation, respiratory depression
Ask client to report any changes in pain or any new pain

Outcome Evaluation

Outcome met: client reports pain as 0–2 at discharge

PRACTICE EXERCISE: DIAGNOSING

The following exercise will give you some practice in using client data to make accurate diagnoses. Read through the client data for each of the examples. Identify the problem area, e.g., nutrition, fluid/hydration, pain, mobility, safety/protection. Then turn to the Data ⇒ Diagnosis Matching Guide for that problem area. Compare the client data to the data for the various diagnoses listed. Select the best match as the client's diagnosis. Complete the nursing diagnosis by writing in the "related to" part. Check your answers at the end of this section.

1. Client data: 55-year-old female receiving radiation and chemotherapy for cancer treatment; low WBC count; weight loss of 12 lb in last 3 weeks; weight 115 lb, height 5 ft 6 in; feels weak; appears emaciated; nauseated with occasional vomiting; feels thirsty; dry loose skin; I = 800 mL/24 h; O = 500 mL concentrated urine; pulse 98 and weak; Hgb 12.

a. What are problem areas?

_____
_____
_____

b. What are the NANDA diagnostic labels?

_____
_____
_____

c. Write the complete nursing diagnosis, i.e., the diagnostic label and related factors.

_____
_____
_____

2. Client data: 76-year-old man admitted for hip replacement surgery; 3 days postoperatively activity restrictions "up with walker, no hip flexion beyond 90 degrees;" says he really feels weak and needs help in and out of bed; states, "I hate to move too much or get out of bed because then it really hurts;" last bowel movement before admission; normal pattern qod; urine output 500 mL; intake 1300 mL; says he feels a constant urge to pass his water but has trouble going; voiding in amounts of 75–150 mL each voiding; using the urinal every hour or less; some distention palpated over lower abdomen above pubic symphysis; no nausea; pain rated at 6 most of time and as a 10 in physical therapy; unable to sleep, states "pain keeping me awake;" two Tylenol #3 ordered every 3–4 hours prn; client has taken five Tylenol #3 over last two shifts (16 hours).

a. What are problem areas?

_____
_____
_____
_____
_____

b. What are the NANDA diagnostic labels?

_____
_____
_____
_____
_____

c. Write the complete nursing diagnosis, i.e. the diagnostic label and related factors.

_____
_____
_____
_____
_____

ANSWERS

1.a. What are problem areas?
    Nutrition

    Fluid/hydration

    Safety/protection

b. What are the NANDA diagnostic labels?
Altered nutrition: less than body requirements

Fluid volume deficit (total body fluid volume deficit)

High risk for infection and high risk for injury (this data could also be appropriate for high risk for trauma)

c. Write the complete nursing diagnosis.
Altered nutrition: less than body requirements related to nausea, vomiting secondary to chemotherapy and radiation

Fluid volume deficit related to vomiting, low fluid intake, nausea

High risk for infection related to malnutrition, low WBC secondary to chemotherapy and radiation for cancer treatment

High risk for injury related to weakness, malnutrition, radiation chemotherapy

2.a. What are problem areas?

Urinary

Bowel

Mobility

Pain

Sleep

b. What are the NANDA diagnostic labels?

Urinary retention

Constipation

Impaired physical mobility

Acute pain

Sleep pattern disturbance

c. Write the complete nursing diagnosis.

Urinary retention related to surgery and anesthesia, decreased activity and abnormal positioning for voiding, and pain

Constipation related to decreased activity, analgesics, surgical experience

Impaired physical mobility related to weakness, pain, ordered limitation on hip flexion

Acute pain related to movement, physical therapy, inadequate analgesics, inadequate sleep

Sleep pattern disturbance related to pain

PART 1

PHYSICAL PROBLEMS

Chapter 1

Bowel Problems

FOCUSED ASSESSMENT GUIDE

Complete this focused assessment if a general nursing assessment indicates a possible problem. Then turn to page 31 of this text for the Data ⇒ Diagnosis Matching Guide for bowel problems to help you select the best nursing diagnosis to match the client's data.

TELL ME IF YOU ARE HAVING ANY OF THESE PROBLEMS

___ involuntary passage of stool
___ decreased frequency
___ increased frequency
___ hard stool
___ loose, fluid stools
___ straining or difficult to pass
___ urgency
___ feeling of rectal fullness/pressure
___ abdominal distention
___ abdominal pain
___ cramping
___ frequent use of laxatives

NORMALS AND INFORMATION

Table 1.1
CHARACTERISTICS OF FECES

Characteristic	Normal Data	Abnormal Data
Color	brown	red or black in bleeding clay-colored when bile is absent green in some infections varied colors caused by some food, medications, or diseases
Odor	characteristic odor due to bacterial decomposition	foul odor due to digestive disorder or intestinal infection
Consistency	soft, formed	watery in diarrhea or impaction hard in constipation
Constituents	shreds of mucous or particles of undigested food	excessive fat (appears frothy) mucous, blood, pus, or parasites

Source: *Fundamentals of Nursing: A Nursing Process Approach,* L.D. Atkinson, M.E. Murray, MacMillan, 1985.

Table 1.2
ALTERATION IN BOWEL ELIMINATION

Characteristic	Constipation	Fecal Impaction	Diarrhea
Stool consistency	excessively hard	seepage of fecal material hard stool in rectum	liquid, unformed
Stool frequency	less often than usual for the individual	no stool passed	more than 3 stools per day
Passage	difficult, requires increased effort may be painful	unable to pass	difficult to control
Related data	rectal pressure headache anorexia possible hemorrhoids	abdominal and rectal discomfort anorexia abdominal distention	cramping in abdomen anorexia irritation of skin around anus possible dehydration

Source: *Fundamentals of Nursing: A Nursing Process Approach,* L. D. Atkinson, M. E. Murray, Macmillan, 1985.

DATA ⇒ DIAGNOSIS MATCHING GUIDE

Compare your client data from the Bowel Focused Assessment to these related bowel nursing diagnoses and abbreviated descriptions. Select the nursing diagnosis which is the best match. Then turn to the page in this section with that specific diagnosis for help in planning care.

1. *Bowel Incontinence: page 32*
   - definition: involuntary passage of stool
   - data: involuntary passage of stool

2. *Constipation: page 34*
   - definition: decrease in frequency and/or passage of hard, dry stool
   - data: decreased frequency; hard, difficult to pass stools; complaints of rectal fullness, pressure

3. *Colonic Constipation: page 36*
   - definition: hard dry stool caused by delay in food movement through bowel
   - data: decreased frequency; hard, dry stool; abdominal distention; abdominal pain

4. *Perceived Constipation: page 38*
   - definition: self-diagnosis of constipation and abuse of laxatives, enemas and suppositories to ensure daily bowel movement
   - data: expectation of bowel movement (BM) same time every day; overuse of laxative, enema, suppositories

5. *Diarrhea: page 40*
   - definition: frequent passage of loose, fluid, unformed stools
   - data: abdominal pain/cramping; loose liquid stools; increased frequency; overactive bowel sounds; urgency

GENERAL OUTCOMES AND NURSING INTERVENTIONS

GENERAL BOWEL OUTCOMES

- Client reestablishes normal bowel pattern.
- Client passes soft, formed stool without straining.

- Client maintains normal bowel pattern.
- Client identifies measures to promote normal bowel function.

GENERAL BOWEL NURSING INTERVENTIONS

- Promote adequate fluid intake.
- Assess and record frequency and consistency of BMs.
- Provide for privacy.
- Administer ordered prn medications.
- Instruct in dietary modifications to promote normal bowel function.

RELATED NURSING DIAGNOSES

BOWEL INCONTINENCE

Definition
A state in which an individual experiences a change in normal bowel habits characterized by involuntary passage of stool.

Defining Characteristics
- involuntary passage of stool

Examples of Specific Nursing Diagnoses
1. Bowel incontinence related to fecal impaction.
   Bowel incontinence related to fecal impaction as manifested by loose diarrhea-like stool and presence of hard, dry stool in rectum. (PES format)
2. Bowel incontinence related to CVA.
   Bowel incontinence related to CVA as manifested by client's inability to communicate need to defecate. (PES format)

Examples of Specific Outcomes
1. Client will have one soft, formed stool in toilet every 1–3 days after breakfast with bowel training program.
2. Client will communicate need to defecate by end of week.
3. Client's perianal skin will remain intact during period of incontinence.

Examples of Specific Nursing Interventions
- See General Bowel Nursing Interventions, page 32.
- Assess for fecal impaction by digital examination.
- If impaction is present, secure physician order for digital stimulation, lubrication, manual removal, glycerine suppositories, oil retention enemas.
- Assess skin integrity of perianal area.
- Wash and dry perianal area after each BM.
- Apply skin barrier cream/lotion after each cleansing.
- Instruct client (post-CVA) in use of communication board to indicate need to defecate.
- Assess nutrition and fluid intake.
- Encourage foods that facilitate bowel elimination, especially diets which include fresh fruit and vegetables. Note that some foods are naturally constipating (cheese) and some naturally facilitate bowel movements (beans, prune juice, hot liquids).
- Encourage fluid intake to 2000 mL daily.
- Establish routine time for evacuation daily.
- Provide privacy for bowel movement.
- Assist with personal hygiene after BM: handwashing and washing of perianal area.

Examples of Specific Evaluations for Outcome 1
1. Outcome met. Client had soft, formed BM at 7:30 A.M. after breakfast.
2. Outcome partially met. Client incontinent of soft, formed BM in wheelchair midmorning.
3. Outcome not met. Client continues to have diarrhea-like stool around fecal impaction.

Key Index Words for Nursing Interventions
Look up these words in the index of fundamentals and medical-surgical nursing textbooks to find page references for additional nursing interventions and rationale for their selection:

- bowel training
- cerebrovascular accident (CVA)
- fecal incontinence
- impaction
- incontinence, bowel
- spinal cord trauma
- ulcerative colitis

CONSTIPATION

Definition
A state in which an individual experiences a change in normal bowel habits characterized by a decrease in frequency and/or passage of hard, dry stools.

Defining Characteristics
- hard, formed stools
- frequency less than usual
- feeling of pressure in rectum
- straining when passing stool

Other Possible Characteristics
- abdominal pain
- appetite impairment
- interference with daily living
- use of laxatives
- back pain
- headache

Related Factors
- decreased activity level
- opioid (narcotic) use for pain management
- dehydration
- reduced fluid intake
- anesthesia; surgery

Examples of Specific Nursing Diagnoses
1. Constipation related to use of narcotic analgesics and decreased activity following surgery.
   Constipation related to decreased activity, and use of narcotic analgesics following surgery as evidenced by absence of BM 3 days post-op. (PES format)
2. Constipation related to inactivity from confinement in total body cast.
   Constipation related to inactivity from confinement in total body cast as evidenced by passage of small amount of hard stool, and by complaints of rectal pressure. (PES format)

Examples of Specific Outcomes

1. Client will have soft BM with assistance of stool softener/enema within 24 hours.
2. Client will state normal BM pattern of every other day has returned by discharge.
3. Client will state feeling of rectal pressure has resolved, no straining with defecation in 24 hours.

Examples of Specific Nursing Interventions

- See General Bowel Nursing Interventions, page 32.
- Listen (auscultate) for bowel sounds in four quadrants.
- Palpate for presence of abdominal mass or gas distention.
- Assess pain on scale of 1 to 10.
- Review medication use and orders.
- Review fluid and diet intake: encourage fluid to 2000 mL 24 h unless contraindicated.
- Assess for dietary preferences and provide if possible.
- Secure physician order for nonnarcotic analgesic.
- Teach alternative method of pain control: imaging, relaxation, transcutaneous nerve stimulation, as appropriate.
- Ambulate with assistance and as tolerated.

Examples of Specific Evaluations for Outcomes 1 to 3

1. Outcome met. Client had soft BM using Colace.
2. Outcome partially met. Client states normal BM pattern of qod has returned, but stool is hard and difficult to pass.
3. Outcome not met. Client reports worsening of rectal pressure and continuous straining at stool.

Key Index Words for Nursing Interventions

Look up these words in the index of fundamentals and medical-surgical nursing textbooks to find page references for additional nursing interventions and rationale for their selection:

- bulk-forming medications
- care of the surgical client
- cathartics
- constipation
- fecal softeners
- impaction, fecal
- laxatives
- pain/pain control

Case Management Example
See Appendix for an example of a nursing diagnosis of constipation within a clinical pathway for DRG 209, Total Hip Replacement, page 474.

COLONIC CONSTIPATION

Definition
The state in which an individual's pattern of elimination is characterized by a hard, dry stool which results from a delay in passage of food residue.

Major Defining Characteristics
- decreased frequency
- straining at stool
- abdominal distention
- hard, dry stool
- painful defecation
- palpable mass

Minor Defining Characteristics
- rectal pressure
- appetite impairment
- headache
- abdominal pain

Related Factors
- less than adequate fluid intake
- less than adequate dietary intake
- less than adequate fiber
- less than adequate physical activity
- immobility
- lack of privacy
- emotional disturbance
- chronic use of medication and enemas
- stress
- change in daily routine
- metabolic problems, for example, hypothyroidism, hypocalcemia, hypokalemia

Examples of Specific Nursing Diagnoses
1. Colonic constipation related to lack of activity of paraplegia.
   Colonic constipation related to lack of activity of paraplegia as evidenced by distended abdomen; hard dry stools, palpable abdominal mass. (PES format)
2. Colonic constipation related to less than adequate dietary intake.
   Colonic constipation related to less than adequate dietary intake as evidenced by 3-day period without passing a stool, straining, rectal pressure. (PES format)

Examples of Specific Outcomes
1. Client reports passage of soft, formed stool with use of stool softeners and cathartics within 48 hours.
2. Client describes bowel training routine which fits own lifestyle within 72 hours.
3. Absence of abdominal distention and absence of palpable abdominal mass within 48 hours.

Examples of Specific Nursing Interventions
- See General Bowel Nursing Interventions, page 32.
- Assess for usual dietary intake, fluid intake, and activity.
- Assess for presence of bowel sounds in all four quadrants.
- Assess for fecal impaction.
- Teach client importance of fluid intake up to 2 quarts/day.
- Teach client high fiber/high roughage diet: increase fruits and vegetables.
- Teach client naturally constipating foods.
- Collaborate with physical therapist to maximize physical activity.
- Establish regular time each day for BM.

Examples of Specific Evaluations for Outcomes 1 to 3
1. Outcome met. Client reports soft, formed stool using Colace and Vacuette suppository.
2. Outcome partially met. Client can describe weekday bowel regimen but has difficulty adapting weekend schedule.
3. Outcome not met. Had small BM but abdominal distention remains.

Key Index Words for Nursing Interventions
Look up these words in the index of fundamentals and medical-surgical nursing textbooks to find page references for additional nursing interventions and rationale for their selection:

- cathartic, laxative
- constipation, colonic
- diet: fiber, bulk, cultural
- enema
- paraplegic
- quadriplegic
- spinal injury
- stool softener

PERCEIVED CONSTIPATION

Definition
The state in which an individual makes a self-diagnosis of constipation and insures a daily bowel movement through abuse of laxatives, enemas, and suppositories.

Major Defining Characteristics
- expectation of a daily bowel movement with the resulting overuse of laxatives, enemas, and suppositories
- expected passage of stool at same time every day

Related Factors
- cultural/family health beliefs
- faulty appraisal
- impaired thought processes

Examples of Specific Nursing Diagnoses
1. Perceived constipation related to inaccurate health belief. Perceived constipation related to inaccurate health belief as evidenced by client statement, "If you don't have a BM every day it turns to cement inside and then you got real problems". (PES format)
2. Perceived constipation related to family health belief. Perceived constipation related to family health belief as indicated by client statement, "My mother taught us that you would be poisoned if you didn't have a BM every day." (PES format)

Example of Specific Outcomes
1. Client will describe a normal bowel elimination pattern by the end of the teaching session.

2. Client will state indications for use of laxative/stool softener and describe potential hazards of prolonged use by discharge.
3. Client will describe foods high in bulk/fiber which enhance bowel movements by end of shift.

Examples of Specific Interventions

■ See General Bowel Nursing Interventions, page 32.
■ Teach the client about normal bowel function, including frequency of stool every 1–3 days; normal stool is soft, formed, and passes without straining; normal stool is brown and does not contain blood, or look black and tar-like.
■ If the client has indicated a use of laxatives or stool softeners, assess knowledge about the medication and teach specifically about each medication. Indicate the side effects of the medication and the hazards of prolonged use.
■ Teach about the alternatives to the use of medications: food, fluid, and exercise. Foods high in bulk include fruits and vegetables, whole grain breads and cereals. Identify specific foods within these groups that are acceptable to the clients and make a written list for the client. Identify amounts of servings.
■ Encourage fluids up to 2 L ($\frac{1}{2}$ gallon) per day unless contraindicated by medical condition.
■ Encourage increased exercise, which may be as simple as parking further out in the parking lot at work or walking around the block. It does not have to be a complicated routine.

Examples of Specific Evaluations for Outcomes 1 to 3

1. Outcome met. Client states, "So I won't worry because I only have a BM every other day as long as it is soft and passes without pain."
2. Outcome partially met. Client states: "I will only use a laxative if I don't have a BM by the fourth day and am uncomfortable. By then I may need a triple dose."
3. Outcome not met. Client states, "I've always been a fussy eater and I don't intend to change now!"

Key Index Words for Nursing Interventions
Look up these words in the index of fundamentals
and medical-surgical nursing textbooks to find page
references for additional nursing interventions and rationale
for their selection:

- cathartic
- constipation, perceived
- diet: fiber, bulk, cultural
- enema
- laxative
- stool softener

DIARRHEA

Definition
A state in which an individual experiences a change in
normal bowel habits characterized by the frequent passage
of loose, fluid, unformed stools.

Defining Characteristics
- abdominal pain
- cramping
- increased frequency
- increased frequency of bowel sounds
- loose liquid stools
- urgency

Other Possible Characteristics
- changes in color

Related Factors
- to be developed by NANDA
- antibiotic therapy
- excessive alcohol intake
- change in diet/water
- food intolerance
- medication side effect
- anxiety, stress
- infection
- AIDS
- fecal impaction
- abuse of laxatives

Examples of Specific Nursing Diagnoses
1. Diarrhea related to use of ampicillin.
   Diarrhea related to use of ampicillin as evidenced by loose, watery stools 24 hours following start of antibiotic therapy. (PES format)
2. Diarrhea related to infection.
   Diarrhea related to infection as evidenced by loose, watery stools every 1–2 hours, frequent crying, and fussiness. (PES format)

Examples of Specific Outcomes
1. Two or fewer diarrhea stools in next 24 hours.
2. Client reports cessation of abdominal cramping/pain by bedtime (hs).
3. Client will state foods to avoid to reduce diarrhea by hs.
4. Bowel sounds will become less active within 24 hours.
5. Soft, formed stool after 72 hours.

Examples of Specific Nursing Interventions
- See General Bowel Nursing Interventions, page 32.
- Record daily weight.
- I&O each shift.
- Assess for dehydration; encourage fluids in small amounts, frequently.
- Assess for perianal skin irritation.
- Clear liquid diet only for 24 hours (obtain physician order).
- Administer antidiarrheal medication (Lomotil) prn.
- Assess knowledge and teach client regarding:
  antidiarrheal medication
  need to report each stool to nurse
  foods which aggravate diarrhea (milk, raw fruits and vegetables, caffeine)
  ordered diet restriction

Examples of Specific Evaluations for Outcome 1
1. Outcome met. Client had only one loose stool in last 24 hours.
2. Outcome partially met. Client had three loose stools in last 24 hours but states much better than yesterday with loose stools very few hours.

3. Outcome not met. Client continues to have four to six loose stools per day.

Key Index Words for Nursing Interventions

Look up these words in the index of fundamentals and medical-surgical nursing textbooks to find page references for additional nursing interventions and rationale for their selection:

- antibiotics
- anxiety disorder
- Crohn's disease
- diarrhea
- electrolyte imbalance
- food poisoning
- gastroenteritis
- radiation therapy
- ulcerative colitis

Circulation Problems

FOCUSED ASSESSMENT GUIDE

Complete this focused assessment if a general nursing assessment indicates a possible problem. Then turn to page 46 of this text for the Data $\Rightarrow$ Diagnosis Matching Guide for circulation problems to help you select the best nursing diagnosis to match the client's data.

TELL ME IF YOU ARE HAVING ANY OF THESE PROBLEMS

___ shortness of breath
___ labored or difficult breathing (dyspnea)
___ needing to be in upright position to breathe easily (orthopnea)
___ fatigue and/or weakness
___ feeling restless
___ feeling faint (syncope) or as though you or your surroundings are rotating (vertigo)
___ edema; weight gain
___ pain in your buttocks, thighs, or calfs with walking; if yes, does pain go away if you rest? (claudication)

PHYSICAL ASSESSMENT FOR

___ Blood pressure (BP): variations in readings, abnormally high or low

___ Pulse: irregular heart rhythm or gallop rhythm (extra heart sounds, S3, S4), abnormally high or low rate

___ Respirations: increased rate; rales/crackles (moist sounds in lung); cough (may be dry cough, usually moist), frothy sputum

___ mechanical compression of circulation (e.g., tourniquet, cast, brace, dressings or restraint, obesity, pregnancy, edema)

___ jugular vein distention

___ slow capillary refill (longer than 3 seconds)

___ pale, dusky, blue color to skin and/or mucous membranes

___ oliguria (decreased urine output related to fluid intake)

___ cold, clammy skin; cool or cold extremities

___ change in mental status; confused, decreased level of consciousness

ASSESS LEGS FOR

___ skin pale on elevation; no return of color on lowering

___ edema (measure calf circumferences with tape measure)

___ diminished peripheral pulses (weaker, hard or impossible to palpate; pulses unequal in strength bilaterally)

___ shining skin quality; lack of hair on extremity

___ slow-growing, dry, brittle nails

___ slow-healing wounds; gangrene

REVIEW CHART FOR RELATED CAUSATIVE FACTORS

___ vascular obstruction; arterial and/or venous insufficiency

___ inadequate cardiac output, heart disease

___ low hemoglobin; abnormal arterial blood gases

___ trauma to extremities; fractures; burns

___ orthopedic surgery

___ immobilization

___ hypovolemia (e.g., dehydration, bleeding, third spacing)

___ history of diabetes mellitus, emboli and/or thrombophlebitis, atherosclerosis, sickle cell disease

ADULT NORMALS AND INFORMATION

- Cardiac output = stroke volume × heart rate
- Normal adult cardiac output is 5 L/min; stroke volume is 70 mL/beat; resting heart rate is 60–80 beats/min
- Normal blood pressure, 120/80 mmHg (range 100/60 to 140/90 mmHg)
- Normal capillary refill occurs within 3 seconds of compression and release of nail bed
- Peripheral pulses should be equal and strong bilaterally: pedal, popliteal, posterior tibial
- Extremities have equal color, movement, and sensation (CMS)
- Body tissues need for oxygen increases with physical activity, elevated body temperature, infection, injury
- Body tissues need for oxygen decreases during rest, therapeutic hypothermia, minimal activity
- Ischemia is an inadequate blood flow to a part of the body because of constriction or obstruction of blood vessels
- Ischemia results in inadequate oxygenation (hypoxia) and nutrition to tissues supplied by the constricted vessels
- Vasodilation increases blood flow to an area; it results from: heat, decreased sympathetic nervous system stimulation, increased tissue metabolism, decreased oxygen concentration in tissues, increased potassium, magnesium, and hydrogen ion concentration in tissues, increased carbon dioxide levels
- Vasoconstriction reduces blood flow to an area; it results from: cold, increased sympathetic nervous system stimulation during stress or fear, increased calcium ion concentration in tissues, vascular disease that narrows vessels (e.g., coronary artery disease, atherosclerosis)
- Skin breakdown, slowed wound healing and gangrene is more likely in ischemic tissue
- Ischemic tissues can die if deprived of oxygen for too long
- Tissue ischemia can stimulate growth of new blood vessels
- Collateral circulation develops in response to tissue ischemia. Small existing vessels dilate within minutes to increase blood flow. Dilation and new growth occurs over weeks or months to replace obstructed or narrowed primary blood vessels.

DATA ⇒ DIAGNOSIS MATCHING GUIDE

Compare your client data from the Circulation Focused Assessment to these related nursing diagnoses and abbreviated descriptions. Select the nursing diagnosis with the best match. Then turn to the page in this section with that specific diagnosis for help in planning care.

1. Altered Peripheral* Tissue Perfusion: page 49
   ■ definition: a decrease in nutrition and oxygen at the peripheral cellular level due to a deficit in capillary blood flow
   ■ data: extremities cold, blue or purple skin color; loss of or decreased motion, loss of or altered sensation; capillary refill takes longer than 3 seconds; uncontrolled pain; skin on leg pale on elevation with no return of color on lowering; weaker arterial pulsations; shining skin quality; slow-growing, dry, brittle nails; slow-healing wounds; leg pain with walking resolves with rest.

2. Decreased Cardiac Output: page 53
   ■ definition: blood pumped by an individual's heart is inadequate to meet the needs of the body's tissues
   ■ data: variations in blood pressure readings; arrhythmias (irregular heartbeats); fatigue; jugular vein distention; color changes in skin and mucous membranes; oliguria (low urine output); decreased peripheral pulses; cold, clammy skin; rales (moist lung sounds); dyspnea (difficulty breathing); orthopnea (breathes easily only in upright position); restlessness.

3. High Risk for Peripheral Neurovascular Dysfunction: page 56
   ■ definition: at risk for a disruption in circulation, sensation, or motion of an extremity
   ■ risk factors: fractures; mechanical compression (e.g., tourniquet, cast, brace, dressing, or restraint); orthopedic surgery; trauma; immobilization; burns; vascular obstruction; arterial/venous insufficiency.

*Further work and development are needed for the subcompartments of renal, cerebral, cardiovascular, and gastrointestinal altered tissue perfusion.

GENERAL OUTCOMES AND NURSING INTERVENTIONS

GENERAL CIRCULATION OUTCOMES

- Tissue perfusion meets tissues' oxygen and nutrient needs as evidenced by normal function, color, temperature, sensation.
- Pulses, color, temperature, movement, and sensation in extremities equal bilaterally and within normal limits.
- Urine output of 40–70 mL/h.
- Clear lung/breath sounds.
- Skin and mucous membranes pink.
- Absence of pain (chest or leg), weakness, and shortness of breath with moderate activity.

GENERAL CIRCULATION NURSING INTERVENTIONS

- Reduce or eliminate factors causing and contributing to the problem (e.g., casts or restraints that are too tight, dehydration, cold stress, smoking, stress, anxiety).
- Assess and record vital signs, heart and lung sounds, level of consciousness, presence of leg/calf edema, strength and bilateral equality of peripheral pulses, color, movement, and sensation (CMS) of extremities, presence of jugular vein distension.
- Monitor arterial blood gases, hemoglobin, and hematocrit.
- Monitor and record I&O; decreased urine output or output less than 30 mL/h indicates inadequate blood flow to kidneys and should be reported.
- Promote arterial and venous blood flow.
    Apply antiembolism stockings if ordered; remove for 30 minutes twice a day.
    Position extremity in dependent position to promote arterial blood flow in arterial insufficiency; elevate to promote venous blood flow in venous insufficiency.
    Encourage moderate daily exercise as condition permits; encourage exercises while in bed (unless contraindicated).
    Quadriceps setting: lying flat with leg straight on bed, push knee down into mattress by contracting anterior

thigh muscle, hold 5–10 seconds and relax; do 10 repetitions per hour.

Gluteal setting: lying flat in bed with leg straight, contract muscles of buttocks and abdomen, hold for 5–10 seconds; do 10 repetitions per hour.

Ankle pumps: flexion and extension of ankle; do 10 repetitions per hour.

Calf pumping exercises: contract and relax calf; do 10 repetitions per hour.

Move extremities: move hands, feet, fingers, and toes hourly.

Active and/or passive range of motion exercises every shift.

Keep client warm; neither chilled nor overheated.

Encourage deep breathing to produce increased negative pressure in the thorax, which helps to empty large veins.

Promote good hydration and nutrition to maintain adequate blood volume and promote healing.

Reduce fluid volume overload (peripheral edema) through medications such as diuretics, rest, reduced sodium diets, and fluid restrictions as ordered by the physician.

Prevent peripheral vasoconstriction by maintaining adequate circulating blood volume, maintaining normal blood pressure, preventing chilling or cold stress, decreasing anxiety, eliminating nicotine (smoking, chewing), assessing for any medications or over-the-counter drugs that may cause vasoconstriction and notifying the physician.

- Maintain or decrease cellular need for oxygen and nutrients by maintaining normal body temperature, promoting rest and sleep, decreasing pain, anxiety, and stress.
- Promote effective respirations by ensuring clear airway, encouraging frequent deep breathing, positioning for maximum chest expansion with head elevated, reducing fluid volume overload.
- Administer oxygen as ordered (correct flow/concentration).
- Teach client and family based on assessment of learning needs about:

    medications and possible side effects;

ways to promote circulation and oxygenation;
factors in lifestyle contributing to circulation problems
(e.g., smoking, inactivity, high fat diet, genetics);
ways to change lifestyle to promote circulation;
dietary restrictions (e.g., fluid, sodium restrictions).
- Problem-solve with the family ways to adapt favorite
foods and recipes to new restrictions; consider referral to
dietician.

RELATED NURSING DIAGNOSES

ALTERED PERIPHERAL* TISSUE PERFUSION

Definition
The state in which an individual experiences a decrease in
nutrition and oxygenation at the peripheral cellular level
due to a deficit in capillary blood flow.

Critical Defining Characteristics: One or More Required for Dx
- skin on leg pale on elevation; no return of color on
lowering
- diminished arterial pulsation (weak, hard to palpate)

Defining Characteristics
- cool or cold extremity; blue or purple skin color
- shining skin quality
- lack of hair on extremity
- slow-growing, dry, brittle nails
- slow-healing wounds; gangrene
- bruits (sound/murmur heard with stethoscope caused by
blood turbulence over narrowed or obstructed vessel)
- blood pressure changes in extremities
- claudication (pain in buttocks, thigh, or calf develops with
walking; resolves with rest)

Other Characteristics
- loss of or changed sensation
- loss of or decreased motion

*Further work and development are needed for the subcompartments of
renal, cerebral, cardiovascular, and gastrointestinal altered tissue perfusion.

- uncontrolled pain (especially related to orthopedic surgery)
- slow capillary refill (longer than 3 seconds after compression of nail bed)

Related Factors
- exchange problems (e.g., low hemoglobin)
- hypovolemia (reduced vascular blood volume)
- hypervolemia (increased vascular blood volume; fluid overload)
- interruption of arterial or venous blood flow due to:
    narrowing of vessels (e.g., peripheral vascular disease as is common in diabetes mellitus, atherosclerosis);
    compression or obstruction from inside the vessel (e.g., vasospasms, emboli, sickle cell crisis, thrombophlebitis);
    compression and/or obstruction from outside vessel (e.g., obesity, pregnancy, casts, tumor, unrelieved pressure from not changing positions, compartment syndrome);
    injury/trauma/surgery (e.g., edema, compartment syndrome);
    vasoconstriction from: cold stress/hypothermia, medications or drugs (e.g., nicotine), sympathetic nervous system stimulation.

Examples of Specific Nursing Diagnoses
1. Altered peripheral tissue perfusion related to surgical repair and casting for fractured left leg.
   Altered peripheral tissue perfusion related to surgical repair and casting for fractured left leg as evidenced by pain, decreased pedal pulse on left, cool, pale, slow capillary refill and edema. (PES format)
2. Altered peripheral tissue perfusion related to peripheral vascular disease secondary to diabetes mellitus for 30 years.
   Altered peripheral tissue perfusion related to peripheral vascular disease secondary to diabetes mellitus for 30 years as evidenced by decreased pedal and posterior tibial pulses on left, intermittent claudication after walking four blocks, nonhealing wound on left foot. (PES format)

Examples of Specific Outcomes
1. Pedal pulses equal and strong in both legs within 6 hours.
2. Wound heals on left foot within 3 weeks.

3. Left leg and foot equal to right in color, temperature, movement and sensation within 24 hours.
4. Walks 1 mile without developing intermittent claudication in 6 weeks.

Examples of Specific Nursing Interventions

■ See General Circulation Nursing Interventions, page 47.
■ Assess for adequate tissue perfusion (compare to opposite extremity for baseline): presence of uncontrolled pain; swelling; feeling of tightness; pale, blue, or dusky color; tingling or numbness; cool; decreased pulse strength; reduced movement; longer capillary refill; positive Homans' sign (pain in calf on dorsiflexion of ankle); abnormal or changed color, motion, sensation (CMS) checks.
■ Recheck any abnormal finding or change; if same findings obtained when rechecked, report them to the charge nurse or physician. Restrictive wraps or casts may need to be loosened or released.
■ Elevate injured extremity to promote venous return and prevent edema after injury, surgery, casting, or in venous insufficiency.
■ Lower extremity below heart level to promote arterial blood flow in arterial insufficiency.
■ Cryotherapy (therapeutic use of cold) may be ordered after injury or surgery to prevent or reduce swelling, thus maintaining circulation (e.g., cold packs, cryocuff for knee surgery).
■ Heat should be applied only with physician's order (causes vasodilation, thus increasing blood flow, but also can burn ischemic tissues; heat increases cellular metabolism, thus increasing need for oxygen and nutrients above baseline, which can worsen ischemia).
■ Administer prophylactic anticoagulants as ordered; monitor for complications of bleeding.
■ Provide postoperative pain management so client more willing to move, exercise, and ambulate.
■ Assist with CPM (continuous passive motion) machine when ordered to promote circulation and joint mobility.
■ Turn and reposition every 1–2 hours; place in correct body alignment.
■ Avoid pressure on affected extremity (e.g., foot cradles,

air or water mattresses, lamb's wool between toes of foot that rub).
- Inspect skin area for signs of damage or breakdown.
- Out of bed as soon as possible; early ambulation.
- Encourage progressive exercise to build collateral circulation.
- Encourage client to stop exercising and rest if pain develops.
- Teach client to avoid positions that restrict blood flow, such as crossed legs, pillows under knees, bed knee gatch-up, sitting for long periods of time, standing in one place with minimal movement. Tight clothing, undergarments or shoes should also be avoided.
- Encourage client to avoid exposure to cold and nicotine (causes peripheral vasoconstriction).
- Teach and encourage daily foot care: inspection for blisters, sores; daily washing, drying, and lubricating; lamb's wool between toes that rub; foot massages; trimming nails; cotton socks; and well-fitting shoes.

Examples of Specific Evaluations for Outcomes 1 to 4

1. Outcome met. Pedal pulses on left improved over several hours with elevation of leg; pain decreased; pulses equal to right and strong by 6 hours.
2. Outcome partially met. Wound has decreased in size by half but has not healed completely after 3 weeks of treatment.
3. Outcome not met. Left leg continues to be cool and pale with decreased sensation compared to right after 24 hours.
4. Outcome met. Walking 1 mile without pain after 6 weeks of progressive exercising.

Key Index Words for Nursing Interventions

Look up these words in the index of fundamentals and medical-surgical nursing textbooks to find page references for additional nursing interventions and rationale for their selection:

- arterial insufficiency
- atherosclerosis
- compartment syndrome
- cryotherapy (cold)
- embolism
- heat, application of
- ischemia, tissue
- peripheral vascular disease
- perfusion, tissue
- venous insufficiency

DECREASED CARDIAC OUTPUT

Definition
A state in which the blood pumped by an individual's heart is sufficiently reduced that it is inadequate to meet the needs of the body's tissues.

Defining Characteristics
- variations in blood pressure readings
- arrhythmias (variations in normal heart rhythm)
- fatigue
- jugular vein distention (elevated venous pressure from right ventricular failure)
- color changes in skin and mucous membranes (pale, dusky, blue)
- oliguria (decreased urine output from inadequate blood flow to kidney)
- decreased peripheral pulses (weak, difficult to palpate)
- cold, clammy skin
- rales (moist sounds in lung); dyspnea (difficult breathing); orthopnea (breathes easily only in upright position); related to pulmonary edema from left-sided cardiac failure
- restlessness

Other Characteristics
- change in mental status (from inadequate cerebral blood flow)
- shortness of breath
- syncope (fainting)
- vertigo (sensation of rotation or movement of self or surroundings)
- edema and weight gain (dependent edema of feet and legs associated with right ventricular heart failure)
- cough (may be dry cough but usually moist) and frothy sputum from pulmonary edema in left ventricular failure)
- gallop rhythm (extra heart sounds, S3, S4)
- weakness

Related Factors
- decreased venous return to heart
- decreased strength of heart contractions (e.g., damaged tissue)

- increased systemic or pulmonary vascular resistance (systemic or pulmonary hypertension from right- or left-sided heart failure)
- problems with heart's electrical conduction to control heart rate and rhythm (e.g., dysrhythmias)
- ineffective heart valves
- cardiac output inadequate for increased need, such as pregnancy or heavy physical exercise (e.g., snow shoveling)

Examples of Specific Nursing Diagnoses

1. Decreased cardiac output related to decreased heart contractility secondary to failure to take medications, increased systemic vascular resistance, and nonadherence to sodium-restricted diet.

   Decreased cardiac output related to decreased heart contractility secondary to failure to take medications, increased systemic vascular resistance, and nonadherence to sodium-restricted diet as evidenced by peripheral edema, moist breath sounds (rales/crackles), BP 188/98, weight gain of 8 lb in one week. (PES format)

2. Decreased cardiac output related to damaged heart valve, third trimester pregnancy.

   Decreased cardiac output related to damaged heart valves, third trimester pregnancy as evidenced by pale bluish skin tone, fatigue, weakness, shortness of breath, moist breath sounds (rales/crackles), uterine height below normal for gestation. (PES format)

Examples of Specific Outcomes

1. Circumference of calfs decreases by 1 cm and weight loss of 5 lb in 48 hours.
2. Clear breath sounds and no shortness of breath within 8 hours.
3. Client states fatigue and weakness improved in 48 hours.
4. Urine output of 50 mL in next hour.

Examples of Specific Nursing Interventions

- See General Circulation Nursing Interventions, page 47.
- Weigh daily and record; be alert for weight gain indicating edema (same time, same scale, same clothing).
- Explain and involve client/family in planning fluid intake if fluid restriction ordered.

- Administer ordered medications and monitor for side effects (e.g., digitalis, diuretics, vasodilators).
- Encourage rest to reduce cardiac workload and promote diuresis.
- Promote sleep through maintenance of sleep habits, rituals, no coffee or nicotine intake, and encourage milk and/or high protein bedtime snack; avoid giving a diuretic before bed if possible since the resulting increased urine output will interrupt sleep if the client has to void frequently.
- Elevate head or bed; support arms with pillows; support client in armchair.
- Provide emotional support to reduce anxiety; encourage family to stay with client.
- Encourage exercise as condition permits; discuss reasons for avoiding excess exercise, fatigue, breathlessness.
- Discuss effects of infection on condition and ways to minimize risk.
- Problem-solve with client and family on ways to adapt and pace activities of daily living to maximize independence and minimize fatigue and breathlessness.

Examples of Specific Evaluations for Outcomes 1 to 4

1. Outcome met. Edema decreased by 2 cm in right calf and 1.5 cm in left; weight loss of 6 lb over last 2 days.
2. Outcome not met. Lungs continue to sound moist with rales in lower lobes; client reports continued shortness of breath on oxygen.
3. Outcome met. Client states feeling stronger and less fatigued after rest and administration of digitalis and diuretic for last 48 hours.
4. Outcome partially met. Urine output has increased from 30 mL/h to 46 mL over last hour.

Key Index Words for Nursing Interventions

Look up these words in the index of fundamentals and medical-surgical nursing textbooks to find page references for additional nursing interventions and rationale for their selection:

- cardiac disorders
- cardiac failure

- cardiac output, decreased
- congestive heart failure
- dysrhythmias
- hypertension, pulmonary, systemic
- peripheral vascular resistance
- pulmonary edema

HIGH RISK FOR PERIPHERAL NEUROVASCULAR DYSFUNCTION

Definition
The state in which an individual is at risk of experiencing a disruption in circulation, sensation, or motion of an extremity.

Defining Risk Factors
- fractures; trauma
- mechanical compression (e.g., tourniquet, cast, brace, dressings, restraint, pregnant uterus obstructing venous return)
- orthopedic surgery (e.g., compartment syndrome, fat emboli)
- immobilization
- burns (e.g., compartment syndrome, hypovolemia, damaged vessels)
- vascular obstruction (e.g., emboli, sickle cell disease)
- arterial and venous insufficiency (e.g., peripheral vascular insufficiency as in diabetes mellitus, thrombophlebitis, atherosclerosis)

Examples of Specific Nursing Diagnoses
1. High risk for peripheral neurovascular dysfunction related to repaired fracture of right leg and casting.
2. High risk for peripheral neurovascular dysfunction related to poorly regulated diabetes mellitus, smoking, inactive lifestyle.
3. High risk for peripheral neurovascular dysfunction related to second-degree burns on legs.

Examples of Specific Outcomes
1. CMS in right leg remains normal and equal to left leg during the postoperative period (as assessed every 2 hours) for 48 hours.
2. Peripheral pulses strong with good CMS at annual physical exam.
3. Pedal pulses remain strong and equal bilaterally for the next 8 hours.

Examples of Specific Nursing Interventions
- See General Circulation Nursing Interventions, page 47.
- See Specific Nursing Interventions for Altered Peripheral Tissue Perfusion, page 51.
- Work with clients and families to identify:
  personal risk factors
  potential outcomes if untreated
  interventions to prevent circulation problems from developing, to slow progression, or to delay onset of symptoms
- Work with clients and family to identify realistic personal outcomes related to lifestyle changes to reduce risk.

Examples of Specific Evaluations for Outcomes 1 to 3
1. Outcome met. CMS strong, equal bilaterally for last 48 hours.
2. Outcome partially met. Peripheral pulses remain strong and equal bilaterally but sensation is slightly less on right foot and pressure rub is present on great toe.
3. Outcome not met. Pedal pulses on right foot became weak, edema and pallor developed, foot is cool to touch 4 hours after admission to burns unit.

Key Index Words for Nursing Interventions
Use key index words listed for the nursing diagnosis Altered Peripheral Tissue Perfusion.

Chapter 3

Fluid/Hydration Problems

FOCUSED ASSESSMENT GUIDE

Complete this focused assessment if a general nursing assessment indicates a possible problem. Then turn to page 60 of this text for the Data ⇒ Diagnosis Matching Guide for fluid/hydration problems to help you select the best nursing diagnosis to match a client's data.

TELL ME IF YOU ARE HAVING ANY OF THESE PROBLEMS

___ weight gain or loss in a short time
___ shortness of breath; difficult breathing
___ weakness
___ nausea or vomiting
___ decreased tearing, dry eyes; decreased salivation, dry mouth
___ increased thirst
___ difficulty swallowing; choking and coughing when swallowing

OBSERVE FOR THE FOLLOWING DATA FROM CHART AND PHYSICAL ASSESSMENT

___ skin: edematous, puffy, tight or dry, loose with poor turgor
___ elevated temperature; diaphoretic (sweaty, perspiring)
___ pulse: elevated rate; full, bounding, or weak
___ blood pressure elevated or decreased from normal

___ more than 3–5 seconds for hand vein filling or emptying; flat or distended neck veins when lying down
___ urine specific gravity 1.030+ for concentrated or 1.003 for dilute
___ I > O or I < O over last several days; urine output above or below expected normal of 1500 mL/24 h
___ elevated or decreased hemoglobin (Hgb), hematocrit (Hct), urea nitrogen concentration (BUN); elevated blood glucose
___ moist breath sounds (rales/crackles)
___ decreased level of consciousness
___ abnormal electrolyte values
___ presence of tubes draining body fluids (NG tubes, wound drains)
___ presence of tubes adding fluids (IVs, feeding tubes)
___ loss of fluids through wounds, burns, diarrhea, vomiting, etc.
___ physical or cognitive limitations preventing free access and consumption of fluid; nonmobile, weak, confused, restraints

NORMALS AND INFORMATION

- One pound weight gain or loss equals 500 mL of fluid
- The swallowing center is located in the brain (medulla and lower pons)
- Movement of food/fluids into the back of the mouth initiates the swallowing reflex, which is under voluntary control
- The swallowing center inhibits the respiratory center so swallowing can occur without food and fluids being inspired into the airway (aspirated)
- Normal daily fluid intake 1300 mL; urine output 1500 mL (range 1000–2000 mL/24 h)
- Normal hourly urine output 40–80 mL/h; less than 30 mL/h is inadequate and should be reported to the physician
- Normal specific gravity of 1.012–1.025; the higher the number, the more concentrated the urine
- Elevated specific gravity usually accompanies low,

concentrated urine output; decreased specific gravity
accompanies increased dilute urine output
■ When adequately hydrated, pinched skin will go back to
normal position immediately; poor skin turgor results in
skin remaining pinched up for several seconds
■ Decreased plasma volume causes hand veins to take
longer than 3–5 seconds to fill when held in a dependent
position; increased plasma volume causes hand veins to
take more than 3–5 seconds to empty when elevated
■ Body temperature of 101–103°F (38.3–39.4°C) increases
fluid needs by 500 mL/24 h; above 103°F fluid needs
increase by 1000 mL/24 h
■ Normal central venous pressure in the vena cava is
4–11 cm of water
■ Elevated blood glucose levels cause dehydration through
excessive urine production; normal range 65–110 mg/dL

DATA ⇒ DIAGNOSIS MATCHING GUIDE

Compare your client data from the Fluid/Hydration
Focused Assessment to these related fluid/hydration nursing
diagnoses and abbreviated descriptions. Select the nursing
diagnosis with the best match. Then turn to the page in this
section with that specific diagnosis for help in planning care.

1. *Fluid Volume Excess: page 68*
    ■ definition: increased fluid retention and edema
    ■ data: I > O; edema; weight gain; increased urine output
      if kidney function normal; breathing difficulty; moist
      breath sounds, rales; distended neck veins; bounding,
      full, rapid pulse; decreased hemoglobin and hematocrit,
      caused by excess fluid intake, excess sodium intake, or
      fluid regulation problems

2. *Fluid Volume Deficit: page 62*
    ■ definition: vascular, cellular, or intracellular dehydration
    ■ general data:* decreased urine output; increased
      specific gravity (1.030 +); weak rapid pulse; decreased
      BP; increased hemoglobin and hematocrit; poor skin

*Authors' division of NANDA diagnosis for clarity and treatment
considerations.

turgor; dry tongue and mucous membranes; weak, thirsty

(a) *Fluid Volume Deficit — Reduced Volume** (total body fluid reduced) I < O; rapid weight loss; clear breath sounds; caused by increased fluid loss, decreased fluid intake, fluid regulation problems

(b) *Fluid Volume Deficit — Third Spacing of Fluids** (no fluid loss) I > O; weight normal or increased; caused by trauma, surgery, burns, sepsis, intestinal obstruction, inflammation

3. *High Risk for Fluid Volume Deficit: page 66*
   - definition: at risk for vascular, cellular, or intracellular dehydration
   - risk factors: extremes of age; extremes of weight; excessive losses through normal/abnormal routes (environmental heat, heavy exercise, fever, wounds, drains, GI suction); conditions that limit access to or absorption and excretion of fluids (e.g., physical immobility; confusion, coma, depression; elevated blood glucose levels; diuretics, laxative abuse); trauma; surgery; burns; sepsis

4. *Impaired Swallowing: page 72*
   - definition: decreased ability to voluntarily pass fluids and/or solids from the mouth to the stomach
   - data: observed evidence of difficulty swallowing; food/fluids remain in mouth, coughing/choking; evidence of aspiration

GENERAL OUTCOMES AND NURSING INTERVENTIONS

GENERAL FLUID/HYDRATION OUTCOMES

- Client's I&O is in normal range.
- Client's body weight will return to normal range.
- Client's intake will equal output.
- Client's urine output will be 1500 mL/24 h.
- Client's skin has good turgor.

*Authors' division of NANDA diagnosis for clarity and treatment considerations.

- Client's vital signs return to normal range.
- Client's edema is resolved.
- Client's urine specific gravity is in normal range.

GENERAL FLUID/HYDRATION NURSING INTERVENTIONS

- Assess swallowing ability; if this is a problem implement interventions to promote swallowing and prevent choking. See Specific Nursing Interventions for Impaired Swallowing, page 73.
- Accurately record I&O; may be done hourly, every 4 hours, every shift, and every 24 hours (24-hour totals usually start and stop at midnight).
- Weigh daily at same time every day; usually before breakfast.
- Assess vital signs and breath sounds; compare to normals and client's previous values.
- Assess skin turgor, moistness of mucous membranes and edema.
- Review hemoglobin (Hbg) and hematocrit (Hct) values if available for changes from normals.
- Assess for and take precautions for altered level of consciousness to prevent injury.
- Administer IV solutions at ordered rate; monitor every 1 hour.
- Encourage fluid intake in normal range of 1300 mL/24 h.

RELATED NURSING DIAGNOSES

FLUID VOLUME DEFICIT

Definition
The state in which an individual experiences vascular, cellular, or intracellular dehydration.

*General Defining Characteristics**
These characteristics apply to both volume deficits: reduced volume and third spacing of fluid. Characteristics specific to each are covered separately.

---

*Authors' division of NANDA diagnosis for clarity and treatment considerations.

- decreased urine output; oliguria (less than 30 mL/h)
- increased specific gravity (1.030+) as urine volume decreases
- weak rapid pulse; decreased BP; postural hypotension (drop in systolic BP of 15 mmHg when moving from lying position to sitting position or standing position)
- decreased central venous pressure
- increased hemoglobin (Hgb), hematocrit (Hct), blood urea nitrogen (BUN); reduced blood volume causes hemo-concentration of these components—no real gain
- poor skin turgor; dry tongue and mucous membranes
- slow hand vein filling (takes longer than 3–5 seconds to fill when held in dependent position); capillary refill takes longer than 3 seconds after nail compressed for color to come back
- flat neck veins when lying down
- decreased tearing and salivation
- weak, thirsty
- decreased level of consciousness

(a) Fluid Volume Deficit — Reduced Volume* (total body fluid reduced)

Specific Characteristics
- total output of all body fluids greater than intake (O > I)
- rapid weight loss (several pounds or more over a few days)
- clear breath sounds
- elevated serum sodium level if dehydration from inadequate water intake versus loss of water and sodium
- elevated body temperature if dehydration due to water deficit and client unable to cool body by sweating

Related Factors
- increased fluid loss (bleeding, vomiting, diarrhea, gastro-intestinal suctioning, draining wounds, abuse of laxatives, sweating with a fever, vigorous exercise, or external heat)
- decreased fluid intake (nausea, trouble swallowing, decreased level of consciousness, depression, confusion, mobility limitations, restraints, fluid out of reach or unavailable)
- fluid regulation problems (e.g., excess urine output (polyurea) due to inadequate antidiuretic hormone,

*Authors' division of NANDA diagnosis for clarity and treatment considerations.

elevated blood glucose levels in diabetics, hyperosmotic tube feedings, IV glucose therapy)

(b) Fluid Volume Deficit — Third Spacing of Fluids*
(no fluid loss)
Blood volume is reduced because fluid is moving out of the vascular space into interstitial spaces, tissues, and cells.

Specific Characteristics
- urine output less than intake (O < I)
- weight normal or increased
- edema in injured part of body, body spaces, joints, inflamed tissue, obstructed bowel

Related Factors
- trauma, surgery, burns
- sepsis
- intestinal obstruction
- inflamed tissues (pancreatitis, peritonitis)

Examples of Specific Nursing Diagnoses
1. Fluid volume deficit, third spacing of fluids, related to trauma and surgery on fractured leg.
   Fluid volume deficit, third spacing of fluids, related to trauma and surgery on broken hip as evidenced by urine output of 200 mL in last 8 hours, infusion of 1000 mL by IV, edema in casted leg and foot, BP of 100/68, pulse 108, slow hand vein filling. (PES format)
2. Fluid volume deficit, reduced volume, related to nausea, and vomiting.
   Fluid volume deficit, reduced volume, related to nausea, and vomiting as evidenced by loss of 5 lb in 2 days, intake of 550 mL in 24 hours; urine output of 800 mL/24 h; emesis × 3. (PES format)

Examples of Specific Outcomes
1. Urine output increases to 40–50 mL/h within 4 hours.
2. Intake of 2000 mL with output of 1500 mL in 48 hours.
3. Resolution of vomiting within 24 hours.
4. Weight gain of 8 lb to normal range of 165–170 lb by discharge.

---

*Authors' division of NANDA diagnosis for clarity and treatment considerations.

Examples of Specific Nursing Interventions
■ See General Fluid/Hydration Nursing Interventions, page 62.
■ Review client's related factors and select interventions to treat cause of fluid deficit.

> Total body fluid reduction: decrease losses, increase intake, promote regulatory function
>
> Third spacing of fluids: promote healing, treat infection, promote bowel function, reduce inflammation

■ Maintain IV fluids until client drinks at least 300–500 mL over 2–3 hours with no nausea or vomiting (doctor's order often reads "discontinue IV when taking PO fluids").
■ Replace fluids by mouth or as ordered by IV route (often start with lactated Ringer's solution or normal saline).

> Assess and teach as needed about dehydration and need for increased intake of fluids or IV therapy.
>
> Ask about and provide preferred fluids at preferred temperatures by preferred method of drinking (e.g., bottle, cup, with straw); offer Popsicles if available.
>
> Encourage consumption of fluid with electrolytes (sodium, potassium, chloride) similar to those being lost rather than water, tea, coffee.
>
> Divide daily oral fluid intake goal by 16 hours (awake time) and encourage client to drink this amount every hour.

■ Provide oral care every 2–4 hours for dry mouth.
■ Relieve nausea as much as possible; gentle fingertip stroking of stomach and abdomen may relieve nausea sensation; small, frequent fluid intake; crackers or toast; upright position; request and administer antiemetic drug from physician.
■ Report inadequate intake/reduced output to physician for possible IV therapy; tube feedings.
■ Report signs of fluid volume deficit worsening to physician: steady or decreasing urine output, increasing pulse, decreasing BP, worsening edema (third spacing), continued weight loss.
■ Assess for indications that treatment is improving fluid volume deficit: increasing urine output, decreasing pulse and increasing BP back to normal range, improved level of consciousness, increasing body weight and improved

skin turgor. If fluid volume deficit from third spacing, notify physician for possible reduction of IV flow rate to prevent hypervolemia as fluid moves out of body tissues into vascular space.

- If fluid volume deficit is caused by third spacing of fluids, watch for signs of fluid volume excess and hypervolemia as condition resolves (2–10 days after causative event/ trauma). See defining characteristics for Fluid Volume Excess, page 68.

- Assess for postural hypertension; if present take precautions to prevent faintness and falls when getting out of bed: support stockings, elevate head of bed several minutes before standing client.

Examples of Specific Evaluations for Outcomes 1 to 4

1. Outcome not met. Urine volume of 30–38 mL over last 3 hours.
2. Outcome partially met. Intake of 2500 mL but output only 1000 mL of urine with specific gravity of 1.028.
3. Outcome not met. Vomiting × 3 this shift after fluid intake.
4. Outcome met. Weight of 167 lb.

Key Index Words for Nursing Interventions

Look up these words in the index of fundamentals and medical-surgical nursing textbooks to find page references for additional nursing interventions and rationale for their selection:

- dehydration
- fluid volume deficit
- hypovolemia
- third spacing of fluids

HIGH RISK FOR FLUID VOLUME DEFICIT

Definition

The state in which an individual is at risk of experiencing vascular, cellular, or intracellular dehydration.

Defining Risk Factors

- extremes of age
- extremes of weight
- excessive losses through normal routes, e.g., vomiting, diarrhea, sweating, evaporation from exposure

- loss of fluid through abnormal routes, e.g., indwelling tubes; drains, fistulas, burns, surgery
- factors preventing or reducing access to or intake of fluids, e.g., nausea, bulimia, physical immobility, restraints, depression, confusion, NPO status prior to surgery/tests
- factors affecting absorption and excretion of fluids, e.g., elevated glucose levels; inadequate antidiuretic hormone, bowel obstructions, paralytic ileus
- factors increasing fluid needs, e.g., hypermetabolic states, fever, environmental heat, exposure of large skin surfaces
- knowledge deficiency related to fluid volume
- medications, e.g., diuretics; laxative abuse

Examples of Specific Diagnoses
1. High risk for fluid volume deficit related to history of repeated episodes of diarrhea; age 6 months.
2. High risk for fluid volume deficit related to confusion, decreased level of consciousness.
3. High risk for fluid volume deficit related to burns over 30% of body.
4. High risk for fluid volume deficit related to surgery, NPO status before and after surgery.

Examples of Specific Outcomes
1. Client maintains body weight within normal range if diarrhea recurs.
2. Fluid intake of 1500 mL or more for each 24-hour period.
3. Pulse and blood pressure remain in normal range during hospitalization.
4. Urine output of 30–50 mL/h in post-op recovery room.

Examples of Specific Nursing Interventions
- See General Fluid/Hydration Nursing Interventions, page 62.
- Reduce or eliminate risk factors.
- Compensate for risk factors by hydrating the body before and/or during events or conditions that lead to dehydration.
- Discuss with clients why they are at risk and consider interventions to prevent dehydration or reduce the severity if it develops.

- Attend to hydration needs of all clients every 2–4 hours, depending on risk factors, to prevent deficit from occurring.
- Teach parents about use of oral glucose and electrolyte solutions to help prevent dehydration in infants and children, especially with diarrhea (e.g., ORS, Rehydralyte, Pedialyte).

Examples of Specific Evaluations for Outcomes 1 to 4

1. Outcome met. Baby seen for diarrhea at age 28 months; weight for length in normal range; weight 17 lb, up 1.5 lb from visit one month ago.
2. Outcome partially met. Intake of 1500–2000 mL/24 h for first week; decreasing level of consciousness and choking episodes have reduced intake to 800–1000 mL over last 3 days.
3. Outcome not met. Hypotension, elevated pulse, and oliguria developed during transfer to burns unit.
4. Outcome met. Urine output of 40–60 mL/h while in postanesthesia recovery (PAR) area after surgery.

Key Index Words for Nursing Interventions

Look up these words in the index of fundamentals and medical-surgical nursing textbooks to find page references for additional nursing interventions and rationale for their selection:

- dehydration
- fluid volume deficit
- hypovolemia
- third spacing of fluids

FLUID VOLUME EXCESS

Definition

The state in which an individual experiences increased fluid retention and edema (isotonic fluid excess).

Defining Characteristics

- total fluid intake greater than total fluid output (I > O)
- edema: peripheral extremities; effusion (escape of fluid into body parts/spaces); anasarca (massive generalized edema)
- pulmonary congestion (chest x-ray); moist rales/crackles heard
- shortness of breath, dyspnea (difficulty breathing);

orthopnea (breathes easily only in upright position); increased rate
- weight gain over brief time period (several days)
- S3 heart sound (associated with cardiac/pumping failure)
- decreased hemoglobin (Hgb), hematocrit (Hct) and blood urea nitrogen (BUN); increased blood volume causes hemodilution of these factors—no real loss
- elevated BP and central venous pressure (above 11 cm water in vena cave)
- pulmonary artery pressure changes
- jugular (neck) vein distension
- positive hepatojugular reflex (if pressure applied over the liver for 30–60 seconds causes neck vein distention, it is a positive test for increased venous pressure)
- altered electrolytes
- azotemia (nitrogen-containing compounds in the blood)
- change in mental status (confusion)
- restlessness and anxiety

Other Characteristics
- full, bounding pulse
- slow-emptying peripheral veins (vascular fluid volume excess causes hand veins to take longer than 3–5 seconds to empty and go flat when hand elevated)
- increased urine production (polyurea) and decreased specific gravity if kidney function is normal or diuretics given (body removes excess fluid by increasing urine output)
- oliguria with increased specific gravity (decreased urine output if regulatory problem causes fluid volume excess)

Related Factors
- fluid regulatory problem (e.g., congestive heart failure, kidney failure, cirrhosis of the liver, use of steroids)
- excess fluid intake (by mouth, tube feeding, or intravenously)
- excess sodium intake (table salt, salty foods, IV solutions)

Examples of Specific Nursing Diagnoses
1. Fluid volume excess related to medication error of rapid unregulated infusion of IV solution by gravity flow.
   Fluid volume excess related to medication error of rapid

unregulated infusion of IV solution by gravity flow as evidenced by 1000 mL of normal saline infusing in 15 minutes or less, rapid bounding pulse, elevated BP, and difficulty breathing. (PES format)
2. Fluid volume excess related to ingestion of foods high in sodium and congestive heart failure.
   Fluid volume excess related to ingestion of foods high in sodium and congestive heart failure as evidenced by I > O, oliguria (25 mL/h), urine specific gravity of 1.035, edema in legs and feet; weight gain of 6 lb in 3 days; pulse 98/min and bounding, BP 178/98 mmHg, difficulty breathing, and moist rales/crackles in lower lobes of lungs. (PES format)

Examples of Specific Outcomes
1. Edema resolved by discharge; weight within 5 lb of normal.
2. Urine output increases to 1800 mL or more by end of day.
3. Two pounds weight loss in 24 hours.
4. Clear breath sounds by end of shift.

Examples of Specific Nursing Interventions
- See General Fluid/Hydration Nursing Interventions, page 62.
- Treat/correct the related factors causing the problem.
- Assess breath sounds every 4 hours or more often, based on status.
- Raise the head of the bed (semi-Fowler's position) for difficult breathing.
- Administer oxygen as ordered for breathing difficulty and altered blood gases; monitor concentration and flow rate every 1 hour.
- Assess for edema in dependent parts: feet, ankles, sacral area.
- Assess for pitting edema and measure circumference of extremity with millimeter tape measure; compare to previous measurements.
- Turn and reposition every 2 hours to prevent skin breakdown of edematous tissue.
- Explain and administer ordered diuretics; observe for increased urine output and record; watch for decreases in blood pressure.

- Assess client's knowledge and teach as needed in area of:
  fluid restrictions (physician's order)
  sodium-restricted diet (physician's order); use of distilled water if community drinking water contains too much sodium
  food seasoning alternatives to salt
  hidden sodium content in over-the-counter drugs
  preventing recurrence of fluid excess
- Collaborate with client to develop an acceptable plan for implementing fluid/diet restrictions.
- Referral to dietician; observe and reinforce teaching.
- Encourage periods of rest (lying down to promote diuresis).

Examples of Specific Evaluations for Outcomes 1 to 4 above
1. Outcome partially met. Edema reduced but still present at discharge in feet and ankles; weight 8 lb over normal.
2. Outcome met. Diuresis occurring and output 2000 mL/24 h.
3. Outcome not met. Weight is unchanged from previous day.
4. Outcome partially met. Rales/crackles in upper lobes have cleared but remain in left lower lobe.

Key Index Words for Nursing Interventions
Look up these words in the index of fundamentals and medical-surgical nursing textbooks to find page references for additional nursing interventions and rationale for their selection:

- diuresis
- edema
- fluid imbalances, excess
- fluid volume excess
- hypervolemia
- isotonic excess
- overhydration
- pulmonary edema

Case Management Example
See Appendix for examples of a nursing diagnosis of Fluid Volume Excess within clinical pathways for DRG 089, Pneumonia, page 460, and DRG 127, Congestive Heart Failure (CHF), page 466.

IMPAIRED SWALLOWING

Definition
The state in which an individual has decreased ability to voluntarily pass fluids and/or solids from the mouth to the stomach.

Major Defining Characteristics
- observed evidence of difficulty swallowing, e.g., stasis of food or fluids in oral cavity, coughing/choking

Minor Defining Characteristics
- evidence of aspiration (inspiration into the airway of foreign material; signs include difficulty breathing, coughing, abnormal breath sounds, x-ray evidence)

Related Factors
- neuromuscular impairment (e.g., decreased or absent gag reflex, as with anesthesia; decreased strength or movement of muscles involved in chewing; perceptual impairment; damage to Vth, IXth or Xth cranial nerves; muscular dystrophy, Parkinson's disease, traumatic brain injury, facial paralysis, CVA/stroke)
- mechanical obstruction (e.g., edema, tracheostomy tube, tumor)
- reddened, irritated oropharyngeal cavity; pain with swallowing; (postoperative irritation and pain from endotrachial tube)
- fatigue
- limited awareness

Examples of Specific Nursing Diagnoses
1. Impaired swallowing related to left-sided paralysis following CVA (stroke).
   Impaired swallowing related to left-sided paralysis following CVA (stroke) as evidenced by loss of liquid from left side of mouth, coughing/choking when trying to swallow. (PES format)
2. Impaired swallowing related to cleft lip and palate.
   Impaired swallowing related to cleft lip and palate as evidenced by formula draining out of nose, repeated sneezing and choking, turning dusky color during feeding attempt. (PES format)

Examples of Specific Outcomes
1. Swallowing of all foods and fluids without choking and coughing within 2 weeks.
2. Sucking and swallowing 30 mL of formula with no choking or dusky spells at next feeding.
3. Client reports no difficulty or pain with swallowing on second postoperative day.
4. Intake of 1300 mL using aseptosyringe and adaptive tubing by 10 P.M. tonight.

Examples of Specific Nursing Interventions
- See General Fluid/Hydration Nursing Interventions, page 62.
- Provide food and fluids when client is most alert and least sedated or drowsy from anesthesia, analgesics, or fatigue.
- Assess ability to swallow before giving food and fluids by asking client to demonstrate swallowing.
- Place client in an upright position with head bent slightly forward for swallowing (decrease risk of aspiration).
- Offer fluids/foods in small amounts, frequently; watch for swallowing before offering more.
- Try alternative methods: use of syringe to deliver fluids into the mouth; adaptive tubing attached to a syringe; straws.
- Allow unhurried and supportive eating and drinking time; encourage client to eat and drink slowly.
- Encourage complete, thorough chewing of food; check fit of dentures and presence of enough teeth to chew.
- If chewing is a problem, provide food in a mechanically altered form from ground to pureed or liquified.
- Encourage client to close lips when swallowing; hold lips closed for clients unable to do this independently.
- If CVA (stroke) is the cause of the swallowing problem:
  instruct client to turn the head to the unaffected side or turn head for client if unable.
  place food, fluids, straw on unaffected side of mouth.
- Provide moisture for dry mouth; artificial saliva; liquids swallowed with food.
- Have suctioning equipment available in case of choking.
- Refer to occupational therapy or dietician.

■ Assess family and client knowledge of the Heimlich maneuver and teach as needed before discharge if the swallowing problem continues.

Examples of Specific Evaluations for Outcomes 1 to 4

1. Outcome partially met. Swallowing without problem except when fatigued or drowsy in evening; then choking recurs.
2. Outcome met. When held upright and using special nipple, feeding of 35 mL taken without difficulty.
3. Outcome met. Client reports no swallowing problems or pain with use of Tylenol #3 1 hour before eating and drinking.
4. Outcome not met. Total intake of 800 mL with difficulty by 10 P.M.

Key Index Words for Nursing Interventions

Look up these words in the index of fundamentals and medical-surgical nursing textbooks to find page references for additional nursing interventions and rationale for their selection:

■ aspiration
■ dysphagia (difficulty swallowing)
■ swallowing; impaired, promoting

Chapter 4

Infant Feeding/ Breast-Feeding Problems

FOCUSED ASSESSMENT GUIDE

Complete this focused assessment if a general nursing assessment indicates a possible problem. Then turn to page 77 of this text for the Data ⇒ Diagnosis Matching Guide for infant feeding problems to help you select the best nursing diagnosis to match a client's data.

OBSERVE AND ASSESS FOR PROBLEMS WITH

Mother
___ preparation and storage of formula; where to buy
___ correct positioning of plastic nipple in mouth and angled so it is filled with formula for bottle-feeding
___ effective burping technique
___ positioning infant at breast
___ helping infant attach correctly to nipple
___ breaking suction before removing baby from breast
___ timing: frequency of feedings (every 2–4 hours), nursing 10–15 minutes on each breast; uses both breasts for each feeding; alternates starting breast
___ maternal fatigue, pain, anxiety, adequacy of diet and fluids
___ expected duration for breast-feeding; knowledge of weaning

Breasts
___ inverted or flat nipples make latch-on difficult or impossible
___ presence of sucking bruises (indicates incorrect positioning of infant on nipple), sore damaged nipples, painful areas (mastitis)
___ poorly fitting support bra
___ presence of milk/colostrum; let down or milk ejection reflex

Infant
___ 6–8 wet diapers per day
___ soft stool, easy to pass
___ weight gain and growth appropriate for age and length
___ satisfaction in between feedings
___ effective latch-on and suck for duration of feeding; frequent swallowing
___ sucking and swallowing coordinated with breathing
___ contented during feeding

NORMALS AND INFORMATION

- If obtaining adequate breast milk, newborn will regain birth weight in 2 weeks or less
- Height and weight appropriate for age are indicators of adequate nutrition in infancy
- The breast takes about 2 hours to refill when lactating
- Nursing mothers have increased metabolic needs, 500 cal/day
- Infants will breast-feed on a 2–5 hour variable schedule; approximately 6–8 feedings in a 24-hour period
- Most of the milk is emptied out of the breast after 5–8 minutes of effective sucking; breast-feeding 10–15 minutes on each breast is common
- Infants usually nurse from both breasts at each feeding
- Stress, anxiety, fatigue, and pain can prevent the let down reflex and the infant will be unable to obtain the mother's milk
- Touching the nipples or infant sucking on the nipples causes the let down reflex, which forces milk out into the

main ducts of the breasts, where the baby can pump it out through sucking

- On average, breast milk comes in on the third day after delivery (range 1–5 days); before then baby receives colostrum
- The average infant sleeps through the night around 3–4 months with great individual variation
- Healthy full-term infants need no awakening to feed
- Breast milk is the best product for infant nutrition and is completely adequate as a food and fluid source until 5–6 months
- Cow milk should not be offered during the first year of life to reduce the risk of allergies; use breast milk or infant formula
- Breast-feeding does not prevent ovulation or pregnancy
- Breast milk averages 20 cal/oz (as does infant formula)

DATA ⇒ DIAGNOSIS MATCHING GUIDE

Compare your client data from the Infant Feeding/Breast-feeding Focused Assessment to these related nursing diagnoses and abbreviated descriptions. Select the nursing diagnosis with the best match. Then turn to the page in this section with that specific diagnosis for help in planning care.

1. *Effective Breast-feeding: page 79*
   - definition: mother and infant show adequate proficiency and satisfaction with breast-feeding process
   - data: mother able to position infant at breast to promote a successful latch-on response; infant is content after feeding; regular and sustained suckling/swallowing at breast; appropriate infant weight patterns for age; effective mother/infant communication patterns (infant cues, maternal interpretation, and response)

2. *Ineffective Breast-feeding: page 82*
   - definition: a mother, infant, or child experience dissatisfaction or difficulty with the breast-feeding process
   - data: unsatisfactory breast-feeding process

3. *Interrupted Breast-feeding: page 85*
    ■ definition: a break in the continuity of the breast-feeding process as a result of inability or inadvisability to put baby to breast for feeding
    ■ data: infant does not receive nourishment at the breast for some or all of the feeding

4. *Ineffective Infant Feeding Pattern: page 88*
    ■ definition: infant demonstrates an impaired ability to suck or coordinate the suck/swallow response
    ■ data: inability to initiate or sustain an effective suck; inability to coordinate sucking, swallowing, and breathing.

GENERAL OUTCOMES AND NURSING INTERVENTIONS

GENERAL INFANT FEEDING/BREAST-FEEDING OUTCOMES

■ Infant's weight is appropriate for age and length.
■ Family states satisfaction with chosen method of infant feeding.
■ Mother/family states confidence in ability to feed infant.
■ Infant eats effectively at breast or bottle.
■ Infant has 6–8 wet diapers per day; soft stools, easy to pass.
■ Infant meets all nutrition/fluid needs through oral feedings at breast or bottle for first 4–6 months of life.

GENERAL INFANT FEEDING/BREAST-FEEDING NURSING INTERVENTIONS

■ Reduce or eliminate any related factors causing the feeding problem whenever possible (e.g., teach mother how to promote a healthy full-term pregnancy, assess for flat or inverted nipples and treat before delivery with breast shields, begin breast-feeding teaching during last months of pregnancy).
■ Assess knowledge and skill level of mother/family in breast or bottle feeding and base teaching on identified learning needs.

- Initiate breast-feeding as soon as possible; within first hour after delivery when newborn is alert and likely to suck.
- Take care of the mother's needs for pain relief, rest, personal grooming, food/fluids.
- Stay with the mother and assist with the first few feedings.
- Reinforce feeding efforts; minimize stress by assuring mother of success as baby becomes more alert and she becomes more rested.
- Provide parents with outcomes to evaluate adequacy of infant feeding: 6–8 wet diapers per day; soft stools, easy to pass; going 2 hours before wanting to eat; contented in between feedings, contented at breast while nursing; sucking and swallowing with no choking; weight gain appropriate for age at next well-baby checkup.

RELATED NURSING DIAGNOSES

EFFECTIVE BREAST-FEEDING

Definition
A state in which a mother/infant dyad or family exhibits adequate proficiency and satisfaction with the breast-feeding process.

Major Defining Characteristics
- mother able to position infant at breast to promote a successful latch-on response
- infant is contented after feeding
- regular and sustained suckling/swallowing at breast
- appropriate infant weight patterns for age
- effective mother/infant communication patterns (infant cues, maternal interpretation, and response)

Minor Defining Characteristics
- signs and/or symptoms of oxytocin release (let down or milk ejection reflex), e.g., milk begins to drip, tingling sensation in breasts/nipples, infant swallowing frequently
- adequate infant elimination patterns for age (e.g., 6–8 wet diapers per day; soft stools, easy to pass)
- eagerness of infant to nurse
- mother states satisfaction with the breast-feeding process

Related Factors
- basic breast-feeding knowledge
- normal breast structure
- normal infant oral structure
- infant gestational age greater than 34 weeks (full term 38–42 weeks)
- support sources
- maternal confidence

Examples of Specific Nursing Diagnoses
1. Effective breast-feeding related to mastering basic knowledge and skills of breast-feeding, and strong support from family.
   Effective breast-feeding related to mastering basic knowledge and skills of breast-feeding, and strong support from family as evidenced by baby nursing 10 minutes per breast at feedings every 2–4 hours and regaining birth weight by 2 weeks. (PES format)
2. Effective breast-feeding related to maternal knowledge, skill, and confidence from successfully breast-feeding last child; full-term, healthy newborn with strong suck.
   Effective breast-feeding related to maternal knowledge, skill, and confidence from successfully nursing last child; full-term, healthy newborn with strong suck as evidenced by good positioning and latch-on for nursing, effective sucking for 10–15 minutes per breast and denial of any problems. (PES format)

Examples of Specific Outcomes
1. Mother demonstrates basic knowledge and skills in breast-feeding by discharge.
2. Infant sucking effectively for 10–15 minutes per breast at all feedings on a 2–5 hour schedule one week after delivery.
3. Infant has 6–8 wet diapers day and stools are soft and easy to pass for the duration of the breast-feeding experience.
4. Baby's weight appropriate for age and length at all well-baby visits during the breast-feeding experience.

Examples of Specific Nursing Interventions
- See General Infant Feeding/Breast-feeding Nursing Interventions, page 78.

- Promote development of all related factors resulting in successful breast-feeding whenever possible (e.g., assess early in pregnancy for use of any medications/drugs that cause birth defects or prematurity, such as alcohol or cocaine, and work with mother to terminate use; begin teaching about breast-feeding in last trimester of pregnancy; initiate use of breast shields/cups during last half of pregnancy for flat or inverted nipples to make nipples protractile by delivery).
- Assess and teach based on the mother's knowledge and skill level.
- Encourage and support at all feedings.
- Meet the mother's physical and psychosocial needs.
- Verbally and physically help the mother with breast-feeding skills during the first few feedings.
- Provide privacy as desired by mothers learning to breast-feed.

Examples of Specific Evaluations for Outcomes 1 to 4

1. Outcome met. At discharge, mother breast-feeds successfully and verbalizes adequate knowledge in response to questions about common breast-feeding problems.
2. Outcome partially met. Infant breast-feeding for 15 minutes on first breast but only a few minutes of effective sucking on second breast on a 2–3 hour schedule.
3. Outcome not met. Infant has 2–3 wet diapers per day, stools are pellet-like from straining to pass and crying in between a strict 4-hour feeding schedule.
4. Outcome partially met. Infant in 90% for weight but only 30% for length at age 3 months. Mother states infant loves to nurse and is nursing every 2–3 hours for 30 minutes around-the-clock.

Key Index Words for Nursing Interventions

Look up these words in the index of fundamentals and medical-surgical nursing textbooks to find page references for additional nursing interventions and rationale for their selection:

- breast-feeding
- breast shields

- inverted nipples, treatment
- prematurity, prevention, risk factors
- teratogens

INEFFECTIVE BREAST-FEEDING

Definition
A state in which a mother, infant, or child experiences dissatisfaction or difficulty with the breast-feeding process.

Major Defining Characteristic
- unsatisfactory breast-feeding process

Minor Defining Characteristics
- actual or perceived inadequate milk supply
- infant inability to attach to maternal breast correctly
- no observable sign of oxytocin release (no tingling sensation in breast/nipples, no milk dripping, minimal infant swallowing, lack of infant satisfaction in between feedings, wanting to nurse every hour or "all the time")
- signs of inadequate infant intake (few wet diapers, hard dry stools with straining, crying in between feedings, demanding to feed frequently, weight loss of more than 10% of birth weight, inadequate weight gain)
- nonsustained suckling at the breast; pulls away or loses nipple (engorgement, flat nipple, inverted nipple, unable to obtain air around breast while sucking), weak suck, fatigue
- insufficient emptying of each breast per feeding (inadequate suck, inadequate sucking time at breasts, failure of let down reflex, nursing at only one breast each feeding)
- persistence of sore nipples beyond the first week of nursing
- insufficient opportunity for suckling at the breast
- infant exhibiting fussiness and crying within the first hour after breast-feeding
- infant unresponsive to other comfort measures
- infant arching and crying at the breast
- infant resists latch-on

Related Factors
- previous history of breast-feeding failure
- infant receiving supplemental feedings with artificial nipple

- poor infant sucking reflex
- nonsupportive partner/family
- knowledge deficit
- interruption in breast-feeding
- maternal anxiety or ambivalence; pain, fatigue, inadequate nutritional and fluid intake
- prematurity
- infant anomaly (e.g., cleft lip, palate)
- maternal breast anomaly (flat or inverted nipples)
- previous breast surgery (breast reduction surgery prevents breast-feeding because of disruption of duct system and movement of nipple; breast-feeding possible with breast augmentation)

Examples of Specific Nursing Diagnoses
1. Ineffective breast-feeding related to lack of knowledge and skill in breast-feeding.
   Ineffective breast-feeding related to lack of knowledge and skill in breast-feeding as evidenced by incorrect positioning of infant at breast, incorrect placement of nipple in mouth for effective sucking, sucking bruises around nipple, sore nipples. (PES format)
2. Ineffective breast-feeding related to fatigue, anxiety, lack of family support.
   Ineffective breast-feeding related to fatigue, anxiety, lack of family support as evidenced by reports of nursing every hour around the clock for last 2 days, no sleep, baby crying all the time, family telling mother to bottle-feed, absence of let down sensation in breasts. (PES format)

Examples of Specific Outcomes
1. Infant nursing 5 minutes per breast with correct sucking hold and position at next feeding.
2. Infant content between breast-feedings and reestablished a 2–5 hour schedule by end of week.
3. Mother states breast-feeding is going well before discharge.
4. Newborn regains birth weight within 2 weeks on breast milk.

Examples of Specific Nursing Interventions
- See General Infant Feeding/Breast-feeding Nursing Interventions, page 78.

- Reduce or eliminate the related factors interfering with breast-feeding (e.g., do not offer breast-feeding newborns supplemental bottle feedings of water or glucose; start mother with inverted or flat nipples on breast shields in last months of pregnancy so nipples are everted by delivery).
- Provide privacy from visitors as mother desires.
- Reassess knowledge/skill level to identify specific problems and teach as needed about:

    positions for nursing: side lying, football hold, cradle

    timing: 5–10 minutes per breast to start, rather than 2–3 minutes, to reduce risk of engorgement and sore nipples; advance to 10–15 minutes by discharge; nurse every 2–4 hours when baby alert in first few days

    nursing at both night feedings to prevent engorgement

    elicit the rooting reflex by stroking down baby's cheek with finger or nipple so baby turns toward breast with open mouth

    correct positioning of nipple in infant's mouth

    provide breathing space for nursing infant with finger or by pulling down on breast close to nose

    stimulate sucking by stroking around lips or bumping under chin

    break suction before pulling breast out of baby's mouth

    air-dry nipples; no plastic liners in bra (prevents drying); avoid use of soap on nipples

    relationship between milk supply, adequate nutrition/fluid intake by mother and infant emptying breasts at each feeding

    let down reflex (milk ejection reflex) and effect of stress, fatigue, pain, anxiety

    expression of milk, manually, with hand pump or electric pump

    storage of milk

    use of occasional supplemental bottle after 2 weeks so baby will take plastic nipple if mother away for a feeding

    weaning

    birth control while lactating

- Encourage mother to keep baby in room and attempt

nursing when baby awake rather than on set time schedule in first few days.

■ Emphasize the need for mother to take good care of herself as the milk producer: rest, increased calorie intake of 500 cal/day, extra fluids, minimal visitors and household responsibilities in first few weeks.

■ Problem-solve with mother how to prevent/manage fatigue, sore nipples, inadequate milk supply, too frequent nursings, or missing a feeding.

Examples of Specific Evaluations for Outcomes 1 to 4

1. Outcome met. Mother and infant nursing well together 8–10 minutes per breast per feeding with nipple and areola positioned back in mouth.
2. Outcome partially met. Infant back on 2–5 hour feeding intervals and is content between but is being supplemented with formula after each breast-feeding.
3. Outcome not met. Mother states husband and in-laws continually questioned the adequacy of her milk supply, making her so tense that she switched to bottle feeding.
4. Outcome met. Weight 3 oz above birth weight at 2 weeks.

Key Index Words for Nursing Interventions

Look up these words in the index of fundamentals and medical-surgical nursing textbooks to find page references for additional nursing interventions and rationale for their selection:

- breast-feeding, ineffective
- breast milk
- engorgement
- lactation
- let down reflex
- milk ejection reflex
- nutrition, newborn, infant
- oxytocin
- prolactin

INTERRUPTED BREAST-FEEDING

Definition

A break in the continuity of the breast-feeding process as a result of inability or inadvisability to put baby to breast for feeding.

Major Defining Characteristic
- infant does not receive nourishment at the breast for some or all of feeding

Minor Defining Characteristics
- maternal desire to maintain lactation and provide (or eventually provide) her breast milk for her infant's nutritional needs
- separation of mother and infant
- lack of knowledge regarding expression and storage of breast milk

Related Factors
- maternal or infant illness
- prematurity
- maternal employment
- contraindications to breast-feeding (e.g., drugs, true breast milk jaundice)
- need to abruptly wean infant

Examples of Specific Nursing Diagnoses
1. Interrupted breast-feeding related to maternal fever of 102°F (38.9°C), 24-hour hold ordered on breast-feeding by pediatrician.
   Interrupted breast-feeding related to maternal fever of 102°F, 24-hour hold ordered on breast-feeding by pediatrician, resulting in bottle-feeding of formula at all feedings for next 24 hours. (PES format)
2. Interrupted breast-feeding related to discovery of cardiac defect in newborn, heart surgery within 24 hours of delivery.
   Interrupted breast-feeding related to discovery of cardiac defect in newborn, heart surgery within 24 hours of delivery as evidenced by IV therapy, and gavage and bottle-feeding of formula for first week after surgery. (PES format)

Examples of Specific Outcomes
1. Newborn nursing 5–10 minutes per breast at all feedings 24 hours after reinitiating breast-feeding.
2. Newborn sucks at least 5 minutes at breast during first feeding after reinitiating breast-feeding.

3. Mother's milk supply adequate to meet total nutritional needs of infant within 1 week of reinitiating breast-feeding.
4. Mother pumps out 1/2 to 1 oz of breast milk from each breast every 4–6 hours until reinitiation of breast-feeding.

Examples of Specific Nursing Interventions

- See General Infant Feeding/Breast-feeding Nursing Interventions, page 78.
- Reduce, treat, or eliminate factors preventing breast-feeding.
- Discuss feeding options with family: continuation of nursing as soon as possible or switching to bottle feeding; reassure mother of likelihood of successful reinitiation if that is what she and family desire.
- Teach mother how to maintain milk supply until breast-feeding reinitiated by pumping each breast every 4 hours using manual expression, manual breast pump, or electric breast pump.
- Feed expressed breast milk to infant whenever possible (e.g., gavage feed breast milk rather than formula).
- If infant being fed by gavage tube, stimulate sucking reflex with clean little finger in mouth while gavage feeding (encourage parents to do this as nurse does gavage).
- Review breast-feeding teaching as needed (see Specific Nursing Interventions for Ineffective Breast-feeding, page 83).
- Stay with mother for first several feedings; encourage and support her efforts; make suggestions for promoting more effective breast-feeding based on observations.
- Have mother express milk onto nipple when trying to get infant to latch on during reinitiation of breast-feeding.
- Encourage frequent feedings, every 2–3 hours when reinitiating breast-feeding to increase mother's milk supply.

Examples of Specific Evaluations for Outcomes 1 to 4

1. Outcome met. Nursing without difficulty for 10 minutes per breast at every feeding since restarting breast-feeding.
2. Outcome not met. Infant very sleepy with weak suck; crying with mother's nipple in mouth and does not suck; sucks poorly on plastic nipple.

3. Outcome partially met. Baby obtaining 3 oz at breast at feedings but demanding to feed every 1–2 hours and mother becoming exhausted.
4. Outcome met. Mother obtaining 2–3 oz of breast milk every 4 hours with the electric breast pump.

Key Index Words for Nursing Interventions
Look up these words in the index of fundamentals and medical-surgical nursing textbooks to find page references for additional nursing interventions and rationale for their selection:

- breast-feeding, interrupted
- breast pump, manual, electric
- lactation
- relactation

INEFFECTIVE INFANT FEEDING PATTERN

Definition
A state in which an infant demonstrates an impaired ability to suck or coordinate the suck/swallow response.

Major Defining Characteristics
- inability to initiate or sustain an effective suck
- inability to coordinate sucking, swallowing, and breathing

Related Factors
- prematurity (weak suck, tires easily, immature gag reflex)
- neurological impairment/delay
- oral hypersensitivity
- prolonged NPO (infant loses sucking reflex/response)
- anatomical abnormality (cleft lip and/or palate; tracheo-esophageal fistula)

Examples of Specific Nursing Diagnoses
1. Ineffective infant feeding pattern related to prematurity. Ineffective infant feeding pattern related to prematurity as evidenced by weak, nonsustained sucking during 30 minutes of attempted bottle feeding. (PES format)
2. Ineffective infant feeding pattern related to prolonged feeding through gastrostomy. Ineffective infant feeding pattern related to prolonged feeding through gastrostomy as evidenced by minimal

response to stimulation of the sucking reflex or absence of effective suck. (PES format)

Examples of Specific Outcomes

1. Baby sucking effectively for all feeding by discharge.
2. Baby sucks several times on pacifier during next gavage feeding.
3. Baby gaining 1/4 to 1/2 oz per day on oral feedings by discharge at end of week.
4. Baby takes 2 oz of feeding in 30 minutes or less at next feeding with no color changes, choking, or bradycardia (slow heart rate).

Examples of Specific Nursing Interventions

- See General Infant Feeding/Breast-feeding Nursing Interventions, page 78.
- Reduce or eliminate the related factors causing the problem as much as possible.
- Use prosthetic or adaptive nipples to overcome anatomical and/or maturational problem (e.g., special nipples available for preterms, for cleft lip/palate).
- Begin or reinitiate nipple feedings as soon as possible (e.g., report spontaneous sucking and gagging response by preterm to physician as a sign of readiness to begin nipple feedings).
- Feed in a more upright position to facilitate swallowing without choking; position on right side with head elevated after feeding to decrease chance of regurgitation.
- Gradually change to oral feedings to prevent fatigue and maintain daily weight gain, especially in preterm (e.g., begin with one nipple feeding a day, advance to one per shift, advance to nipple feeding every other feeding); advance number of nipple feedings based on infant response and daily weight gain (usually a doctor's order).
- Prevent formula or breast milk from flowing too rapidly if infant choking is a problem (smaller hole in nipple if bottle feeding, removing baby from breast briefly as let down occurs if reflex too forceful).
- If baby forgets to breathe (turns dusky, bluish gray color) during feeding, remove nipple and stimulate to breathe.
- Try to elicit sucking reflex with pacifier or clean little finger whenever feeding by gavage or through gastrostomy

to maintain reflex and pair sucking with satiation of hunger.

Examples of Specific Evaluations for Outcomes 1 to 4

1. Outcome partially met. Infant being discharged with fairly strong suck but tires at the end of feeding; mother works nipple up against the palate and uses preterm nipple to feed.
2. Outcome met. Baby showed sucking activity × 2 during gavage feeding with stimulation of upper palate using pacifier.
3. Outcome not met. Infant unable to maintain weight gain on all oral feedings by end of week.
4. Outcome met. Obtained 45 mL of formula during 30 minutes of sucking with no color or vital sign changes.

Key Index Words for Nursing Interventions

Look up these words in the index of fundamentals and medical-surgical nursing textbooks to find page references for additional nursing interventions and rationale for their selection:

- cleft lip, palate
- gag reflex
- gavage feeding
- infant feeding, ineffective pattern
- prematurity
- rooting reflex
- sucking reflex

Chapter 5

Mobility/Activity Problems

FOCUSED ASSESSMENT GUIDE

Complete this focused assessment if a general nursing assessment indicates a possible problem. Then turn to page 94 of this text for the Data ⇒ Diagnosis Matching Guide for mobility/activity problems to help you select the best nursing diagnosis to match the client's data.

TELL ME IF YOU ARE HAVING ANY OF THESE PROBLEMS

___ a decrease in your usual type or amount of exercise/physical activity because of health problems
___ pain/discomfort generally or with movement
___ fatigue or weakness generally or with activity
___ difficult or labored breathing with activity
___ current restrictions or limitations on movement/activity, joint flexion, weight bearing, positioning in bed or elevation of the bed (ordered by physician; for comfort; for physical problems) Describe:

AND ASK THESE QUESTIONS

___ If on bed rest or limited activity, how long has it been?
___ Do you use any assistive devices like a brace, walker, crutches, or cane?

___ What kind of help do you need to turn and reposition in bed, get out of bed to a chair, and to walk?

___ What kind of exercise/physical activity do you usually do each week? (Look for evidence of sedentary life style.)

___ Are you feeling bored or wishing there was something to do?

ASSESS CLIENT/CHART/PHYSICIAN'S ORDERS FOR

___ activity order; movement/flexion/weight-bearing restrictions

___ presence of treatment-related obstacles to mobility such as drains, urinary catheters, IVs, braces, casts, prostheses

___ new mobility skill such as use of crutches, walker

___ relearning mobility skills or performing them in a new way because of injury, trauma, treatment, activity restrictions

___ abnormal heart rate or BP response to activity (e.g., orthostatic hypotension—increased pulse, decreased BP, dizzy, faint when moved from lying to standing position)

___ presence of arrhythmias (irregular heart rhythm) with activity

___ deconditioned status (decreased muscle strength, endurance, control and/or mass)

___ impaired coordination and/or ability to move, reposition, transfer, ambulate unassisted

___ limited range of joint motion

___ lack of diversional activities in room or immediate environment

___ presence of circulatory/respiratory problems

___ perceptual/cognitive impairment (orientation, level of consciousness, thinking ability)

___ neuromuscular impairment (e.g., paralysis, MS, MD, Parkinson's disease)

___ musculoskeletal impairment (e.g., fractures, contractures)

___ depression/severe anxiety

ADULT NORMALS AND INFORMATION

- Energy (ATP) is needed for muscle contractions and relaxation
- Muscles are attached to bones by connective tissue (tendons)
- Body movement is caused by simultaneous contraction of antagonistic muscles on opposite sides of joints (coactivation)
- Purposeful movement of skeletal muscles is controlled by the brain and spinal cord
- Resting muscles are slightly contracted; this is called muscle tone and is controlled by the brain, spinal nerves, and muscles; muscles with decreased tone are called flaccid; muscles with increased tone are called spastic
- Muscles are constantly being remodeled to match their use
- Muscle hypertrophy (increased muscle mass) occurs over time when muscles are contracting at maximum or near maximum strength; three or four strong contractions every day will cause muscle hypertrophy in 6–10 weeks and increased strength
- Muscle atrophy (decreased muscle mass) occurs in response to disuse of the muscle or loss of the muscle's nerve supply; atrophy begins almost immediately; muscle degeneration (destruction of muscle tissue and replacement with fibrous and fatty tissue) occurs over several months; if nerve supply is reestablished within 3 months, full return of function will occur; after 1–2 years without nerve stimulation return of muscle function will not occur
- Contractures are shortening of muscles occurring during disuse from muscle atrophy and degeneration
- Rigor mortis occurs several hours after death when all the muscles of the body contract and become rigid from loss of ATP needed for relaxation; 15–25 hours after death the muscle proteins have been destroyed and rigor mortis ends
- Interruption of blood flow through a contracting muscle will lead to complete muscle fatigue in about one minute because of loss of nutrients and oxygen
- Isotonic muscle contractions result in muscle shortening and movement (bending an arm)

- Isometric muscle contractions do not result in much muscle shortening or movement but cause increased muscle tension

DATA ⇒ DIAGNOSIS MATCHING GUIDE

Compare your client data from the Mobility/Activity Focused Assessment to these related mobility/activity nursing diagnoses and abbreviated descriptions. Select the nursing diagnosis with the best match. Then turn to the page in this section with that specific diagnosis for help in planning care.

1. *Activity Intolerance: page 98*
   - definition: insufficient physiological or psychological energy to endure or complete required/desired daily activity
   - data: verbal report of fatigue, weakness with activity; difficult, labored breathing and BP and pulse changes with activity
2. *High Risk for Activity Intolerance: page 101*
   - definition: at risk for insufficient physiological/ psychological energy to endure or complete required/ desired daily activity
   - data: deconditioned status; previous intolerance; presence of circulatory/respiratory problems; bed rest, immobility or reduced mobility for a period of time
3. *Diversional Activity Deficit: page 103*
   - definition: decreased interest, participation or stimulation from recreational or leisure activities
   - data: patient statements of boredom, wishing there was something to do; unable to engage self in usual hobbies/activities
4. *Impaired Physical Mobility: page 109*
   - definition: limited ability for independent physical movement
   - data: inability to move purposefully within physical environment; reluctant to attempt movement; limited range of motion; decreased muscle strength/mass; imposed movement restrictions; impaired coordination

5. *High Risk for Peripheral Neurovascular Dysfunction: page 56*
   - definition: at risk for disruption in circulation, sensation, or motion of an extremity (see Circulation Problems, page 43)
   - risk factors: fractures; mechanical compression (e.g., tourniquet, cast, brace, dressings or restraint); orthopedic surgery; trauma; immobilization; burns; vascular obstruction

6. *High Risk for Disuse Syndrome: page 106*
   - definition: at risk for deterioration of body systems as the result of prescribed or unavoidable musculoskeletal inactivity (complications of immobility)
   - risk factors: paralysis; mechanical or prescribed immobility; severe pain; altered level of consciousness

7. *Fatigue: page 205*
   - definition: overwhelming sustained sense of exhaustion and decreased capacity for physical and mental work (see Rest and Sleep Problems, page 202)
   - data: report of overwhelming, continuing lack of energy; inability to maintain usual routines

8. *Self-Care Deficit:*
   Bathing/Hygiene: page 217
   Dressing/Grooming: page 220
   Feeding: page 222
   Toileting: page 225
   - definition: an impaired ability to perform or complete any of the above activities for oneself

GENERAL OUTCOMES AND NURSING INTERVENTIONS

GENERAL MOBILITY/ACTIVITY OUTCOMES

- Client will reestablish independent physical mobility.
- Client will return to prior level of activity or mobility following period of healing and imposed limitations.
- Client will experience no complications of immobility.
- Client will use mobility aids correctly and consistently.

- Client will perform activities of daily living safely, independently, and without excessive fatigue or weakness.
- Client will participate in activities for mental and physical stimulation, enjoyment, and relaxation.

GENERAL MOBILITY/ACTIVITY NURSING INTERVENTIONS

- Reduce or eliminate any related factors causing/contributing to the mobility/activity problem whenever possible.
- Review any activity/mobility restriction ordered by physician with client and family; document in large print in client's room for other health care providers to follow.
- Assess client's abilities and responses to activity/mobility (vital signs, BP, skin color; development of any pulse irregularities, sweating, angina/chest pain; report of fatigue, dizziness, faintness, weakness).
- Manage current pain; anticipate painful activities and medicate to prevent pain (e.g., physical therapy, turning, transfers).
- Promote good fluid and nutrition intake (see General Nutrition Nursing Interventions, page 117, and Fluid/Hydration Nursing Interventions, page 62).
- Promote optimal respiratory functioning (see General Respiratory/Breathing Nursing Interventions, page 179).
- Promote rest and sleep (see General Rest/Sleep Nursing Interventions, page 204).
- Anticipate fear/anxiety associated with decreased mobility, loss of independence, confinement in cast, traction, circle bed, etc.; provide support, explanations, call light, and consistent nursing personnel to decrease anxiety.
- Explain all treatments and interventions to client/family; demonstrate and teach based on assessment of current knowledge and skills (e.g., transfers, crutch walking, isometric exercises, activities to prevent complications of immobility).
- Turn and reposition in good alignment every 2 hours (minimum).
- Exercise muscles and joints (unless contraindicated):
  Range of motion to joints: move through full range of

motion or to point of discomfort every shift; active range of motion (AROM) if client able to move independently; passive range of motion (PROM) to assist or replace AROM to achieve full joint movement.

Promote strength and independent movement: use of bed trapeze; encourage client to use muscles during turning, repositioning and self-care to maintain strength; encourage participation in activities of daily living within limits of treatment or condition.

Use machines, aids as ordered to maintain joint mobility, improve circulation and healing (e.g., continuous passive motion machine (CPM) following knee surgery; electrical muscle stimulators.

Encourage isometric exercise of extremities, including immobilized part (10 repetitions per hour while awake):
  —quadriceps setting exercises: lying flat with leg straight on bed, push knee down into mattress by contracting anterior thigh muscle, hold 5–10 seconds and relax (can be done with leg cast, brace).
  —gluteal setting exercises: lying flat in bed with leg straight, contract muscles of buttocks and abdomen, hold for 5–10 seconds and relax.

Encourage isotonic movement of extremities, hands, feet, fingers, and toes as condition permits; ankle pumps 10 repetitions per hour while awake (flexion and extension of ankles).

■ Out of bed as soon as possible; up in chair for meals; early ambulation; encourage weight-bearing activity.

■ Progressive ambulation; progress slowly if client has been on bed rest to prevent orthostatic hypotension, weakness, fatigue or falls; advance only if client reports no dizziness or faintness and enough strength to continue.

  Before Getting Out of Bed
  —isometric leg exercises (several repetitions)
  —elevate head of bed for 20–30 minutes
  —put on support hose, if available, and any required braces
  —dangle at side of bed with legs hanging over for 1–2 minutes

—put on transfer belt and supportive, nonslip shoes
Out of Bed
—position any assistive devices for client use
—assist to standing position using transfer belt and support for 1–2 minutes
—assist with transfer to chair or commode
—assist with ambulating in room and back to bed/chair
—assist with ambulating in hall and back to bed/chair

- Encourage rest before and after exercise and activity.
- Apply braces and pillows to limit movement of affected joint or extremity while allowing safe turning, repositioning, ambulation (e.g., abductor pillow for turning, raised toilet seat to prevent excessive flexion at hip when toileting following hip replacement; leg brace for knee surgery).
- Use of transfer belts, good body mechanics and help from other personnel during client repositioning, transfers, and ambulation to provide client safety and prevent injury to the nurse.
- Coordinate nursing efforts with those of physical therapy; provide rest and anticipatory pain relief before scheduling PT treatments; review and clarify client teaching done by therapist and reinforce.

RELATED NURSING DIAGNOSES

ACTIVITY INTOLERANCE

Definition
A state in which an individual has insufficient physiological or psychological energy to endure or complete required or desired daily activity.

Critical Defining Characteristic
- verbal report of fatigue or weakness

Defining Characteristics
- abnormal heart rate or blood pressure response to activity (e.g., increased pulse and respiratory rates; drop in BP when moving from lying to standing position)
- exertion discomfort or dyspnea (difficult, labored breathing)

- electrocardiographic changes reflecting arrhythmias (irregular heart rhythm) or ischemia (inadequate blood flow to heart tissues)

Related Factors
- decreased mobility/bed rest/immobility caused by progressive chronic diseases, injury, surgery, treatment regimens, obesity, pain
- generalized weakness caused by such things as poor nutrition, endocrine and fluid/electrolyte disturbances, neurological problems, kidney and liver disease
- sedentary lifestyle as may occur with depression, lack of knowledge, learned behaviors, confusion, use of restraints for disoriented clients, lack of people to assist with ambulation, inadequate sleep, medications, alcohol consumption
- imbalance between oxygen supply/demand (inadequate oxygenation) as occurs in chronic respiratory or cardiac disease, anemia

Examples of Specific Nursing Diagnoses
1. Activity intolerance related to bed rest and general weakness secondary to fracture of hip and surgical repair.
   Activity intolerance related to bed rest and general weakness secondary to fracture of hip and surgical repair as evidenced by report of weakness, increased heart rate, decreased BP, and faintness when attempting ambulation. (PES format)
2. Activity intolerance related to sedentary lifestyle, emphysema (smoker for 30 years), 50 lb overweight for height.
   Activity intolerance related to sedentary lifestyle, emphysema (smoker for 30 years), 50 lb overweight for height as evidenced by hard breathing with increased rate and depth and elevated pulse after walking two blocks. (PES format)

Examples of Specific Outcomes
1. Client reports no abnormal fatigue or weakness after walking length of hall before discharge.
2. Client reports no faintness or dizziness and maintains pulse below 90 beats per minute and BP above 130/70 mmHg during next attempt to ambulate in room.

3. Client reports no difficult, labored breathing after walking 1 mile following 6 weeks of progressive exercise.
4. Client performs activities of daily living without excessive fatigue 6 weeks after surgery for fractured hip.

Examples of Specific Nursing Interventions

- See General Mobility/Activity Nursing Interventions, page 96.
- Assess for types and amount of activities causing problem.
- Assess for presence of factors which may be causing or contributing to the intolerance (e.g., pain, activity after eating, inadequate nutritional intake, alcohol consumption, insomnia, inadequate sleep, medications, chronic cardiac, or respiratory conditions).
- Teach client and family about factors causing or contributing to the activity intolerance; select realistic interventions with them to eliminate, reduce or compensate for these factors.
- Help client develop activity/exercise plan to improve general physical status; consider individual physical abilities and lifestyle; include conditioning, exercise, scheduling, rest, employment/family demands, leisure interests, and adaptations of daily activities to make plan acceptable and achievable.
- Provide support and encouragement as client begins conditioning plan; involve family and friends to encourage client and participate with client in exercises and activity.
- Teach and assist with oxygen support when ordered.

Examples of Specific Evaluations for Outcomes 1 to 4

1. Outcome met. Client ambulating length of hall and back × 2 without experiencing fatigue or weakness before discharge.
2. Outcome not met. Client reporting faintness with pulse of 110 beats per minute and BP of 90/60 mmHg when standing at bedside; relieved after lying back in bed for several minutes.
3. Outcome partially met. Client walking 1 mile every day with some "huffing and puffing" but much less than 6 weeks ago.
4. Outcome met. Client feels like old self 6 weeks after surgical repair of fractured hip; reports no fatigue during daily activities and is eager to start gardening.

Key Index Words for Nursing Interventions
Look up these words in the index of fundamentals and
medical-surgical nursing textbooks to find page references
for additional nursing interventions and rationale for their
selection:

- activity: intolerance of, promoting
- ambulation: assisting with, progressive
- body mechanics
- exercise
- hypoxia
- ischemia
- orthostatic hypotension

Case Management Example
See Appendix for an example of a nursing diagnosis of
Activity Intolerance within a clinical pathway for DRG 089,
Pneumonia, page 460, and DRG 127, Congestive Heart
Failure (CHF), page 466.

HIGH RISK FOR ACTIVITY INTOLERANCE

Definition
A state in which an individual is at risk of experiencing
insufficient physiological or psychological energy to endure
or complete required or desired daily activity.

Defining Risk Factors
- history of previous intolerance
- deconditioned status
- presence of circulatory/respiratory problems
- inexperience with activity (e.g., crutch walking)
- bed rest, immobility, reduced/limited movement and/or
  activity

Examples of Specific Nursing Diagnoses
1. High risk for activity intolerance related to general
   deconditioned status and lack of experience with crutch
   walking.
2. High risk for activity intolerance related to presence of
   chronic obstructive pulmonary disease (COPD) and
   medically ordered restriction to bed rest for last 4 days.

3. High risk for activity intolerance following left hip replacement related to previous history of faintness, weakness, orthostatic hypotension when attempting transfers and ambulation following right hip replacement.

Examples of Specific Outcomes

1. Client demonstrates crutch walking for first time at 10 A.M. in physical therapy without excessive fatigue, faintness, or dyspnea (difficult, labored breathing).
2. Client tolerates ambulation to bathroom for next voiding as evidenced by report of enough strength to continue, respirations below 35 per minute, no facial pallor or cyanosis.
3. Client assists nurse with transfer to chair and tolerates sitting for 1 hour to eat breakfast on second postoperative day.

Examples of Specific Nursing Interventions

- See General Mobility/Activity Nursing Interventions, page 96.
- See Specific Nursing Interventions for Activity Intolerance, page 100.
- Intervene to prevent problem from occurring, rather than to treat activity intolerance after it happens, by promoting muscle tone, activity, strength, good nutrition and hydration, optimum circulation and respirations, and positive mental attitude.

Examples of Specific Evaluations for Outcomes 1 to 3

1. Outcome not met. Became very weak and faint in physical therapy (PT) and had to go back to room for rest.
2. Outcome partially met. Ambulated to bathroom and back; color good and reported feeling strong enough but pulse 110 per minute and respirations 42 per minute when back in bed.
3. Outcome met. Did isometric leg exercises while stting up in bed for 30 minutes before transfer, elastic stockings on, transfer to chair achieved without problems; in chair for 1 hour and ate breakfast before requesting help to return to bed.

Key Index Words for Nursing Interventions

- See index words for Activity Intolerance, page 101.

DIVERSIONAL ACTIVITY DEFICIT

Definition
A state in which an individual experiences a decreased stimulation from, interest in, or engagement with recreational or leisure activities.

Defining Characteristics
- patient's statements regarding boredom, wishing there was something to do, to read, etc.
- usual hobbies cannot be undertaken in hospital

Other Characteristics
- activities limited/prevented by physical or health limitations (e.g., confinement, loss or reduced vision/hearing, mobility problems, disease, or illness)
- absence of leisure/diversional activities in schedule; all of time given to work/career-related activities
- large amount of unoccupied time

Related Factors
- environmental lack of diversional activity, as in long-term hospitalization, frequent lengthy treatments

Other Related Factors
- major life change (e.g., retirement, children moving out, moving to new home in unfamiliar area, death of spouse, development of physical/mobility limitations, illness, injury)
- lack of knowledge of value of diversional activities to health and stress reduction; unavailable in current environment
- cultural beliefs which devalue leisure activity and value work

Examples of Specific Nursing Diagnoses
1. Diversional activity deficit related to confinement to circle bed, minimal movement of arms and fingers secondary to cervical spine injury.
   Diversional activity deficit related to confinement to circle bed, minimal movement of arms and fingers secondary to cervical spine injury as evidenced by inability to do any of usual diversional activities, statements of being bored. (PES format)

2. Diversional activity deficit related to dialysis treatments secondary to kidney failure.

Diversional activity deficit related to dialysis treatments secondary to kidney failure as evidenced by statements of boredom, inability to do knitting, gardening, and take care of granddaughter. (PES format)

Examples of Specific Outcomes

1. Client states enjoyment from listening to CD collection several times each week.
2. Client selects and engages self in one enjoyable activity during next dialysis treatment.
3. Client states that playing TV video games during next chemotherapy treatment is fun.

Examples of Specific Nursing Interventions

- See General Mobility/Activity Nursing Interventions, page 96.
- Assess diversional activities client normally engages in for possible adaptation to hospital or long-term care environment; identify interests, hobbies that client enjoys or has enjoyed in the past.
- Discuss the role that diversional activities play in healthy living and stress reduction; explain concern that client has too much unoccupied time (or too little recreation time) because of excessive work schedule and ask for client's perception.
- Help overworked clients begin to fit in leisure activities.
  Discuss value of leisure activities to client's mental and physical health and to social/family relationships.
  Encourage client to examine their priorities (personal, work, social, and family).
  Problem-solve with clients on ways to rearrange small parts of their schedules or delegate/eliminate low priority work responsibilities/jobs to allow time and energy for activities.
- Help client with excess unoccupied time match abilities and interests to diversional activities; have client describe the parts of prior activities that were enjoyed and discuss how some sort of participation may still be possible.
- Brainstorm with client and family for interesting, safe, realistic activities appropriate for age group; consider

client's visual, auditory, tactile, physical, and mental abilities; encourage activities that use a range of abilities to occupy and enrich mind and body.

■ Encourage family and friends to visit, talk on phone, assist with activities, bring in media, books, and magazines which client enjoys.

■ Refer to:

occupational therapy for activities, aids to facilitate participation, new ways of doing things necessitated by treatments, injury, illness, disease conditions;

social services for resources available to help purchase/ rent aids, make environmental adaptations, arrange transportation, physically assist client, modify client's car, boat, etc. to enable client to participate in preferred activities;

recreational therapist for help matching possible new and previous activities/hobbies to client's current interests and abilities.

Examples of Specific Evaluations for Outcomes 1 to 3

1. Outcome met. Client had parents bring in CD player and has been listening to music for several hours each afternoon this week and states he really loves his music.

2. Outcome not met. Client withdrawn and depressed during dialysis, and has refused to do anything but sleep; "I'm no good to myself or anyone else".

3. Outcome partially met. Client played favorite video game during chemotherapy treatment and stated it was fun, but movement in hands and arms resulted in irritation at IV site and arm had to be elevated, restricting movement.

Key Index Words for Nursing Interventions

Look up these words in the index of fundamentals and medical-surgical nursing textbooks to find page references for additional nursing interventions and rationale for their selection:

■ diversional activity deficit
■ hobbies
■ occupational therapy
■ recreation
■ recreational therapy

■ self-actualization
■ self-esteem
■ social service
■ stimulation, lack of
■ stress reduction

HIGH RISK FOR DISUSE SYNDROME
(Complications of Immobility)

Definition
A state in which an individual is at risk for deterioration of body systems (complications of immobility) as the result of prescribed or unavoidable musculoskeletal inactivity.

Complications of immobility can include pressure ulcer, constipation, stasis of pulmonary secretions, thrombosis, urinary tract infection/retention, decreased strength/endurance, orthostatic hypotension, decreased range of joint motion, disorientation, body image disturbance, and powerlessness.

Defining Risk Factors
- paralysis
- mechanical or prescribed immobilization
- severe pain
- altered level of consciousness

Examples of Specific Nursing Diagnoses
1. High risk for disuse syndrome related to prescribed bed rest secondary to preterm labor and elevated blood pressure.
2. High risk for disuse syndrome related to pain, bed rest, inability to change positions independently secondary to fracture of hip and surgical repair.
3. High risk for disuse syndrome related to spinal cord injury, surgery, pain, and medically ordered bed rest in supine or prone positions only.

Examples of Specific Outcomes
1. Client returns to previous level of mobility and range of motion following period of medically ordered bed rest.
2. Client demonstrates none of the signs and symptoms indicating complications from immobility while on bed rest for fractured hip and surgical repair.
3. Client maintains normal bowel function, intact skin, clear breath sounds, spontaneous urine output of 1000 mL/day, full range of motion in joints during hospitalization in rehabilitation unit following spinal cord injury.

Examples of Specific Nursing Interventions
■ See General Mobility/Activity Nursing Interventions, page 96.
■ Promote healing and resolution of conditions placing client at risk for disuse syndrome: relieve pain, provide good hydration and nutrition, assess for and prevent oversedation, maintain oxygenation through chest physiotherapy (pulmonary hygiene).
■ Assess for complication of immobility: VS, BP (lying, sitting, standing), abnormal breath sounds, abnormal CMS (color, motion, sensation) in extremities, weak or unequal peripheral pulses, dizziness with sitting/standing, inadequate or abnormal I&O, deviation from normal bowel pattern, date of last bowel movement, presence of burning or hesitancy with urination, inability to void, voiding in small amounts, distended bladder, large residual urine volumes, red or pale skin areas, blisters or skin abrasions over pressure areas, reduced or painful range of motion in joints, disorientation, decreased level of consciousness.
■ Take preventive measures to avoid complication of immobility:
  constipation: stool softener, laxative, suppository as needed to restore/maintain function, good fluid intake, fruits, vegetables, activity as permitted (see Specific Nursing Interventions for Constipation, page 35, and General Bowel Nursing Interventions, page 32).
  skin breakdown: turn and reposition at least every 2 hours (see Specific Nursing Interventions for Impaired Skin Integrity, page 245, High Risk for Impaired Skin Integrity, page 247, and General Skin/Mucous Membrane Nursing Interventions, page 240).
  stasis of lung secretions; atelectasis (collapse of sections of alveoli in the lung): turn and reposition at least every 2 hours, cough, deep breathe, sustained maximal inspirations, use of inspirometer (see Specific Nursing Interventions for Ineffective Airway Clearance, page 197, Ineffective Breathing Patterns, page 200, and General Respiratory/Breathing Nursing Interventions, page 179).

thrombosis formation: movement and exercise of extremities, early ambulation (see Specific Nursing Interventions for Altered Peripheral Tissue Perfusion, page 51, High Risk for Peripheral Neurovascular Dysfunction, page 56, and General Circulation Nursing Interventions, page 47).

urinary tract infection/retention: fluid intake of 2000 mL/day, provide privacy, prevent overdistention of bladder (see Specific Nursing Interventions for Urinary Retention, page 291, and General Urinary/ Voiding Nursing Interventions, page 272).

decreased strength and endurance, orthostatic hypotension, decreased range of joint motion: exercises, AROM, PROM, isometric exercises, use of support hose when transferring and ambulating, early ambulation, progressive ambulation (see Specific Nursing Interventions for Impaired Mobility, page 110, and General Mobility/Activity Nursing Interventions, page 96).

disorientation: meet oxygenation needs; view of windows; calendars; visual, auditory, and tactile stimulation; night light; reorient as needed; assess for over-medication/side effects.

Examples of Specific Evaluations for Outcomes 1 to 3

1. Outcome not met. Foot drop on left noted during first attempt to ambulate after 3 weeks on bed rest.
2. Outcome partially met. Assessment parameters all within normal limits except for bowel function; constipation continues to be a problem 8 days postoperatively.
3. Outcome met. During 3 weeks on rehabilitation unit, bowel function occurred every 1–2 days with use of BID stool softener, skin intact, breath sounds clear, voiding into urinal every 2–4 hours in amounts of 250–350 mL, full range of motion in joints.

Key Index Words for Nursing Interventions

Look up these words in the index of fundamentals and medical-surgical nursing textbooks to find page references for additional nursing interventions and rationale for their selection:

- chest physiotherapy, TCH
- constipation

- contractures
- decubitus (pressure) ulcers
- exercises: AROM/PROM, isometric/isotonic, breathing
- foot drop
- immobility: hazards of, care during
- inspirometer, inspiratory spirometer
- orthostatic hypotension
- sustained maximal inspirations
- thrombus: causes, prevention
- urine: infection, retention

IMPAIRED PHYSICAL MOBILITY

Definition
A state in which an individual experiences a limitation of ability for independent physical movement.

*Suggested Functional Level Classification**
0 = Complete independence
1 = Requires use of equipment or device
2 = Requires help from another person, for assistance, supervision, teaching
3 = Requires help from another person and equipment or device
4 = Dependent, does not participate in activity

Defining Characteristics
- inability to move purposefully within the physical environment, including moving and repositioning in bed, transfers, ambulation
- reluctance to attempt movement
- limited range of motion
- decreased muscle strength, control and/or mass
- imposed restrictions of movement, including mechanical, medical protocol (e.g., casts, braces, traction, bed rest/log-roll only)
- impaired coordination

*Code adapted by NANDA from E. Jones et al., *Patient Classification for Long-Term Care: User's Manual*, HEW, Pub. No. HRA-74-3107, Nov. 1974.

Related Factors

- intolerance to activity/decreased strength and endurance
- pain/discomfort
- perceptual/cognitive impairment
- neuromuscular impairment
- musculoskeletal impairment
- depression/severe anxiety

Examples of Specific Nursing Diagnoses

1. Impaired physical mobility, level 2, related to fatigue, weakness, visual disturbances, numbness in legs and poor coordination secondary to multiple sclerosis.

   Impaired physical mobility, level 2, related to fatigue, weakness, visual disturbances, numbness in legs and poor coordination secondary to multiple sclerosis as evidenced by needing help to get out of bed and when walking. (PES format)

2. Impaired physical mobility, level 3, related to lack of knowledge of methods of ambulation, use of prosthesis, care of stump, secondary to below-the-knee amputation of right leg.

   Impaired physical mobility, level 3, related to lack of knowledge of methods of ambulation, use of prosthesis, care of stump, secondary to below-the-knee amputation of right leg as evidenced by inability to transfer or walk unassisted. (PES format)

Examples of Specific Outcomes

1. Client experiences return of independent physical mobility and steady gait after 2 days of drug therapy.
2. Client manages independent ambulation with prosthetic leg and cane by discharge.
3. Client ambulates length of hall and goes up and down four stairs with use of walker on sixth postoperative day.
4. Client achieves 30-degree flexion in right knee this shift using a continuous passive motion (CPM) machine.

Examples of Specific Nursing Interventions

- See General Mobility/Activity Nursing Interventions, page 96.

■ Discuss and teach about mobility restriction to client/family:

> what movement, activity client can and cannot do
> reasons for restrictions
> expected duration of restrictions
> how client and staff will help client with daily living needs
> activities client and family can perform to maintain strength and function in extremities while mobility is limited

■ Teach client and family how to regain maximum mobility:

> provide information on realistic outcomes on an estimated time frame for regaining mobility based on progress made by most clients with similar mobility impairments
> use of analgesics if pain is experienced with movement
> exercises to maintain or regain strength and joint mobility: isometric, isotonic, AROM, PROM
> use of assistive devices (e.g., bed trapeze, crutches, walkers, canes, wheelchairs, lifts) for moving in bed, transferring, ambulating
> use of medically ordered therapeutic devices (e.g., braces, casts, splints, traction, positioning pillows, abductor pillows, CPM machine, cryocuff) to maintain good alignment, treat/prevent injury, and to promote healing

■ Discuss risk of injury and/or falls with impaired mobility and ways client can reduce risk (see General Physical Safety/Protection Nursing Interventions, page 150).

■ Teach transfer techniques and assist.

■ Teach progressive ambulation and assist.

■ Discuss feelings related to impaired mobility; emphasize ability and progress already made; praise efforts; maintain hope.

Examples of Specific Evaluations for Outcomes 1 to 4

1. Outcome met. Client has steady gait, increased strength and is ambulating independently 24 hours after finishing drug therapy.

2. Outcome partially met. Client ambulating independently with prosthetic leg at discharge but continues to use crutches rather than cane for stability.

3. Outcome not met. Client has developed a fever and possible infection and has been unable to attend physical therapy to learn walking and stair climbing with walker.
4. Outcome met. Client flexing knee 35 degrees on CPM machine by end of shift.

Key Index Words for Nursing Interventions

Look up these words in the index of fundamentals and medical-surgical nursing textbooks to find page references for additional nursing interventions and rationale for their selection:

- active range of motion (AROM)
- amputation
- braces
- casts
- CPM machine
- crutch walking
- exercise, isometric/isotonic
- fractures, effect on mobility
- immobility
- mobility: impaired, of joints
- musculoskeletal disorders/trauma, mobility and
- neurologic/neuromuscular disorders, mobility
- passive range of motion exercises (PROM)
- spinal cord injury, mobility and
- traction

Case Management Example

See Appendix for an example of a nursing diagnosis of Impaired Physical Mobility within a clinical pathway for DRG 209, Total Hip Replacement, page 474.

Chapter 6

Nutrition/Eating Problems

FOCUSED ASSESSMENT GUIDE

Complete this focused assessment if a general nursing assessment indicates a possible problem. Then turn to page 116 of this text for the Data ⇒ Diagnosis Matching Guide for nutrition/eating problems to help you select the best nursing diagnosis to match a client's data.

OVER THE LAST 24 HOURS, WHAT HAVE YOU HAD TO EAT AND DRINK

Breakfast _____
Snack/drink _____
Lunch _____
Snack/drink _____
Supper _____
Snacks/drink _____
Alcoholic drink _____

TELL ME IF YOU ARE HAVING ANY OF THESE PROBLEMS OR CONCERNS

___ changes in your diet because of health problems
___ eating less (or more) than you think you need
___ recent weight loss (or gain)
___ dissatisfaction with your weight

___ trouble or soreness when chewing or swallowing your food
___ difficulty feeding yourself
___ loss of appetite or loss of interest in eating
___ loss or decreased sense of taste
___ nausea or vomiting
___ diarrhea or constipation
___ difficulty getting food from the store or cooking it
___ problems affording the kind of food you think you should eat
___ food allergies, food intolerances, or restrictions (by doctor)

OBSERVE CLIENT/CHART FOR

___ diet ordered by physician
___ body weight 20% or more above or below ideal (based on client's actual weight and height/weight graph)
___ triceps skin fold greater than 15 mm in men, 25 mm in women
___ inadequate food intake; less than recommended daily allowance (RDA)
___ changes in body weight from admission weight or reported normal
___ reported or observed obesity in one or both parents
___ rapid transition across growth percentiles in infants/children
___ inability to bring food from a receptacle to the mouth
___ evidence of difficulty swallowing

ADULT NORMALS AND INFORMATION

- Eating center located in the hypothalamus of the brain
- Mechanics of eating and swallowing controlled in the brain stem
- Clients can be overweight and malnourished at the same time
- Eating patterns and food choices are learned cultural responses and must be interpreted based on cultural norms

- Food guide pyramid (US Department of Agriculture 1992)
  6–11 servings from breads, cereals, pasta per day
  3–5 servings from vegetables per day
  2–4 servings from fruit per day
  2–3 servings from milk, cheese, yogurt per day
  2–3 servings from meat, eggs, fish, dry beans per day
  fats, oils, sweets, use sparingly
- Starvation leads to death at 66% of ideal body weight
- Factors increasing metabolic (caloric) need: exercise (daily muscular activity uses one-third of calories or more); growth; young age (especially first few years, adolescence); injury; infection; fever (increase metabolic rate); cancer; AIDS (increased resting energy expenditure); being male (testosterone increases metabolic rate); pregnancy, breast-feeding (lactation); cool climates (more calories needed to maintain temperature)
- Factors decreasing metabolic (caloric) need: inactivity; sleep; aging (metabolic rate decreases over time with aging)
- One pound of body fat equals 3500 calories
- To maintain weight (whether underweight, normal weight, or overweight) calorie intake will equal calorie utilization

TO CALCULATE DAILY CALORIC REQUIREMENT TO MAINTAIN WEIGHT

Ideal (Not Actual) Body Weight × Activity Level from Table = Calorie Requirements

| | Calories per Pound | |
	Male	Female
heavy	28	22
moderate	21	18
sedentary	16	14

Examples: 180-lb male construction worker at ideal weight: 180 lb × 28 cal/lb = 5040 cal
140-lb female night nurse whose ideal weight is 120 lb: 120 lb × 18 cal/lb = 2160 cal

TO GAIN WEIGHT Calorie Intake Must Exceed Calorie Utilization
To gain 1 lb in 1 week:

- intake must increase by 500 cal/day (500 cal/day × 7 days = 3500 cal) if activity remains constant.
- activity level must go down to the next level in the table for most of the week if calorie intake remains constant.

TO LOSE WEIGHT Calorie Intake Must be Less Than Calorie Utilization
To lose 1 lb in 1 week:

- intake must decrease by 500 cal/day if activity remains constant.
- activity must go up to the next level in the table for most of the week if calorie intake remains constant.
- a combination of calorie reduction and increased activity for weight loss is most effective.

DATA ⇒ DIAGNOSIS MATCHING GUIDE

Compare your client data from the Nutrition/Eating Focused Assessment to these related nursing diagnosis and abbreviated descriptions. Select the nursing diagnosis with the best match. Then turn to the page in this section with that specific diagnosis for help in planning care.

1. Altered Nutrition: Less Than Body Requirements: page 118

- definition: an intake of nutrients insufficient to meet metabolic needs
- data: body weight 20% or more under ideal; reported inadequate food intake, less than recommended daily allowance (RDA); loss of weight with adequate food intake

2. Altered Nutrition: More Than Body Requirements: page 121

- definition: an intake of nutrients which exceeds metabolic needs
- data: weight 20% over ideal for height and frame; triceps skin fold greater than 15 mm in men, 25 mm in women.

3. *Altered Nutrition: Potential for More Than Body Requirements: page 124*
- definition: at risk of an intake of nutrients which exceeds metabolic needs
- risk factors: reported or observed obesity in one or both parents; rapid transition across growth percentiles in infants or children; dysfunctional eating patterns; using food as a reward or for comfort

4. *Feeding Self-Care Deficit: page 222*
- definition: an impaired ability to perform or complete feeding activities for oneself
- data: inability to bring food from a receptacle to the mouth.

5. *Impaired Swallowing: page 72*
- definition: decreased ability to voluntarily pass fluids and/or solids from the mouth to the stomach
- data: observed evidence of difficulty swallowing

GENERAL OUTCOMES AND NURSING INTERVENTIONS

GENERAL NUTRITION/EATING OUTCOMES
- Client will maintain nutritional balance.
- Client will maintain current weight within 5-lb range.
- Client will restore nutritional balance.
- Client will achieve weight appropriate for height/body frame.
- Client will consume recommended daily servings from the food group pyramid.

GENERAL NUTRITION/EATING NURSING INTERVENTIONS
- Reduce or eliminate the related factors causing the problem whenever possible (e.g., identify and correct dysfunctional eating patterns, decrease or increase calorie intake to match metabolic need).

■ Assess client and family for:

food intake using a 3–5 day written record of types and amounts of food consumed (consider age, sex, activity level, calorie intake and servings per day from each recommended food group when assessing appropriateness of intake).

understanding of good nutrition; knowledge of relationship between caloric needs, activity levels, body weight, and health.

cultural or religious factors affecting current food intake; any potential conflicts with recommended daily allowances and recommended servings or with diet restrictions or suggestions.

psychological factors affecting food consumption; desire to gain or lose weight; depression; eating for comfort or as a reward.

social factors: financial constraints affecting purchase of foods; timing of food intake; pairing food with activities, TV watching, social gatherings.

physical factors: chewing, swallowing ability; ability to shop for and prepare foods; ability to feed self; fatigue, pain, loss of appetite, nausea, loss of sense of taste.

■ Help clients/families select realistic outcomes for improving nutrition and/or changing their weight.
■ Teach based on assessment of client/family knowledge, ability, and needs.
■ Initiate daily food intake record/calorie count.
■ Encourage daily exercise/activity.
■ Refer to social service, dietician, occupational therapy.

RELATED NURSING DIAGNOSES

ALTERED NUTRITION: LESS THAN BODY REQUIREMENTS

Definition
A state in which an individual experiences an intake of nutrients insufficient to meet metabolic needs.

Defining Characteristics
■ loss of weight with adequate food intake

- body weight 20% or more under ideal
- reported inadequate food intake, less than recommended daily allowance (RDA)
- weakness of muscles required for swallowing or chewing
- perceived inability to ingest food
- reported or evidence of lack of food
- aversion to eating; lack of interest in food
- reported altered taste sensation
- satiety immediately after ingesting food
- abdominal pain with or without pathology; abdominal cramping
- sore, inflamed buccal cavity
- capillary fragility (resulting from inadequate nutrition)
- diarrhea and/or steatorrhea (excess fat in the feces from malabsorption because of disease of intestinal mucosa)
- hyperactive bowel sounds
- pale conjunctival and mucous membranes
- poor muscle tone
- excessive loss of hair
- lack of information, misinformation; misconceptions

Related Factors

- inability to ingest food or absorb nutrients due to biological, psychological, or economic factors
- increased metabolic needs (caloric needs above normal because of greatly increased activity level or increased nutritional drain on body, e.g., pregnancy/lactation, cancer, AIDS, trauma, fever)

Examples of Specific Nursing Diagnoses

1. Altered nutrition: less than body requirements related to clear liquid diet restrictions, nausea, decreased bowel activity, abdominal distention secondary to surgical experience.
   Altered nutrition: less than body requirements related to clear liquid diet restrictions, nausea, decreased bowel activity, abdominal distention secondary to surgical experience as evidenced by inadequate intake of calories and nutrients over last 3 days. (PES format)
2. Altered nutrition: less than body requirements related to inaccurate self-image as overweight, skipping meals, abuse of laxatives.

Altered nutrition: less than body requirements related to inaccurate self-image as overweight, skipping meals, abuse of laxatives as evidenced by weight 15 lb under normal for height; reported intake averages 800 cal/day. (PES format)

Examples of Specific Outcomes
1. Client's weight gain of 1 lb/week for next 4 weeks.
2. Client's calorie intake is 2000 cal by end of day.
3. Infant's weight changes from below 25% for age to between 25–50% in 4 weeks.
4. Client eats 50% or more of food on lunch tray today.

Examples of Specific Nursing Interventions
- See General Nutrition/Eating Nursing Interventions, page 117.
- Provide good oral hygiene.
- Provide feeding help as needed.
- Assess for preferred foods, food temperatures, times to eat.
- Allow client to rest before meals.
- Assess and medicate for pain and/or nausea 1 hour before meals.
- Provide small frequent feedings, in between snacks, calorie-containing drinks.
- Encourage family to bring in favorite foods unless contraindicated by diet order for medical reasons.
- Provide more time to eat; reheat foods that become cool.
- Discuss ways to reduce energy and metabolic needs to promote weight gain (e.g., keeping client warm, naps, decreasing pain and stress, reducing physical activity that tires/fatigues client)

Examples of Specific Evaluations for Outcomes 1 to 4
1. Outcome not met. First-week weight gain of 2 lb but became nauseated after chemotherapy and has been unable to eat enough for any further weight gain.
2. Outcome met. Client consumed 2200 cal today by eating small meals with snacks in between every few hours.
3. Outcome partially met. Infant's weight at 50% for age with weight gain of 2 lb but length increased to 90%.
4. Outcome met. Client "feels like old self" 6 weeks after surgical repair of fractured hip; reports no fatigue during daily activities and is eager to start gardening.

Key Index Words for Nursing Interventions
Look up these words in the index of fundamentals and medical-surgical nursing textbooks to find page references for additional nursing interventions and rationale for their selection:

- anorexia
- antiemetics
- calories
- diet, promoting adequate
- dietician
- feeding
- food group pyramid, recommended daily servings
- malnutrition
- nausea
- nutrition
- recommended daily allowance (RDA)
- weight: ideal, gain, loss
- undernourished

Case Management Example
See Appendix for examples of a nursing diagnosis of Altered Nutrition; Less Than Body Requirements within clinical pathways for DRG 089, Pneumonia, page 460.

ALTERED NUTRITION: MORE THAN BODY REQUIREMENTS

Definition
A state in which an individual is experiencing an intake of nutrients which exceeds metabolic needs.

Critical Defining Characteristics (one or more must be present)
- weight 20% over ideal for height and frame
- triceps skin fold greater than 15 mm in men, 25 mm in women

Defining Characteristics
- weight 10% over ideal for height and frame
- sedentary activity level
- reported or observed dysfunctional eating pattern: pairing food with other activities; concentrating food intake at the end of the day; eating in response to external cues

such as time of day, social situation; eating in response to internal cues other than hunger, such as anxiety, fatigue, drowsiness; using food for comfort or as a reward

Related Factors
■ excessive intake in relation to metabolic need

Examples of Specific Nursing Diagnoses
1. Altered nutrition: more than body requirements related to increased consumption of high calorie foods at frequent social functions and decreased activity since retirement.
   Altered nutrition: more than body requirements related to increased consumption of high calorie foods at frequent social functions and decreased activity since retirement as evidenced by weight gain of 15 lb over last year; 5 ft 3 in; 140 lb; female with small body frame. (PES format)
2. Altered nutrition: more than body requirements related to maintenance of previous level of food intake with decreased physical activity.
   Altered nutrition: more than body requirements related to maintenance of previous level of food intake with decreased physical activity as evidenced by weight gain of 20 lb in 3 months; 230 lb; 6 ft 1 in; male with large frame. (PES format)

Examples of Specific Outcomes
Weight loss of more than 2 lb a week in an adult often results in inadequate nutrient intake; total weight loss desired, divided by 2 lb would equal minimum number of weeks to set as time frame in outcome statement, e.g., 18-lb total desired weight loss divided by 2 lb = 9 weeks to achieve.
1. Client loses one pound by the end of the week.
2. Client reaches ideal weight at the end of 8 months.
3. Client weights 156 lb or less (down from 160 lb) at the end of this month.
4. Infant's weight appropriate for length (same percentage on height/weight growth graph) at next well-baby visit.

Examples of Specific Nursing Interventions
■ See General Nutrition/Eating Nursing Interventions, page 117.

- Identify the sources of the excess intake, e.g., types of food, preparation of food, timing most food intake late at night; alcohol, sweets, snacks, fast foods because of work schedule.
- Discuss ways for client to increase activity level if caloric intake remains constant.
- Develop a plan with the client to reduced daily calorie intake if activity level remains constant. Suggest smaller servings; no second helpings; eating only at the kitchen table; using small plates; drinking liquids before and during the meal; eating slowly; choosing crunchy, chewy foods, high fiber; selecting foods lower in both calories and fats; eliminating high calorie drinks, e.g., pop, powdered sugar drinks.
- Help client combine increased activity and decreased caloric intake for best results.
- Identify cooking and eating patterns which are contributing to excess calorie consumption and suggest alternatives: limit fat intake; largest meal during the day rather than late in evening; reduce or eliminate alcohol intake (adds nonnutritive calories and tends to decrease activity); use cooking spray rather than oil; rematch activities associated with eating to other activities such as knitting instead of snacking while watching TV, or a hot bath instead of several glasses of wine before supper.
- Work with client and family to develop a daily exercise program that is realistic, rewarding, and replaces more sedentary activities (e.g., 1-mile walk after dinner while kids clean up the kitchen; going out dancing rather than to dinner on the weekend; parking car at far end of parking lot and walking; encouraging after-school or community sports activity for children; walking the shopping mall every day).
- Encourage client to join support groups for weight loss and active social groups such as walking clubs and swimming pool exercise sessions.

Examples of Specific Evaluations for Outcomes 1 to 4
1. Outcome met. Client lost 2 lb by end of week.
2. Outcome not met. Client lost and regained weight several times over the last 8 months; weighs 187 lb (approximately the same as when weight loss interventions started).

3. Outcome partially met. Weight 157 lb at the end of the month with 3 lb weight loss.
4. Outcome not met. Infant's weight in 50%; height in 25%.

Key Index Words for Nursing Interventions
Look up these words in the index of fundamentals and medical-surgical nursing textbooks to find page references for additional nursing interventions and rationale for their selection:

- calorie intake, excess
- diet
- dietician
- food group pyramid, recommended servings
- nutrition, altered

- obesity
- overeating
- overweight
- recommended daily allowances (RDA)
- weight: ideal, gain, loss

ALTERED NUTRITION: POTENTIAL FOR MORE THAN BODY REQUIREMENTS

Definition
A state in which an individual is at risk of experiencing an intake of nutrients which exceeds metabolic needs.

Critical Defining Characteristics (one or more must be present)
- reported or observed obesity in one or both parents
- rapid transition across growth percentiles in infants or children

Defining Risk Factors
- reported use of solid food as major food source before 5 months of age
- observed use of food as a reward or comfort measure
- reported or observed higher baseline weight at beginning of each pregnancy
- dysfunctional eating pattern:
  pairing food with other activities;
  concentrating food intake at the end of the day;
  eating in response to external cues, e.g., time of day, social situation, watching TV;

eating in response to internal cues other than hunger, e.g., anxiety, fatigue, drowsiness.

Examples of Specific Nursing Diagnoses

1. Altered nutrition: potential for more than body requirements related to family history of obesity in mother, father, and sister.
2. Altered nutrition: potential for more than body requirements related to decreased activity following head injury, parental use of candy and snacks for rewards, eating behavior whenever food is in visual field independent of hunger.
3. Altered nutrition: potential for more than body requirements related to enrollment in college nursing program, decreased physical activity, using food as a reward for studying and to help stay awake, snacking and increased use of fast foods rather than cooking.

Examples of Specific Outcomes

1. Client's weight remains appropriate for age and height in 6 months.
2. Client's weight remains constant within 5 lb of admission weight during stay at teenage rehabilitation facility.
3. Client maintains current weight during enrollment in nursing program.
4. Client's weight is within 110–115 lb every Friday morning at weekly weigh-in on school nurse's scale.

Examples of Specific Nursing Interventions

- See Specific Nursing Interventions for Altered Nutrition: More than Body Requirements, page 122, and General Nutrition/Eating Nursing Interventions, page 117.
- Discuss concerns about client becoming overweight related to personal risk factors.
- With client and family devise ways to maintain lifelong nutritional balance between caloric intake and metabolic utilization through types and amounts of foods eaten, reduction of fats in diet, activity and exercise.
- Develop an assessment program for client to use on a weekly basis to measure progress toward weight maintenance.

- Select interventions with client to initiate when weight increases in a week, so excess intake is recognized and managed early.
- Suggest joining weight maintenance support programs, healthy cooking classes, exercise groups, walking clubs.

Examples of Specific Evaluations for Outcomes 1 to 4

1. Outcome met. Weight appropriate for age and height.
2. Outcome partially met. Weight has increased by 10 lb during 6-month stay in rehabilitation facility but growth of 2 in occurred and gain is appropiate for height.
3. Outcome not met. Weight gain of 10 lb after first year in nursing program.
4. Outcome met for month of February. Weight remains 110–115 lb with height constant at 5 ft 2 in.

Key Index Words for Nursing Interventions

Look up these words in the index of fundamentals and medical-surgical nursing textbooks to find page references for additional nursing interventions and rationale for their selection:

- calorie intake, excess
- diet
- dietician
- food group pyramid, recommended servings
- nutrition, altered
- obesity
- overeating
- overweight
- recommended daily allowances (RDA)
- weight: ideal, gain, loss

Chapter 7

Pain Problems

FOCUSED ASSESSMENT GUIDE

Complete this focused assessment if a general nursing assessment indicates a possible problem. Then turn to page 129 of this text for the Data ⇒ Diagnosis Matching Guide for pain problems to help you select the best nursing diagnosis to match the client's data.

ASK THESE QUESTIONS

___ Where is the pain located?
___ How long have you had the pain?
___ Do you know what is causing the pain?
___ Is your pain constant or does it come and go?
___ When is it better and when is it worse?
___ Has your pain gotten better or worse with time?
___ What words would you use to describe your pain? For example, hurt, ache, sharp, dull, shooting, crushing, searing, burning.
___ How bad is the pain right now?
     0 = no pain
     10 = worst pain imaginable
___ Rate your pain at its worst and at its best.
___ How often are you taking pain medication? How effective is it? How long does the pain relief last?
___ Do you do anything else to relieve or deal with the pain? How well does it work?

____ How has the pain affected your physical, social, work, and family activities?

____ On a scale of 0–10 what level of pain control would you like to have?

____ Are you having any side effects from the pain medication, like constipation, dizziness, or nausea?

ASSESS CLIENT/CHART FOR

____ grimacing, guarding of area, groaning, crying (pain behavior)

____ pain behavior related to movement

____ analgesics ordered/given over last 2 days (drug/dose/frequency)

____ analgesics ordered/given as needed (prn) or around-the-clock (ATC) (e.g., every 3 hours day and night)

NORMALS AND INFORMATION

- Pain prevention is better than pain treatment
- Client's report of pain should be basis of treatment; believe the client
- Pain is frequently undertreated
- Pain can be present when pain behavior is absent and client seems relaxed and resting, with normal vital signs
- Some clients will not report pain unless asked about it
- Pain relief from IM analgesics should occur in 15–30 minutes and in 1 hour after oral administration
- Effective pain management is associated with earlier mobility, decreased length of hospital stay, and reduced costs
- Opioids (narcotics) are analgesics used to manage moderate pain or severe pain; most are compared to morphine
- Long-term use of opioids to treat pain results in tolerance and physical dependence; this is different from psychological dependence (addiction) which rarely occurs in pain treatment
- Opioids probably relieve pain by acting at the central nervous system level by attaching to the body's opiate

receptors; there are three types of opioids: full agonists, partial agonists, mixed agonists-antagonists; full agonists, such as morphine, have no maximum daily dose; dosage can be increased until pain relief achieved

- Nonsteroidal antiinflammatory drugs (NSAIDs) probably relieve pain at the peripheral nervous system level at the site of the injury; each drug has a maximum daily dose; most are compared to aspirin for effectiveness
- Meperidine (Demerol) is short-acting 2.5–3.5 hours, has toxic side effects, and should be used for only brief treatment in clients who have had negative reactions to opioids
- Analgesic doses are similar for IM, IV, and SQ routes; the oral route generally requires a higher dose for the same effect
- Equianalgesic charts are available to compare the dose of various drugs needed to achieve the same pain relief
- Clients abusing narcotics often have drug tolerance and will need higher doses of opioid analgesics for pain relief

DATA ⇒ DIAGNOSIS MATCHING GUIDE

Compare your client data from the Pain Focused Assessment to these related pain nursing diagnoses and abbreviated descriptions. Select the nursing diagnosis with the best match. Then turn to the page in this section with that specific diagnosis for help in planning care.

1. Acute Pain:* page 133
   - definition: severe discomfort or an unpleasant sensation; it follows injury to the body and generally disappears when the bodily injury heals or painful event resolves
   - data: communication (verbal or coded) of pain descriptors; guarded behavior; presence of pain behavior (moaning, crying, pacing, rubbing the area); focused on the pain; autonomic (sympathetic) responses of sweating, pallor, increased BP and pulse, dilated pupils; shallow rapid breathing; anxiety, restlessness

*Authors' adaptation of NANDA diagnoses, Pain and Chronic Pain (References: AHCPR 1992; American Pain Society 1992; Jacox et al., 1994).

2. *Chronic Nonmalignant Pain:* page 140
   - definition: pain that continues for more than 6 months in duration related to a nonmalignant health condition
   - data: verbal report or observed evidence of pain for more than 6 months; pain continues beyond time expected for healing of injury; may not mention pain unless asked; pain behavior absent; absence of autonomic (sympathetic) responses; fear of reinjury; physical and social withdrawal; decreased ability to continue previous activities; may be consciously focusing on distracting activities; fatigue; anorexia; weight changes; changes in sleep patterns; facial mask, expressionless

3. *Chronic Malignant Pain (Cancer Pain):* page 136
   - definition: report of pain associated with malignant health condition and its treatment; pain may be acute, chronic, or intermittent
   - data: see data for Acute Pain and Chronic Nonmalignant Pain; related to tumor progression, operations and other invasive diagnostic or therapeutic procedures, effects of chemotherapy and radiation, infection, muscle soreness from decreased activity; pain tends to worsen as disease progresses; pain ends with death or control of the disease

GENERAL OUTCOMES AND NURSING INTERVENTIONS

GENERAL PAIN OUTCOMES

- Client will report pain was prevented.
- Client will report adequate relief of pain.
- Client will state pain management is/was effective.
- Client will state confidence in own ability to manage pain.
- Client will identify and demonstrate several pain management techniques.
- Client will maintain role within the family and work productively.

*Authors' adaptation of NANDA diagnoses, Pain and Chronic Pain (References: AHCPR 1992; American Pain Society 1992; Jacox et al., 1994).

- Client will report absence of side effects or manageable side effects from analgesics.
- Client will state pain maintained at or below desired level.

GENERAL PAIN NURSING INTERVENTIONS

- Assess client regularly (every 3–4 hours) for pain, changes in pain and effectiveness of pain management interventions.
- Accept client's self-report of pain; use it to guide treatment.
- Individualize pain management strategies and pharmacologic interventions to each client's report of pain.
- Assess and teach as needed (based on client's knowledge level) principles of pain management, pharmacologic interventions, and nonpharmacologic interventions available to client to manage pain.
- Anticipate the possibility of pain with diagnostic and treatment procedures, physical therapy, ambulation, etc., and treat prophylactically to prevent pain (e.g., analgesics 30–60 minutes before physical therapy or turning and repositioning).
- Document pain treatment and effectiveness of interventions; review with client, family, and other care providers.
- Use least invasive pain management strategies first.
- *Nonpharmacologic interventions* for mild to moderate pain or to potentiate effect of analgesics in moderate or severe pain.

  Teach client what to expect; how it will feel; pain relief options; how to take active role in management.

  Provide reassurance/support; encourage presence of supportive family with client; hold client's hand, rock a baby.

  Relaxation techniques: slow rhythmic breathing; jaw relaxation; progressive muscle relaxation; simple imagery (helpful to practice before painful event so client familiar with technique and better able to use it during pain).

  Music distracts, relaxes, and may release body's own opiates.

  Distraction behavior/activity: blowing, breathing exercises, singing, sucking, listening, games, TV, video games, hugging, cuddling, humor and laughter before painful procedure release body's natural opiates.

Cutaneous stimulation: hot/cold applications to skin; massage, effleurage, pressure, vibrator, transcutaneous electrical nerve stimulator (TENS); have client focus attention on the tactile stimulation.

Reposition; maintain good body alignment and support.

Exercise: range of motion exercises; leg exercises; continuous passive motion (CPM) machine, ambulation.

Rest or immobilization for injured tissues; provides alignment for healing.

Hypnosis, biofeedback, acupuncture (done by specialists).

■ *Pharmacologic interventions,* Step Approach, require a physician's order for drug options, dose range, route, frequency of administration but nurses indicate client's need to physician, make choices within the ordered analgesic options, and assess effectiveness of analgesics given.

Step 1 Nonsteroidal Antiinflammatory Drugs: For mild to moderate pain, give nonsteroidal antiinflammatory drugs (NSAIDs) unless contraindicated (e.g., aspirin, acetaminophen, ibuprofen, naproxen); do not exceed recommended daily doses of NSAIDs.

Step 2 Opioid Analgesic + NSAIDs: If pain persists or increases, supplement (not substitute) the NSAIDs with an opioid analgesic such as codeine or hydrocodone (e.g., Tylenol # 3, Empirin # 3, Vicodin, Lorcet); one pill combines opioid and NSAID. For moderate to severe pain on initial assessment, start at this step giving both an opioid and NSAIDs if ordered.

Step 3 Higher Dose/More Potent Opioid: If pain persists, more potent opioids are used (e.g., morphine, hydromorphine, methadone, fentanyl). The opioid dose/potency is increased slowly (titrated up) until pain relief is achieved with minimal or acceptable drug side effects, increasing by one-quarter to one-half the previous dose until relief is obtained.

Adjuvant drugs: adjuvant drugs may be added at any step to enhance the effectiveness of opioids, to treat symptoms that intensify pain, to treat specific types of pain, and to counteract the likely side effects of opioids (e.g., hydroxyzine for anxiety and nausea; coffee to potentiate analgesic and counter sedation; antiemetic for N&V; anticonvulsants for neuropathic pain).

■ Administer analgesics around-the-clock (ATC) versus as needed (prn) when pain is highly likely; move to prn administration as pain becomes less likely or intermittent (e.g., postoperatively give opioids and/or NSAIDs around-the-clock for 2 days then move to prn)

■ Use the oral route whenever possible; when clients cannot take oral medications, use IV, SQ, rectal, transdermal route; avoid IM route (IM routes are painful; clients may not report pain for fear of shot; absorption is unreliable).

■ Assess for side effects of opioid analgesics; prevent and treat as needed (constipation, N&V, sedation, respiratory depression, dry mouth, urinary retention, pruritus (itching), sleep disturbances).

■ Opioid analgesics should not be given if respirations less than 10 breaths per minute; encourage client to breathe deeply and consciously increase rate; increase physical stimulation; treat respiratory depression with naloxone with dose titrated to increase respiratory rate and depth without reversing analgesic effect.

■ Teach clients to report changes in their pain or any new pain; reassess (new pain may indicate new medical problems so report to physician); change pain treatment plan as needed.

RELATED NURSING DIAGNOSES

ACUTE PAIN*

Definition
A state in which an individual experiences and reports the presence of severe discomfort or an unpleasant sensation which follows injury to the body and generally disappears when the bodily injury heals or painful event resolves.

*Authors' adaptation of NANDA's Pain diagnosis for clarity and for treatment considerations.

Defining Characteristics
- communication (verbal or coded) of pain descriptors
- guarded behavior, protective
- self-focusing; narrowed focus (altered time perception, withdrawal from social contact, impaired thought process)
- pain behavior (moaning, crying, grimace, pacing, rubbing)
- restlessness, anxious
- increased muscle tone, tense
- autonomic (sympathetic) responses present: diaphoresis (sweating), BP and pulse elevated, dilated pupils, shallow rapid breathing, pallor

Other Characteristics
- intensity may range from mild (1–3) to severe (7–10)
- reduced movement; unwilling to move
- minimal coughing; refusing to cough and deep breathe
- build-up of lung secretions; moist breath sounds, rales
- unable to sleep; fatigue
- loss of appetite
- elevated blood glucose level
- decreased GI motility
- well-defined onset
- resolves when injury heals, event resolved, treatment over

Related Factors
- injury from biological, chemical, or physical agents (trauma, surgery, medical procedures, treatments)

Examples of Specific Nursing Diagnoses
1. Acute pain related to joint replacement surgery, movement.

   Acute pain related to joint replacement surgery, movement as evidenced by client's rating of pain at 8, groaning and crying out with movement, P 100, BP 156/88 mmHg, R 28 and shallow. (PES format)

2. Acute pain related to fracture of right arm while roller-blading.

   Acute pain related to fracture of right arm while roller-blading as evidenced by crying, holding arm immobile, refusing to let anyone touch arm, reporting pain as 10, dilated pupils, P 110, BP 120/70 mmHg, R 34. (PES format)

Examples of Specific Outcomes

1. Client states pain at an acceptable level within 1 hour.
2. Client states pain does not exceed ability to cope with it during labor and delivery.
3. Client states pain maintained at level of 3 or less during first 24 hours post-op.
4. Client states no increase in pain level during physical therapy.

Examples of Specific Nursing Interventions

- See General Pain Nursing Interventions, page 131.
- Promote healing of injury or resolution of event causing pain.
- Assess pain every 2 hours; increase frequency of assessment if pain poorly controlled.
- If pain severe or poorly controlled:
  give maximum dose ordered of opioid analgesic on an around-the-clock schedule.
  administer a NSAID, if ordered, in addition to opioid.
  add complementary nonpharmacologic interventions.
  if pain continues, contact physician and discuss pain management and need to modify plan or possibility of undiagnosed complications as cause of unresponsive pain.
- As tissue trauma heals, move back down the step approach to pain, titrating the opioid analgesic down as long as adequate pain control is maintained; try using prn dosing.
- Record pain intensity, interventions and pain response.
- Review pain management options the client may use at home during discharge planning.

Examples of Specific Evaluations for Outcomes 1 to 4

1. Outcome met. Client rates pain at 4 some 45 minutes after receiving 30 mg morphine orally.
2. Outcome partially met. Client stated pain was manageable with breathing exercises until 6 cm dilated. Received IV Nubain analgesic, stated pain control was much better, and resumed breathing exercises until delivery.
3. Outcome not met. Client states pain back up to 7–8 some 3 hours after receiving Demerol 100 mg.

4. Outcome met. Client given two Tylenol #3 tablets 1 hour before physical therapy and reports minimal pain.

Key Index Words for Nursing Interventions
Look up these words in the index of fundamentals and medical-surgical nursing textbooks to find page references for additional nursing interventions and rationale for their selection:

- acute pain
- adjuvant drugs, therapy
- analgesics
- cryotherapy
- distraction techniques
- equianalgesic
- nonsteroidal antiinflammatory drugs (NSAIDs)
- opioids (term preferred to *narcotic*)
- opioid: agonist, mixed agonist-antagonist, partial agonist
- pain: acute, intensity scale, management, threshold
- patient-controlled anesthesia (PCA)
- relaxation techniques/exercises
- transcutaneous electrical nerve stimulator (TENS)

Case Management Example
See Appendix for an example of a nursing diagnosis of Acute Pain within a clinical pathway, DRG 209, Total Hip Replacement, page 474.

CHRONIC MALIGNANT PAIN (CANCER PAIN)*

Definition
A state in which an individual experiences pain which may be acute, chronic, or intermittent and is associated with a malignant disease process and its treatment.

Defining Characteristics
- See defining characteristics for Acute Pain, page 134, or Chronic Nonmalignant Pain, page 140.

---

*Authors' adaptation of NANDA's Chronic Pain diagnosis for clarity and for treatment considerations.

■ varied descriptors of pain: constant, intermittent; mild to severe in intensity, tight, constricting, aching, headache, abnormal sensation as burning, prickling, pain with gentle touching
■ weight loss
■ weakness; fatigue
■ pain tends to worsen as disease progresses
■ ends with death or control of the disease

Related Factors
■ tumor progression in cancer, AIDS
■ operations and other invasive diagnostic or therapeutic procedures
■ peripheral nerve damage from tumor, surgery, radiation, chemotherapy, AIDS
■ effects of chemotherapy and radiation
■ infection; HIV positive/AIDS
■ muscle soreness from decreased activity, muscle wasting
■ depression; suicidal thinking, planning

Examples of Specific Nursing Diagnoses
1. Chronic malignant pain related to progression of cancerous tumor near the spine.
   Chronic malignant pain related to progression of cancerous tumor near spine as evidenced by report of radiating pain on left side of body, burning, prickling sensation along arm. (PES format)
2. Chronic malignant pain related to Karposi's sarcoma and peripheral sensory neuropathy.
   Chronic malignant pain related to Karposi's sarcoma and peripheral sensory neuropathy as evidenced by report of aching pain in arms affected by tumors, burning, and numbness in left leg. (PES format)

Examples of Specific Outcomes
1. Client reports no recurrence of pain for the rest of the day.
2. Client reports continuous control of pain at 0–2 rating on revised pain management plan by the end of the week.
3. Client reports pain at 3 or less and normal bowel pattern while on maintenance morphine dose by next clinic visit.
4. Client reports pain management adequate during stay in hospice.

Examples of Specific Nursing Interventions

- See General Pain Nursing Interventions, page 131.
- Titrate dose of opioid to prevent and control pain; manage aggressively; no maximum daily dose for full opioid agonists such as morphine.
- Referral to support groups for client; for caregivers.
- Keep client informed of disease and its treatment, options for managing pain and living with the disease; offer free hot lines for questions: (1-800-342-AIDS) for Center for Disease Control National AIDS Hot Line, (1-800-4-CANCER) for Cancer Information Service.
- Offer support, encouragement, and reassurance of adequate pain management as disease progresses
- Administer analgesics around-the-clock rather than prn for persistent cancer pain to maintain a constant drug blood level and prevent recurrence of pain.
- Administer additional analgesic doses on a prn basis to the around-the-clock schedule as needed for breakthrough pain.
- When clients report decrease in duration of effectiveness of usual opioid dose, suspect drug tolerance; increase opioid dose based on physician's orders; need for higher dose usually related to progression of disease, which causes more pain; stable disease usually does not need increasing opioid doses to prevent pain.
- Use oral route for analgesics whenever possible; rectal or transdermal route is second choice; SQ or IV; patient-controlled analgesia (PCA); avoid IM; intraspinal may be used when other routes unsuccessful; a combination of routes may be needed in terminal stages.
- Monitor for potential side effects of opioid therapy:
  - Anticipate constipation as complication of long-term opioid use; start preventive interventions; daily bowel assessment.
  - Sedation is a common side effect; often treated by giving opioids more frequently but in smaller doses or by switching to different drug; try adding coffee or caffeine-containing drinks.
  - Nausea and vomiting are treated with antiemetics; may be administered around-the-clock for several days followed by prn.

Respiratory depression as an opioid side effect is rare in clients on maintenance doses of opioid to control pain.
- Explain purpose and administer adjuvant drugs for pain:
  Antidepressants or anticonvulsants for tingling or burning pain from damaged nerves; antidepressants may improve sleep.
  Steroids for relief of bone pain, pain from central nervous system tumors and inflammation; may improve appetite.
- Document pain management plan; give the client a copy and review with both client and family; review with new caregiver if client transferred to new setting or new health provider.
- Assess for feelings of hopelessness, suicidal thinking, and rule out uncontrolled pain as the cause.
- If pain decreases or resolves, withdraw the opioid on a slow schedule to prevent withdrawal symptoms (e.g., reduce total daily dose by one-half for first 2 days and by one-quarter every 2 days until client maintained for 2 days on total daily dose of 30 mg morphine, or its equianalgesic equivalent dose; at this level discontinuance will not cause withdrawal S&S).
- An unconscious client near death may continue to receive opioid to prevent withdrawal symptoms; drug may be gradually reduced and client left on one-quarter of original opioid dose for comfort.

Examples of Specific Evaluations for Outcomes 1 to 4
1. Outcome not met. Client reports return of pain at bedtime.
2. Outcome partially met. Client reports pain at 1–2 for most of week but riding in car increased pain to 3–5 rating.
3. Outcome partially met. Client called in to report no BM for 4 days but has had good pain control on morphine using around-the-clock schedule.
4. Outcome met. Daily review of pain management with client and family reflect their satisfaction with pain treatment; report good control.

Key Index Words for Nursing Interventions
Look up these words in the index of fundamentals and
medical-surgical nursing textbooks to find page references
for additional nursing interventions and rationale for their
selection:

- acute pain, management
- adjuvant: drugs, therapy
- analgesics
- cancer pain, management
- chronic pain, management
- cryotherapy
- distraction techniques
- equianalgesic
- malignant pain
- nonsteroidal antiinflammatory drugs (NSAIDs)
- opioids
- opioid: agonist, mixed agonist-antagonist, partial agonist
- pain: acute, intensity scale, management, threshold
- patient-controlled anesthesia (PCA)
- relaxation technique or exercises
- transcutaneous electrical nerve stimulator (TENS)

CHRONIC NONMALIGNANT PAIN*

Definition
A state in which an individual experiences pain that
continues for more than 6 months in duration related to a
nonmalignant health condition.

Major Defining Characteristics
- verbal report or observed evidence of pain experienced
  for more than 6 months
- absence of autonomic/sympathetic responses; normal
  vital signs

Minor Defining Characteristics
- fear of reinjury
- physical and social withdrawal

*Authors' adaptation of NANDA's Chronic Pain diagnosis for clarity and
treatment considerations.

- altered ability to continue previous activities
- anorexia; weight changes
- changes in sleep patterns
- facial mask (eyes lack luster, "beaten look," fixed or scattered eye movement, grimace)
- guarded movement

Other Characteristics
- intensity may range from mild (1–3) to severe (7–10)
- absence of pain behaviors (they do not look like they hurt)
- may not report pain unless asked about it
- may be engaging in distractional activities

Related Factors
- chronic physical/psychological disability or conditions (e.g., arthritis, degenerated joint disease, back pain, phantom limb pain)
- depression; suicidal thinking

Examples of Specific Nursing Diagnoses
1. Chronic nonmalignant pain related to movement secondary to arthritis.
   Chronic nonmalignant pain related to movement secondary to arthritis as evidenced by client report of daily pain rated as 5 in hands and fingers; joint swelling in wrist and digits. (PES format)
2. Chronic nonmalignant pain related to back injury from motor vehicle accident 2 years ago.
   Chronic nonmalignant pain related to back injury from motor vehicle accident 2 years ago as evidenced by statements of daily headaches, shooting pain when turning head, aching at night which disrupts sleep. (PES format)

Examples of Specific Outcomes
1. Client states pain maintained at 4 or less during activity and at 1–2 when inactive by next clinic visit.
2. Client states no return of pain over next month on around-the-clock administration of NSAID.
3. Client states pain has not led to a decreased activity level by next doctor's visit.
4. Client demonstrates and describes correct use of TENS unit by end of home visit.

Examples of Specific Nursing Interventions
- See General Pain Nursing Interventions, page 131.
- Select interventions to relieve or improve the underlying chronic condition causing the pain whenever possible.
- Intervene to reduce problems caused by the pain (e.g., sleep disturbances, family problems, financial problems, depression, drug and alcohol abuse).
- Communicate to the client in a way that conveys that you believe the report of pain and its severity.
- Assess how client copes with pain; promote feelings of control over pain by keeping client well informed about pain, its cause, and its treatment plan.
- Encourage involvement in family, work, and social activities.
- Encourage daily exercise such as walking and swimming in a heated pool.
- Encourage use of nonpharmacologic interventions.
- Review maximum daily doses of any NSAIDs client is taking: encourage around-the-clock dosing schedule for continuous pain to prevent recurrence of pain.
- Review how client is using opioid analgesics if ordered by physician and assess for side effects (long-term opioid therapy more controversial for chronic nonmalignant pain).
- Assess for acute pain episodes and adapt pain management plan as needed in collaboration with client's physician.
- Avoid sudden discontinuance of opioids if pain relief needs decreasing to prevent withdrawal symptoms.
- Support and reinforce client/family efforts to manage and live with the chronic condition and the pain.
- Suggest local support group for specific chronic problem.
- Refer to pain management specialist or pain support groups.
- Assess for suicidal risk when pain is poorly managed.

Examples of Specific Evaluations for Outcomes 1 to 4
1. Outcome not met. Client states pain is very bad with movement and up to 4–5 when resting.
2. Outcome partially met. Client states pain is nonrecurring when occupied during the day; aching in joints present at night.

3. Outcome met. Client states pain management is more effective than she originally thought and has increased her activity to include daily walking.
4. Outcome met. Client correctly demonstrated use of TENS unit for back pain during home visit.

Key Index Words for Nursing Interventions

Look up these words in the index of fundamentals and medical-surgical nursing textbooks to find page references for additional nursing interventions and rationale for their selection:

- acupuncture
- adjuvant therapy
- analgesics
- chronic pain
- cryotherapy
- distraction techniques
- equianalgesic
- heat, application of
- nonsteroidal antiinflammatory drugs (NSAIDs)
- opioid (term preferred to *narcotic*)
- pain: chronic, management, threshold
- phantom limb pain
- placebo
- relaxation techniques or exercises
- transcutaneous electrical nerve stimulator

Chapter 8

Physical Safety/Protection Problems

FOCUSED ASSESSMENT GUIDE

Complete this focused assessment if a general nursing assessment indicates a possible problem. Then turn to page 147 of this text for the Data ⇒ Diagnosis Matching Guide for physical safety/protection problems to help you select the best nursing diagnosis to match a client's data.

ARE ANY OF THE FOLLOWING PRESENT IN THE CLIENT OR IN THE CLIENT'S ENVIRONMENT?

Factors Present in Client

____ inadequate primary defenses (e.g., broken skin, traumatized tissue, decrease in ciliary action, stasis of body fluids, change in pH of secretions, altered peristalsis, rupture of amniotic membranes during pregnancy)

____ inadequate secondary defenses (e.g., abnormal blood profile, suppressed inflammatory response, immunosuppression, inadequate acquired immunity, slow to heal injuries/sores)

____ neurosensory alteration (e.g., reduced vision, hearing; decreased temperature and/or tactile sensation; change in sensory acuity, change in usual response to stimuli; altered sensory reception, transmission and/or integration; consistent inattention to stimuli on an affected side; spinal cord injury)

___ altered mobility (e.g., weakness, dizziness, debilitation, reduced large or small muscle coordination; reduced hand/eye coordination, balancing difficulties; requires help/aids

___ immature or decreased cognitive/thinking ability (e.g., unable to identify or anticipate dangers; disoriented; decreased level of consciousness

___ insufficient knowledge to avoid exposure to hazard; lack of safety or drug education; lack of proper precautions to prevent harm (e.g., lack of protective gear for activities, not using seat belts, unsafe positioning of paralyzed arm, leg)

___ psychological stress, emotional difficulties, apathy, depression

___ history of previous trauma, injury, falls, infection, poisoning

___ insufficient finances

___ communication difficulties; inability to use call light

___ invasive procedures (e.g., indwelling catheter, IVs, surgery)

___ chemical alterations (e.g., medications, drug or alcohol abuse, electrolyte disturbances)

___ chronic disease

___ biochemical or regulatory dysfunction

___ malnutrition; anorexia

___ extremes of age

Hazards Present in Client's Environment

___ biological, chemical (e.g., pollutants, poisons, poisonous plants, lead paint chips, drugs, alcohol, caffeine, nicotine, preservatives, dyes)

___ physical (design, structure and arrangement of community buildings and/or equipment); any factors/obstacles which could cause slipping or falling; inadequate call for aid equipment for bed-resting clients; any practice or setting that could lead to burns, explosions; potentially injurious instruments or equipment; occupational setting without adequate safeguards; altered environmental stimuli (excessive or insufficient)

___ mode of transport/transportation (e.g., unsafe operation of a motor vehicle including not wearing seat belts; any

setting where motorized vehicles could injure pedestrians or result in collision with other vehicles
—— people/provider (e.g., nosocomial agents because of poor aseptic technique by health care providers; staffing patterns resulting in heavy work assignment, call lights answered slowly, unfamiliar with client)

NORMALS AND INFORMATION

- Newborn: at risk for birth trauma, infection, choking (aspiration), effects of drugs used by mother during pregnancy
- Infant: at risk for suffocation, falling, burns, poisoning, electric shock, infection, choking (aspiration), strangulation from things hung around neck, injury in car accidents, child abuse, sudden infant death syndrome
- Toddler and preschool child: at risk for traffic and motor vehicle accidents, poisoning, choking, burns, electrical shock, drowning, falls, playground injury, respiratory and ear infections
- School-age child: at risk for sports injuries, traffic and motor vehicle accidents, tools and machinery injury, injury from guns, drug and alcohol abuse
- Adolescent: at risk for motor vehicle accidents, sports and recreational activities, injury from guns, drug and alcohol abuse, suicide, pregnancy, inadequate nutrition, sexually transmitted infections
- Young adult: at risk for accidents, suicide, drug and alcohol abuse, unwanted pregnancy, sexually transmitted infection
- Middle adult: at risk for motor vehicle accidents, occupational accidents, suicide, obesity, drug and alcohol abuse
- Older adult: at risk for falls, injury, motor vehicle accidents, burns, suicide, drug and alcohol abuse
- Cycle of infection: infectious agent, reservoir, portal of exit, means of transmission, portal of entry, susceptible host
- Inflammatory and immune responses protect the individual from infection by destroying the invading pathogen and promoting tissue repair

DATA ⇒ DIAGNOSIS MATCHING GUIDE

Compare your client data from the Physical Safety/Protection Focused Assessment to these related nursing diagnoses and abbreviated descriptions. Select the nursing diagnosis with the best match. Then turn to the page in this section with that specific diagnosis for help in planning care.

1. *Altered Protection: page 152*
   - definition: a decrease in the ability to guard the self from internal or external threats such as illness or injury
   - data: deficient immunity; impaired healing; altered clotting; maladaptive stress response; neurosensory alteration

2. *Dysreflexia: page 155*
   - definition: a life-threatening, uninhibited, sympathetic response (flight/fight response) of the nervous system to a noxious stimulus in a client with a spinal cord injury at T7 or above
   - data: individual with spinal cord injury (T7 or above) with sudden periodic elevated BP above 140/90 mmHg; pulse above 100 or below 60 beats per minute, sweating above the injury; red splotches on skin above the injury, pallor below; headache

3. *High Risk For Infection: page 158*
   - definition: at risk of being invaded by pathogenic organisms
   - risk factors: inadequate primary defenses, e.g., broken skin, traumatized tissue, decreased ciliary action, stasis of body fluids, change in pH of secretions, altered peristalsis; inadequate secondary defenses, e.g., decreased hemoglobin, leukopenia (decreased number of leukocytes in the blood to 5000 or less), suppressed inflammatory response; immunosuppression; inadequate acquired immunity; chronic disease; invasive procedures; malnutrition; pharmaceutical agents; rupture of amniotic membranes during pregnancy; inadequate knowledge to avoid exposure to pathogens

4. High Risk For Injury: page 162
  ■ definition: at risk of injury from environmental conditions interacting with client's adaptive/defensive resources
  ■ risk factors: internal factors may be biochemical, regulatory, physical, psychological, sensory, or developmental; external hazards may be biological, chemical, nutritional, structural, transportation, or people/provider

5. High Risk For Poisoning: page 164
  ■ definition: at risk of accidental exposure to or ingestion of drugs cr dangerous products in doses able to cause poisoning
  ■ risk factors: internal/individual factors may be decreased vision, inadequate safeguards in occupational setting, lack of safety or drug education, lack of proper precautions, cognitive or emotional difficulties, insufficient finances; external/environmental factors may be a supply of unlocked drugs, medications, cleaning solutions or poisons in the environment of children and confused persons, the presence of atmospheric pollutants, poisonous vegetation, or flaking lead paint, and exposure to paint or lacquer in inadequate ventilation

6. High Risk For Trauma: page 166
  ■ definition: at risk of accidental tissue injury
  ■ risk factors: internal/individual factors may be coordination problems, weakness, altered sensations, lack of safety education and/or safety precautions, cognitive or emotional difficulties, history of previous trauma; external/environmental factors may be dangerous items, structures, neighborhoods, vehicles, work settings, or result from unsafe use of automobiles, fire, machinery, from exposure to sun, cold, heat, gas, explosives, etc., from failure to use safety gear, and from use of alcohol

7. Sensory/Perceptual Alterations: visual, auditory, kinesthetic, gustatory, tactile, olfactory: page 168
  ■ definition: a change in the amount or patterning of oncoming stimuli accompanied by a diminished,

exaggerated, distorted, or impaired response to such stimuli
- data: disoriented in time, in place, or with persons; altered thinking/problem-solving abilities; change in sensory acuity; change in behavior pattern; change in usual response to stimuli; indication of body image alteration; altered communication patterns; restlessness, irritability, anxiety, apathy

8. *Unilateral Neglect: page 171*
- definition: perceptually unaware of and inattentive to one side of the body
- data: consistent inattention to stimuli on an affected side

OTHER SAFETY-RELATED DIAGNOSES

Respiratory/Breathing Diagnoses: page 174
  High Risk For Aspiration: page 181
- definition: at risk for entry of GI secretions, oropharyngeal secretions, or solids/fluids into tracheobronchial passages

  High Risk For Suffocation: page 184
- definition: increased risk of accidental suffocation (inadequate air available for inhalation)

Mobility/Activity Diagnoses: page 91
  High Risk For Disuse Syndrome: page 106
- definition: at risk for deterioration of body systems as the result of prescribed or unavoidable musculoskeletal inactivity (complications of immobility)

Communication, Thinking, and Knowledge Diagnoses: page 295
  Altered Thought Processes: page 298
- definition: a disruption in cognitive operations and activities

Health Management Diagnoses: page 387
  Altered Health Maintenance: page 390
- definition: inability to identify, manage, and/or seek out help to maintain health

Impaired Home Maintenance Management: page 395
- definition: inability to independently maintain a safe growth-promoting immediate environment

Ineffective Management of Therapeutic Regimen: page 398
- definition: unsatisfactory integration of treatment program into daily living for meeting specific health goals

Noncompliance: page 401
- definition: informed decision not to adhere to a therapeutic recommendation

Violence Diagnoses: page 433
  High Risk For Self-Mutilation: page 436
- definition: at risk to perform an act upon the self to injure, not kill, which produces tissue damage and tension relief

  High Risk For Violence to Self or Others: page 439
- definition: behaviors that can be physically harmful either to the self or others

GENERAL OUTCOMES AND NURSING INTERVENTIONS

GENERAL PHYSICAL SAFETY/PROTECTION OUTCOMES

- Client will maintain current status.
- Client will experience no harmful outcomes.
- Client will decrease risk of negative outcomes.
- Client will remain free of harm.

GENERAL PHYSICAL SAFETY/PROTECTION NURSING INTERVENTIONS

- Increase nursing knowledge of potential hazards for:
    developmental age group(s) in clinical practice (e.g., hazards for preterm infants, toddlers, teens, pregnant women, postmenopausal women, elderly).
    high frequency illness/health problems in personal practice (e.g., hip replacement surgery, burns, chemotherapy).

- Assess each client's risk by assessing sensory/perceptual ability, mobility, safety knowledge and precautions being taken, ability to communicate, previous injuries/illnesses, hazards within environment (home or health care facility), lack of safety aids within environment, immune status, blood values/clotting factors, orientation.
- Assess for practices/behaviors that increase risk of harm and explain them to client/family and suggest alternatives.
- Protect client from the hazard by preventing contact with it.

  Move client out of environment containing the hazard.

  Move hazard out of client's environment or eliminate hazard.

  Provide a barrier preventing interaction of client and hazard.

  Make the hazard less of a threat by interventions to strengthen the client and/or to weaken or change the hazard.

- Teach client and family about the hazard and how to reduce their risk of contact or harm.
- Protect the community by working with other citizens, professional nursing groups, and government officials to:

  reduce or eliminate health risks/hazards in the environment (e.g., pollution control, putting up stop signs at dangerous intersections, removing asbestos from school buildings).

  reduce vulnerability of community to health hazards (e.g., immunizations for all children, requiring protective gear/mouthguards for school and community sports programs).

  provide community education to reduce risk or contact with hazard (e.g., antismoking/drug programs in school, sex education, parenting classes and support groups, safe driving courses for seniors).

- Promote good nutrition and hydration. See General Nutrition Nursing Interventions, page 117, and Fluid/Hydration Nursing Interventions, page 62.
- Promote clear lungs. See General Respiratory/Breathing Nursing Interventions, page 179.
- Encourage exercise as condition permits.
- Promote rest and sleep. See General Rest/Sleep Nursing Interventions, page 204.

- Promote client comfort; manage pain. See General Pain Nursing Interventions, page 131.
- Encourage anxiety and stress reduction techniques. See General Coping/Adjustment Nursing Interventions, page 311.
- Use good handwashing before and after client contact.
- Use universal precautions as identified by the Center for Disease Control (CDC); use gloves, gowns, masks, goggles as needed to prevent contact with body fluid of client.
- Use siderails as needed; use wheel locks on beds, commodes, wheelchairs, carts; keep bed in low position.
- Orient to room, bathroom and call light; keep call light within reach and answer promptly.
- Provide good lighting; placement of phone and personal articles within reach.

RELATED NURSING DIAGNOSES

ALTERED PROTECTION

Definition
A state in which an individual experiences a decrease in the ability to guard themselves from internal or external threats such as illness or injury.

Major Defining Characteristics
- deficient immunity
- impaired healing
- altered clotting
- maladaptive stress response
- neurosensory alteration

Minor Defining Characteristics
- chilling; perspiring
- dyspnea (labored or difficult breathing); cough
- itching
- restlessness
- insomnia
- fatigue; weakness
- anorexia (lack of or loss of appetite)
- immobility

■ disorientation
■ pressure sores

Related Factors
■ extremes of age
■ inadequate nutrition
■ alcohol abuse
■ abnormal blood profiles (leukopenia—decreased leukocytes in the blood to 5000 or less; thrombocytopenia—decrease in number of platelets; anemia—inadequate or abnormal erythrocytes in blood; abnormal clotting factors)
■ drug therapies (e.g., antineoplastic, corticosteroid, immune, anticoagulant, thrombolytic)
■ treatments (e.g., surgery, radiation)
■ diseases (e.g., cancer and immune disorders)

Examples of Specific Nursing Diagnoses
1. Altered protection related to prematurity, IV therapy, fragile skin, inadequate nutritional intake.
   Altered protection related to prematurity, IV therapy, fragile skin, inadequate nutrition as evidenced by immaturity of all systems. (PES format)
2. Altered protection related to radiation for cancer, inadequate nutrition.
   Altered protection related to radiation for cancer, inadequate nutrition as evidenced by anemia, leukopenia, and thrombocytopenia, weakness, weight loss, anorexia, nausea, and vomiting. (PES format)

Examples of Specific Outcomes
1. Newborn will experience no signs and symptoms of infection, skin will remain intact; newborn will regain birth weight by 2 weeks.
2. Client will experience no excessive bleeding or infection during period of abnormal blood profile.
3. Client will have fluid intake of 1500 mL/day and caloric intake of 1800 cal/day tomorrow.
4. Client will not injure self while being treated for cancer.

Examples of Specific Nursing Interventions
■ See General Safety/Protection Nursing Interventions, page 150.

- See Specific Nursing Interventions for High Risk for Infection, page 159, and High Risk for Injury, page 162.
- Discuss altered protection status with client and family; identify what types of injury/illness client is at risk for and interventions to reduce risks.
- Reduce or alleviate the client's signs and symptoms (defining characteristics) and related factors as much as possible.
- Every 4 hours assess vital signs, I&O, skin integrity, orientation, wounds; check daily weight and blood work for changes; observe for signs of infection, or bleeding (e.g., dark colored stools; blood in vomitus, sputum, urine; bruising)
- Implement extra measures to guard client from injury, bleeding, infection, fatigue, malnutrition, dehydration, and stress.
- Promote rest, sleep, comfort/pain control (physical and emotional), hydration, nutrition and activity/exercise. (Refer to these individual nursing diagnoses for general and specific interventions).

Examples of Specific Evaluations for Outcomes 1 to 4

1. Outcome met. Preterm has intact skin, no signs of infection, and has regained birthweight at age 12 days.
2. Outcome partially met. No signs/symptoms of infection but accidental cut to finger bled excessively.
3. Outcome not met. Client's nausea and vomiting worse today; intake minimal and needed IV therapy for hydration.
4. Outcome not met. Client weak and faint when getting up to bathroom at night and fell; extensive bruising and swelling over left hip and thigh.

Key Index Words for Nursing Interventions

Look up these words in the index of fundamentals and medical-surgical nursing textbooks to find page references for additional nursing interventions and rationale for their selection:

- bleeding: prevention of, increased risk for
- healing, promotion of
- immunity, promoting

- infection: prevention of, risks of
- injury: prevention of, risks of
- isolation, protective
- protection, altered

DYSREFLEXIA

Definition
A state in which an individual with a spinal cord injury at T7 or above experiences a life-threatening, uninhibited, sympathetic response (flight/fight response) of the nervous system to a noxious stimulus.

Major Defining Characteristics
- paroxysmal hypertension (sudden periodic elevated BP above 140/90 mmHg; BP may go high enough to cause a rupture of cerebral blood vessels, increased intracranial pressure)
- bradycardia (pulse below 60 beats per minute)
- tachycardia (pulse above 100 beats per minute)
- diaphoresis (sweating) above the injury
- red, splotchy skin above injury; pallor below the injury
- headache (severe, pounding)

Minor Defining Characteristics
- chilling
- conjunctival congestion
- Horner's syndrome (contraction of the pupil, partial drooping of the eyelid, a backward displacement of the eyeball into the orbit, and sometimes a loss of sweating over the affected side of the face)
- paresthesia (altered tactile sensation)
- pilorection (gooseflesh)
- blurred vision
- chest pain
- metallic taste in the mouth
- nasal congestion

Related Factors
Spinal cord injury at T7 or above and:

- bladder distention (most common cause); bladder irritation from infections

- bowel distention/constipation/impaction (second most common cause)
- skin irritation/stimulation (third most common cause), e.g., thermal, tactile, or painful stimulation; skin lesions
- lack of client and caregiver knowledge about dysreflexia, its causes, prevention and treatment

Examples of Specific Nursing Diagnoses

1. Dysreflexia related to urinary retention with bladder distention.

   Dysreflexia related to urinary retention with bladder distention as evidenced by sudden rise in BP to 178/90 mmHg, P 120, profuse sweating, and severe headache. (PES format)

2. High risk for dysreflexia related to lack of knowledge of condition, signs, symptoms, and preventive management.

Examples of Specific Outcomes

1. Client's vital signs within normal limits 15 minutes after emptying urine from bladder.

2. Client shows absence of any complication resulting from this episode of dysreflexia.

3. Client shows absence of bladder distention, constipation, impaction, and defining characteristics of dysreflexia during next year.

Examples of Specific Nursing Interventions

- Prevent dysreflexia from occurring.

  Assess frequently for any of the defining characteristics or related factors associated with dysreflexia; assess for any previous episodes of dysreflexia and causative stimuli.

  Prevent bladder/bowel overdistention (See General Nursing Interventions for Bowel Problems, page 32, and Urinary Problems, page 272. See Specific Nursing Interventions for Constipation, page 35, and Urinary Retention, page 291.)

  Encourage fluid intake of 2000 mL/day.

  Practice good hygiene/catheter care to prevent urinary tract infections or catheter obstructions; aseptic technique.

Prevent skin irritation, injury: eliminate drafts, avoid hot/cold skin stimuli and exposure to extremes in room or outside temperatures; control pain; use loose clothing or bedding; encourage frequent position changes to alleviate pressure on the skin.

- If signs and symptoms of dysreflexia begin to occur, identify and remove the triggering stimulus immediately.

    Assess the bladder for distention.

    —Empty distended bladder by inserting urinary cathether using topical anesthetic ointment to prevent further stimulation and to lubricate the catheter; drain bladder (follow hospital guidelines for amount to empty initially, e.g., empty 500 mL, clamp, and wait 15 minutes).

    —Unkink tubing preventing urine from draining.

    —Irrigate obstructed catheter.

    Assess bowel for constipation/distention/impaction if bladder distention is not the problem.

    —Use topical anesthetic ointment to anus and rectum first.

    —Gently remove fecal impaction or insert rectal suppository.

    Assess for skin irritation if neither bladder nor bowel problem is found.

    —Remove skin irritation, remove object from skin.

    —Eliminate cold draft on skin.

    —Spray with topical anesthetic if ordered.

- Treat the signs and symptoms of dysreflexia.

    Raise the head of the bed or place client in a sitting position to lower the blood pressure.

    Assess vital signs, especially BP, every few minutes.

    Notify physician immediately if client is hypertensive; administer medications as ordered by the physician.

    Reassure the client and family to decrease anxiety.

- If stimuli cannot be identified and removed or if hypertension does not resolve with their removal, notify physician immediately for medical management.

- Teach the client and family about dysreflexia, signs and symptoms, possible causes and preventive home management; explain that this condition can be life-threatening; explain when and how to get immediate medical help.

Examples of Specific Evaluations for Outcomes 1 to 3

1. Outcome met. BP down to 110/80 mmHg, P 88, R 18 within 15 minutes of emptying 700 mL from bladder.
2. Outcome not met. BP elevated rapidly and cerebral hemorrhage occurred.
3. Outcome partially met. No signs and symptoms of dysreflexia developed but client has had no bowel movement for 3 days and has a distended abdomen.

Key Index Words for Nursing Interventions

Look up these words in the index of fundamentals and medical-surgical nursing textbooks to find page references for additional nursing interventions and rationale for their selection:

- autonomic hyperreflexia (dysreflexia)
- constipation: prevention of, treatment of
- decubitus ulcers (pressure sores), prevention of
- dysreflexia, autonomic
- hyperreflexia, autonomic
- spinal cord injury
- urinary retention: prevention of, treatment of

HIGH RISK FOR INFECTION

Definition

A state in which an individual is at increased risk for being invaded by pathogenic organisms.

Defining Risk Factors

- inadequate primary defenses (e.g., broken skin, traumatized tissue, decrease in ciliary action, stasis of body fluids, change in pH of secretions, altered peristalsis, rupture of amniotic membranes during pregnancy/labor)
- inadequate secondary defenses (e.g., decreased hemoglobin, leukopenia (reduced leukocyte count in blood to 5000 or lower), suppressed inflammatory response, immuno-suppression)
- inadequate acquired immunity (e.g., children not being immunized)
- tissue destruction (e.g., radiation, burns)

- increased environmental exposure (e.g., hospitalization, multiple sexual partners, travel, attending school/day care)
- chronic disease (e.g., AIDS, aplastic anemia, cancer, diabetes mellitus, leukemia, congestive heart failure)
- invasive procedures (e.g., suction, wound drains, chest tubes, IVs, urinary catheters, injections, surgery)
- malnutrition
- pharmaceutical agents (e.g., steroids, chemotherapy, extensive antibiotic therapy can destroy natural flora, which increases susceptibility to invasion by pathogens)
- trauma
- insufficient knowledge to avoid exposure to pathogens

Examples of Specific Nursing Diagnoses
1. High risk for infection related to cancer, malnutrition, and IV administration of chemotherapy.
2. High risk for infection related to premature rupture of amniotic membrane at 32 weeks of gestation during pregnancy.
3. High risk for infection related to failure to receive any childhood immunizations.

Examples of Specific Outcomes
1. Client shows no signs of infection, temperature normal during course of chemotherapy.
2. Client is afebrile, no chills for next 4 weeks of pregnancy.
3. Client is free of infection from measles, mumps, rubella, hepatitis B, diphtheria, tetanus, pertussis for rest of life.

Examples of Specific Nursing Interventions
- See General Physical Safety/Protection Nursing Interventions, page 150.
- Interrupt the sequence of infection by eliminating one or more of the necessary components: infectious agent, reservoir, portal of exit, transmission, portal of entry, susceptible host.
- Teach client/family personal risk factor for infection or reinfection; suggest alternatives to risky practices/habits/routines; indicate signs and symptoms of infection to watch for, interventions to decrease risk of infection, and when to contact physician/nurse.

- Isolate infected clients to protect others from exposure; isolate very high risk clients to protect them from exposure to infectious agents in environment.
- Use aseptic (sterile) technique when working with wounds, IV therapy, injections, drains, urinary catheters or other potential portals of entry to the client.
- Identify and remedy any breach in handwashing, aseptic technique, cleaning, disinfecting, or sterilizing equipment or client care articles observed in other health care providers.
- Assess client for signs of infection every 4 hours.
     Systemic infection: elevated temperature, (pulse and respirations usually elevated if temperature elevated), elevated white cell count, chills, perspiration, aching, fatigue, loss of appetite, nausea, vomiting; pathogens in blood culture.
     Respiratory infection: congestion, cough, increased sputum, congested nose, chills, fever, increased respiratory rate, decreased depth, weakness; pathogens in sputum culture.
     Urinary infection: burning and/or frequency; pathogens in urine culture.
     Localized infection: swelling, redness, pain, warmth and impaired function of the infected area, presence of pathogens in wound drainage.
- Intervene to prevent client contact with sick visitors/health care workers (or prevent transmission through use of handwashing, masks, no direct contact).
- Teach new parents about childhood immunizations: when, where, why, and cost; send literature home with them.
- Administer antibiotic therapy as ordered; teach clients how to take ordered antibiotics and importance of taking all of medication.
- Assist client to maintain intact skin and mucous membranes (see General Skin/Mucous Membrane Nursing Interventions, page 240, and Specific Nursing Interventions for High Risk for Impaired Skin Integrity, page 247).
- Provide fresh water and clean drinking cup every shift.
- Assist client in personal hygiene.
- Avoid or remove invasive therapies as soon as possible,

e.g., IVs, urinary catheters, wound drains, nasogastric tubes.
- Change dressing, bandages, clothing, and linen when wet and/or soiled; remove and dispose according to institutional policy.
- Empty drainage collection containers as needed or at least once every 8 hours; empty urinals after each voiding and rinse out; keep indwelling urinary drainage systems closed to air and below the level of bladder to prevent backflow of urine; change IV solution containers every 24 hours; change IV tubing every 24–72 hours based on hospital policy.
- Provide bedside receptacle for tissues; replace as needed.

Examples of Specific Evaluations for Outcomes 1 to 3
1. Outcome partially met. IV site became red, warm, and painful with some drainage 2 days after finish of chemotherapy treatments. No signs of systemic infection; afebrile.
2. Outcome not met. Temperature elevated to 101°F (38.3°C) at 34 weeks with chills; group B streptococcus cultured from amniotic fluid.
3. Outcome met. Client received all immunizations for communicable diseases by fourth pediatric visit.

Key Index Words for Nursing Interventions
Look up these words in the index of fundamentals and medical-surgical textbooks to find page references for additional nursing interventions and rationale for their selection:

- asepsis: medical, surgical
- bacteria
- body fluid precautions
- immunizations
- infection: control, cycle of, prevention, risk of
- isolation
- microorganisms, preventing transfer
- nosocomial infection
- pathogen
- sterile
- universal precautions

HIGH RISK FOR INJURY

Definition
A state in which an individual is at risk of injury as a result of environmental conditions interacting with the individual's adaptive and defensive resources.

Defining Risk Factors
Client
biochemical, regulatory dysfunction; malnutrition; auto-immune; abnormal blood profile; physical (broken skin, altered mobility); developmental age; psychological (affective, orientation)

Environment
biological, chemical (pollutants, poisons, drugs, alcohol, caffeine, nicotine, preservatives, dyes), nutrients; physical (design, structure and arrangement of community, buildings and/or equipment); mode of transport/transportation; people/provider (nosocomial agents, staffing patterns, cognitive, affective, and psychomotor factors)

Examples of Specific Nursing Diagnoses
1. High risk for injury related to altered mobility secondary to arthritis.
2. High risk for injury related to age of 89 years, poor vision, unsteady gait, and icy walkway and steps.
3. High risk for injury related to school-age children in home with handgun in unlocked drawer in parent's bedroom.

Examples of Specific Outcomes
1. Client will not experience a fall in her home environment.
2. Client will not fall or injure self while engaging in activities of daily living this winter.
3. Children to remain free of gunshot injuries.

Examples of Specific Nursing Interventions
■ See General Safety/Protection Nursing Interventions, page 150.
■ Identify risk factors with client/family; implement changes that eliminate, reduce, or compensate for risk factors:
　　Remove or fix hazards in environment; uncluttered walkways; wheels locked, bed in low position.

Promote optimum mental clarity, functioning; room calendars, wall clocks, windows, appropriate environmental stimuli, explanations (see Specific Nursing Interventions for Altered Thought Processes, page 299).

Promote optimum mobility, strength, stability through exercises, progressive ambulation, assistive aids for mobility, nonskid slippers or shoes when walking (see Specific Nursing Interventions for Impaired Physical Mobility, page 111).

Promote optimum sensory functioning by adequate lighting, night lights, use of glasses or hearing aids, reducing extraneous sounds that may interfere with understanding communication; raise window shades, position client to see environmental activity; interpret what client sees, hears, feels; clarify misconceptions.

Explore possibility that risk factors could be caused by medication (side effects, incorrect use), drugs, or alcohol.

■ Reassess client frequently for increasing or decreasing risk of injury as changes occur in mental, physical, or environmental status; alter interventions based on new assessment of risk.

■ Use physical restraints only to protect the client from likely injury (e.g., mental confusion with unsteady gait, previous falls) obtain physician's order to implement restraints; assess and reposition or ambulate every 2 hours.

■ Use siderails to prevent independent ambulation based on risk of falling.

■ Consult with client about which personal articles should be within reach and arrange room to meet individual needs; phone, water, TV/radio controls, and bed controls should be in easy reach.

■ Demonstrate use of call light and place within reach; tell client when to use call light for help rather than attempting activity independently; answer call light promptly.

Examples of Specific Evaluations for Outcomes 1 to 3

1. Outcome not met. Client fell while going down the steps to walk the dog: client has broken hip.

2. Outcome partially met. Client experienced no injury but has become unable to move around without a wheelchair and needs help with daily living activities.
3. Outcome met. Children have not had any gunshot injuries over the last 5 years; parents locked handgun in closet safe.

Key Index Words for Nursing Interventions
Look up these words in the index of fundamentals and medical-surgical textbooks to find page references for additional nursing interventions and rationale for their selection:

- accidents, prevention of
- burns: prevention of, risks of
- falls: prevention of, risks of
- hazards: environmental, in home
- injury: prevention of, risks of,
- level of awareness, injury and
- mobility: altered, injury and
- protection
- restraints
- safety: knowledge of, providing for
- sensory-perceptual alterations

HIGH RISK FOR POISONING

Definition
Accentuated risk of accidental exposure to or ingestion of drugs or dangerous products in doses sufficient to cause poisoning.

Defining Risk Factors
Client
reduced vision; verbalization of occupational setting without adequate safeguards; lack of safety or drug education; lack of proper precaution; cognitive or emotional difficulties; insufficient finances

Environment
large supplies of drugs in house; medicine stored in unlocked cabinets accessible to children or confused persons; dangerous products placed or stored within the reach of

children or confused persons; availability of illicit ⌐ ﹏ potentially contaminated by poisonous additives; flaking, peeling paint or plaster in presence of young children; chemical contamination of food and water; unprotected contact with heavy metals or chemicals; paint, lacquer, etc., in poorly ventilated areas or without effective protection; presence of poisonous vegetation; presence of atmospheric pollutants.

Examples of Specific Nursing Diagnoses

1. High risk for poisoning of child related to car care products, antifreeze stored in unlocked cabinets, open buckets in attached garage.
2. High risk for poisoning related to depression, multiple drug use of alcohol and cocaine, history of previous overdose.
3. High risk for poisoning of preschooler related to parent's lack of knowledge of poisons, unlocked cupboards containing toxic household substances, and medicines kept out on counter by kitchen sink.

Examples of Specific Outcomes

1. Child does not ingest any toxic/poisonous products.
2. Client terminates drug abuse behavior within 6 months.
3. Parents prevent contact of toddler with poisonous/toxic household substances by "childproofing" their home within the next week.

Examples of Specific Nursing Interventions

- See General Safety/Protection Nursing Interventions, page 150.
- Assess family environment for risks; discuss possible poisons in their environment and ways to eliminate them or prevent contact.
- Provide clients at risk with phone number for community poison control center.
- Teach parents of young children about state's poison control center; provide samples of 'Mr. Yuk' labels and encourage parents to stick them on phone (poison center phone number on label) and on toxic household substances; encourage them to teach their children about poisons and Mr. Yuk as toddlers and preschoolers;

encourage parents to keep syrup of ipecac in house (nonprescription emetic) to use if poison control center instructs them to do so.

■ If possible ingestion of poison occurs instruct client/family to call poison control center immediately; do not use home remedies.

■ Inform client that all poisonous materials have antidotes or action printed on label; discourage removal of labels, or storage of toxic substances in food or other containers.

■ Assess client ability to read labels on medications and follow directions for dosage; request large-print labels as needed.

■ Assess client/family use of drugs and/or alcohol, over-the-counter drugs, overuse of vitamin/mineral supplements.

■ Encourage clients to destroy all old medicines.

Examples of Specific Evaluations for Outcomes 1 to 3

1. Outcome met. Childhood free of poison ingestion.
2. Outcome not met. Client does not accept that drug behavior has poison risk factor and claims to understand own actions.
3. Outcome partially met. Parents did place all cleaning fluids in cabinet with childproof latch; aspirins and allergy medications remain on counter because parents do not believe child can reach them.

Key Index Words for Nursing Interventions

Look up these words in the index of fundamentals and medical-surgical nursing textbooks to find page references for additional nursing interventions and rationale for their selection:

■ emetics
■ poison control center
■ poison: types of, treatment of, prevention of, antidotes
■ poisoning, high risk for

HIGH RISK FOR TRAUMA

Definition

Accentuated risk of accidental tissue injury, e.g., wound, burn, fracture.

Defining Risk Factors
Client

weakness; poor vision; balancing difficulties; reduced temperature and/or tactile sensation; reduced large or small muscle coordination; reduced hand-eye coordination; lack of safety education and/or precautions; insufficient finances to purchase safety equipment or effect repairs; cognitive or emotional difficulties; history of previous trauma.

Environment

any factors which could cause slipping or falling; inadequate call for aid equipment for bed-resting clients; any practice or setting that could lead to burns, explosions; any setting with potentially injurious instruments or equipment; unsafe operation of a motor vehicle including not wearing seat belts; lack of protective gear for activities; any setting where motorized vehicles could injure pedestrians or result in collision with other vehicles.

Examples of Specific Nursing Diagnoses
1. High risk for trauma (burns) related to smoking in bed, cast on fractured leg, and alcohol consumption at night.
2. High risk for trauma (wound) related to activity of splitting and cutting wood for winter heating needs, 78 years old, previous injury with chain saw, works alone.
3. High risk for trauma (fall/fracture) related to being 75 years old, 5 ft tall, overweight, and walking two large dogs three times daily in winter on icy walks and roads, with dogs pulling at leash.

Examples of Specific Outcomes
1. Client will experience no burns.
2. Client will remain free of trauma during activities of wood cutting/splitting.
3. Client will not experience a fall while walking dogs.

Examples of Specific Nursing Interventions
■ See General Safety/Protection Nursing Interventions, page 150, and Specific Nursing Interventions for High Risk for Injury, page 162.

Examples of Specific Evaluations for Outcomes 1 to 3
1. Outcome partially met. Client did not burn self but did set bed linens and papers on fire while smoking in bed.

2. Outcome not met. Client dropped log on right hand and broke middle finger.
3. Outcome met. Client has experienced no falls while walking dogs during winter months.

Key Index Words for Nursing Interventions
Look up these words in the index of fundamentals and medical-surgical textbooks to find page references for additional nursing interventions and rationale for their selection:

- accidents, prevention of
- burns: prevention of, risks of
- falls: prevention of, risks of
- hazards: environmental, in home
- injury: prevention of, risks of,
- mobility: altered, injury and
- protection
- restraints
- safety: knowledge of, providing for
- sensory-perceptual alterations
- trauma, high risk for

SENSORY/PERCEPTUAL, ALTERATIONS (specify as visual, auditory, kinesthetic, gustatory, tactile, or olfactory)

Definition
A state in which an individual experiences a change in the amount or patterning of oncoming stimuli accompanied by a diminished, exaggerated, distorted, or impaired response to such stimuli.

Defining Characteristics
- disoriented in time, place, or with persons
- altered abstraction, altered conceptualization
- change in problem-solving abilities
- reported or measured change in sensory acuity
- change in behavior pattern
- anxiety; restlessness; irritability; apathy
- change in usual response to stimuli
- indication of body image alteration
- altered communication patterns

Other Possible Characteristics
- complaints of fatigue
- alteration in posture; change in muscular tension
- inappropriate responses
- hallucinations

Related Factors
- altered environmental stimuli (excessive or insufficient)
- altered sensory reception, transmission and/or integration
- chemical alterations; endogenous/electrolyte, exogenous/drugs
- psychological stress

Examples of Specific Nursing Diagnoses
1. Sensory/perceptual alterations (visual, auditory, tactile, kinesthetic) related to altered sensory transmission and integration and confinement to a circle bed in cervical traction secondary to a cervical spinal cord injury.
   Sensory/perceptual alterations (visual, auditory, tactile, kinesthetic) related to altered sensory transmission and integration and confinement to a circle bed in cervical traction secondary to a cervical spinal cord injury, as evidenced by absence of sense of touch or position sense in lower arms/hands and below chest level, disorientation and hallucinations at night. (PES format)
2. Sensory/perceptual alterations (visual, auditory) related to alcohol withdrawal.
   Sensory/perceptual alterations (visual, auditory) related to alcohol withdrawal as evidenced by disorientation, hallucinations, nonreality-based thinking. (PES format)

Examples of Specific Outcomes
1. No further hallucinations while on circle bed and traction.
2. Orientated to time, place, and person during next 8 hours.
3. Injury-free during period of alcohol withdrawal.
4. Return of some sensory ability in arms/hands in 2 weeks.

Examples of Specific Nursing Interventions
- See General Safety/Protection Nursing Interventions, page 150, and Specific Nursing Interventions for High Risk for Injury, page 162.

- Correct or reduce related factors causing the altered sensation/perception.
- Eliminate or reduce the signs and symptoms (defining characteristics) of the sensory/perceptual alteration; if this is not possible help client cope with the alterations.
- Orient initially and as needed to room and health care providers; reorient to time, place, and person as needed; provide consistent personnel and room arrangement; clarify what is real and what is imagined/hallucinated and reassure client of safety; stay with client.
- Provide increased or decreased environmental stimulation based on assessment of client's need (e.g., lighting, sounds, information, visual variety, window to maintain sense of day/night, familiar people, communication, position changes).
- Discuss the sensory/perceptual alteration with the client and family: why it is occurring, the signs and symptoms, how long it may last, risk of injury, and interventions to help client deal with the changes; interpret what the client sees, hears, and feels to help make sense of new or distorted stimuli.
- Involve client and family in decision-making and choices related to care to promote sense of control.
- Encourage the use of familiar routines, personal clothing and grooming practices, usual activities, and familiar objects such as pictures of family.
- Explain all treatments; adapt pace, content, and depth of explanations to assessment of client's ability; stay in client's visual field when speaking; if client cannot see, identify yourself as you enter the room.

Examples of Specific Evaluations for Outcomes 1 to 4

1. Outcome met. With low room light and radio on at night, client has remained oriented with no further hallucinations.
2. Outcome partially met. Client oriented until administration of IM analgesic; some disorientation to time and place occurred 30 minutes later lasting for 2 hours.
3. Outcome not met. Client climbed out of bed waist restraint and over siderail; found on floor moaning and holding left arm; physician notified and diagnosed fracture of left arm.

4. Outcome met. Client has regained sharp and dull sensation in both arms and hands; position sense intact with movement returning.

Key Index Words for Nursing Interventions
Look up these words in the index of fundamentals and medical-surgical nursing textbooks to find page references for additional nursing interventions and rationale for their selection:

- alcohol: intoxication, withdrawal
- blindness
- deafness
- disorientation
- drug: depressants, mind-altering, overdose, stimulants
- electrolyte imbalances
- hallucinations
- hearing, alterations in
- paralysis, sensation and paresthesia
- perception, alterations in
- sensation, alterations in
- sleep deprivation
- stimulation, deprivation
- vision, alteration in

UNILATERAL NEGLECT

Definition
A state in which an individual is perceptually unaware of and inattentive to one side of the body.

Major Defining Characteristics
- consistent inattention to stimuli on an affected side

Minor Defining Characteristics
- inadequate self-care
- inadequate positioning and/or safety precautions in regard to the affected side
- does not look toward the affected side
- leaves food on plate on affected side

Related Factors
- effects of disturbed perceptual abilities, e.g., defective vision or blindness in half of the visual fields
- one-sided blindness
- neurologic illness or trauma (e.g., cerebral vascular accident/stroke; brain trauma or tumors, cerebral hemorrhage)

Examples of Specific Nursing Diagnoses

1. Unilateral neglect related to loss of sensation and movement on right side secondary to recent CVA/stroke.

   Unilateral neglect related to loss of sensation and movement on left side secondary to recent CVA/stroke as evidenced by no response to stimuli on left, unsafe positioning of arm and leg. (PES format)

2. Unilateral neglect related to loss of left half of visual field in both eyes.

   Unilateral neglect related to loss of left half of visual field in both eyes as evidenced by inattention to any visual stimuli on left. (PES format)

Examples of Specific Outcomes

1. Client performs dressing/grooming self-care including affected right side by discharge from rehabilitation unit.
2. Client demonstrates safety precautions to protect affected side from injury by end of teaching session today.
3. Client adapts head movement to scan visual stimuli in left visual field during activities of daily living.

Examples of Specific Nursing Interventions

- See General Safety/Protection Nursing Interventions, page 150.
- Assess effect deficit has on ability to perform activities of daily living, general physical safety and orientation; assess daily for changes in deficit.
- Reorient client as needed; explore and clarify client's overestimation of abilities and underestimation of the extent of the deficit when appropriate.
- Discuss client's risk of injury/trauma because of the deficit.
- Consider with client/family ways to protect the affected side, prevent general injury, increase independence, and promote return of function (based on medical prognosis).

  Adapt environment to deficit (e.g., rearranging room furniture to allow client to transfer out of bed using unaffected side).

  Help client adapt own behavior to consciously attend to affected side (e.g., using unaffected side to give range of motion exercise to affected side).

Provide lap boards, overbed tables, pillows, arm slings for client to use to support affected side and to elevate it when in bed to prevent dependent edema.

Encourage activities that use both sides of the body.

Assist staff and family to adapt their behavior to use client's unaffected side/visual field, e.g., place all food on one side of plate, approach client from unaffected side.

- Referrals to occupational and physical therapy for adaptive aids to compensate for lost function and for activities to promote return of function.
- Referral to community resources for emotional support, physical help, and financial assistance.

Examples of Specific Evaluations for Outcomes 1 to 3
1. Outcome met. Client using left side and adaptive aids to dress and groom affected right side by discharge.
2. Outcome partially met. States correct safety precautions to take but fails to protect/position affected side when getting back into bed after teaching session.
3. Outcome not met. Client refuses to make any adaptive efforts with eyes or head movement to compensate for loss of left visual field.

Key Index Words for Nursing Interventions
Look up these words in the index of fundamentals and medical-surgical nursing textbooks to find page references for additional nursing interventions and rationale for their selection:

- hemiparesis
- hemiplegia
- unilateral neglect

Chapter 9

Respiratory/Breathing Problems

FOCUSED ASSESSMENT GUIDE

Complete this focused assessment if a general nursing assessment indicates a possible problem. Then turn to page 177 of this text for the Data ⇒ Diagnosis Matching Guide for respiratory/breathing problems to help you select the best nursing diagnosis to match the client's data.

TELL ME IF YOU ARE HAVING ANY OF THESE PROBLEMS

___ feeling short of breath at rest; with activity
___ pain with coughing, deep breathing, or movement
___ coughing; productive/unproductive cough; describe sputum
___ decreased energy/fatigue
___ feeling anxious or afraid
___ Are you doing any breathing exercises to help keep your lungs clear? If yes, have client show you.

OBSERVE CLIENT/CHART FOR

___ abnormal skin/nail bed color: pale, dusky, bluish
___ abnormal respirations (rate, depth, pattern); labored respirations; prolonged exhale through pursed lips; shallow respirations

____ short of breath with talking or activity

____ abnormal breath sounds (rales/crackles or rhonchi/ wheezes); absence of breath sounds in areas of lung

____ decreased ability to remove lung secretions/sputum with coughing; depressed or absent cough, choke, gag reflex

____ labored breathing; retractions (substernal, suprasternal, intercostal), use of accessory muscles; nasal flaring

____ fremitus (vibration felt on chest when palpating/ ascultating)

____ assumption of three-point position (hands rest on bed or chair to elevate shoulders)

____ abnormal hemoglobin and hematocrit values

____ oxygen ordered by physician; frequency of use by client; flow rate, concentration

____ elevated TPR, BP values from client's baseline or from normal

____ abnormal arterial blood gases; decreased pO_2 (below 80 mmHg); increased pCO_2 (above 45 mmHg); O_2 saturation below 95%)

____ frequency of repositioning, up in chair, ambulation

____ increased anterior-posterior chest diameter (barrel-chested); asymmetrical chest movement

____ presence of tracheostomy or endotrachial tube; mechanical ventilation

____ gastrointestinal tubes; tube feedings

____ increased metabolic rate from infection, fever, pregnancy

____ surgery with anesthesia

____ trauma or surgery to lungs, chest, face, neck; wired jaws

____ confusion; somnolence; restlessness; irritability; apprehension; decreased cooperation; agitation

____ perceptual/cognitive impairment; head injury

____ neuromuscular and/or musculoskeletal impairment or immaturity; reduced breathing and movement abilities because of disease, trauma, treatments, age

____ situations hindering elevation of upper body

____ increased intragastric pressure; increased gastric residual; decreased gastrointestinal motility; delayed gastric emptying

____ impaired swallowing

___ practices that could lead to suffocation/strangulation (restraints, pacifier hung around infants neck, plastic bags)

ADULT NORMALS AND INFORMATION

- Respiratory center located in medulla and pons of brain
- Relaxed breathing is accomplished by movement of the diaphragm down during inspiration and its relaxation up during exhalation
- Normal adult respirations are silent, effortless, regular with rate of 12–20 breaths per minute; accessory muscles of chest not used; no retractions or nasal flaring
- No shortness of breath, dyspnea with talking/normal activity
- Normal coughing occurs only occasionally with no secretions
- Normal blood gas values reflecting adequate ventilations:

  pH = 7.35–7.45; below 7.35 is acidosis; above 7.45 is alkalosis

  pO_2 = 80–100 mmHg; pO_2 of 60–80 mmHg = mild hypoxemia; a pO_2 of 40–60 mmHg = moderate hypoxemia; below 40 mmHg is severe hypoxemia

  pCO_2 = 35–45 mmHg; above 45 mmHg = inadequate alveolar ventilations and respiratory acidosis; below 35 mmHg = alveolar hyperventilation

  Oxygen saturation (SaO_2) is 95–98%; an SaO_2 of 90% correlates with a pO_2 of 60 mmHg; pulse oximetry is a method of continuous, noninvasive monitoring of SaO_2

- Normal breath sounds:

  present over entire lung field

  absence of adventitious (abnormal) breath sounds

- Abnormal breath sounds:

  crackles (rales) are heard on inspiration caused by delayed reopening of small airways and alveoli; coarse crackles are louder and sound moist; indicate inflammation or congestion

  wheezes (rhonchi) are heard on inspiration, expiration, or continuously as air passes through airways constricted

from secretions, swelling, bronchoconstriction
absent or diminished breath sounds in an area
indicate inadequate ventilation of that area
- Tidal volume is the amount of air inspired or expired in a normal, relaxed breath; approximately 500 mL in adult
- Anterior-posterior chest diameter is approximately one-half of lateral chest diameter

DATA ⇒ DIAGNOSIS MATCHING GUIDE

Compare your client data from the Respiratory/Breathing Focused Assessment to these related nursing diagnoses and abbreviated descriptions. Select the nursing diagnosis with the best match. Then turn to the page in this section with that specific diagnosis for help planning care.

1. *Impaired Gas Exchange: page 186*
   - definition: a decreased passage of oxygen and/or carbon dioxide between the alveoli of the lungs and the vascular system
   - data: confusion; somnolence; restlessness; irritability; inability to move secretions; hypercapnia (elevated pCO_2); hypoxia (inadequate tissue oxygenation)

2. *Ineffective Airway Clearance: page 196*
   - definition: unable to clear secretions or obstructions from the respiratory tract to maintain airway patency
   - data: rales/crackles or rhonchi/wheezes; changes in rate or depth of respirations; very rapid respirations; cough with or without sputum; cyanosis; labored, difficult breathing

3. *Ineffective Breathing Pattern: page 199*
   - definition: inhalation and/or exhalation pattern does not enable adequate pulmonary inflation or emptying
   - data: labored, difficult breathing; shortness of breath; rapid rate; shallow depth; fremitus (vibrations palpated or auscultated over the chest wall); abnormal arterial blood gases; cyanosis; cough; nasal flaring; respiratory depth changes; three-point positioning; pursed lip breathing/prolonged expiratory phase; increased

anterior-posterior diameter; use of accessory muscles; altered chest movement

4. *Inability to Sustain Spontaneous Ventilations: page 189*
   - definition: decreased energy reserves result in an inability to maintain breathing adequate to support life
   - data: difficult, labored breathing; increased metabolic rate; restlessness; apprehension; more use of accessory muscles; increased heart rate, pCO_2 levels; decreased pO_2, O_2 saturation

5. *Dysfunctional Ventilatory Weaning Response (DVWR): page 192*
   - definition: unable to adjust to lowered levels of mechanical ventilator support, which interrupts/ prolongs weaning process
   - data: responds to lowered levels of ventilator support with restlessness, agitation; increased respiratory rate, heart rate, and BP; deterioration in arterial blood gases

6. *High Risk for Suffocation: page 184*
   - definition: accentuated risk of accidental suffocation (inadequate air available for inspiration)
   - risk factors: reduced sense of smell; reduced motor abilities; lack of safety education, safety precautions; cognitive or emotional difficulties; disease or injury process; pillow or propped bottle in an infant's crib; vehicle warming in closed garage; children playing with plastic bags or inserting small objects into their mouths or noses; discarded or unused refrigerators or freezers without removed doors; children unattended in bathtubs or pools; household gas leaks; smoking in bed; unvented, fuel-burning heaters; low-strung clothesline; pacifier hung around infant's head; eating large mouthfuls of food

7. *High Risk for Aspiration: page 181*
   - definition: at risk for entry of oropharyngeal or GI secretions, solids or fluids into the tracheobronchial passage
   - risk factors: reduced level of consciousness; depressed cough and gag reflexes; presence of tracheostomy or endotrachial tube; incomplete lower esophageal

sphincter; GI tubes; tube feedings; medication administration; situations hindering elevation of upper body; increased intragastric pressure; increased gastric residual; decreased GI motility; delayed gastric emptying; impaired swallowing; facial/oral/neck surgery or trauma; wired jaws

GENERAL OUTCOMES AND NURSING INTERVENTIONS

GENERAL RESPIRATORY/BREATHING OUTCOMES

- Client will have vital signs in normal range.
- Client will have blood gases in normal range.
- Client will be alert and oriented to time, place, and person.
- Client will maintain a patent airway.
- Client will have a clear airway and clear breath sounds.
- Client will perform activities of daily living without dyspnea or signs of hypoxia.

GENERAL RESPIRATORY/BREATHING NURSING INTERVENTIONS

- Reduce or eliminate related factors causing or contributing to the respiratory problem whenever possible.
- Assess vital signs, depth of respirations, breath sounds, type and amount of secretions, effectiveness of cough, effort and use of accessory muscles, presence of retractions, nasal flaring, feeling short of breath or having difficulty breathing, color, level of consciousness.
- Monitor blood gases, hemoglobin values, pulse oximetry (measures oxygen saturation); report abnormals to physician.
- Maintain good nutrition and hydration, > 2000 mL/24 h (unless contraindicated) to keep lung secretions thin and loose, to promote healing, and to provide energy.
- Record I&O and daily weights.
- Perform Chest Physiotherapy (Pulmonary Hygiene) Assess and record VS, breath sounds before and after treatment to evaluate effectiveness.

Postural drainage as ordered (2–4 times per day) to remove lung secretions by gravity and coughing efforts.

Chest percussion and vibration to shake loose secretions which can then be removed by client's coughing efforts.

Teach deep breathing exercises:

Sustained maximal inspirations (SMI): deep breath in, hold for 3 seconds to force open alveoli followed by relaxed exhale; repeat 3–4 times every hour while awake.

Use of incentive spirometer: 10 breaths per hour while awake.

Coughing to remove bronchial secretions: teach client to take several deep breaths, cough several times, repeat; end with several SMIs to reopen alveoli that may have collapsed during forceful coughing; provide tissues for mucus and waste bag.

- Suction airway to remove secretions as needed.
- Teach breathing retraining: pursed-lip breathing, diaphragmatic breathing; three-point positioning; relaxation breathing.
- Administer oxygen as ordered; check tubing patency, flow, concentration every 1–2 hours, to ensure correct administration; assess and record client response to oxygen therapy.
- Provide humidity as ordered or as needed.
- Administer ordered medications (antibiotics, bronchodilators, antiinflammatory drugs, nebulizations) to treat primary disease and resulting respiratory problems; explain to client reason for medication and possible side effects.
- Assist client to turn and reposition every 2 hours while in bed to prevent accumulation of secretions and promote drainage.
- Assist client out of bed as soon as possible; early ambulation.
- Encourage rest in between activity.
- Manage pain effectively so client is more willing to cough, deep breathe, turn and reposition, ambulate; teach

splinting and use of pillows when coughing to support incision and reduce pain; assess for signs of respiratory depression (decreasing rate and depth) if managing acute pain with opioid analgesics.

- Provide for safety needs if client confused, uncooperative.
- Provide emotional support, reassurance to reduce anxiety.
- Coordinate efforts with respiratory therapy to make client's treatments consistent and as effective as possible (e.g., client in upright position, rest before and after treatments).
- Teach home management of respiratory problem/ preventive care: medications, oxygen use, avoiding infections, promoting clearance of secretions, promoting general muscle tone and respiratory muscle function; maintaining good hydration and nutrition; reducing oxygen need through rest and more effective breathing patterns; ways to stop smoking.

RELATED NURSING DIAGNOSES

HIGH RISK FOR ASPIRATION

Definition
A state in which an individual is at risk for entry of gastrointestinal secretions, oropharyngeal secretions, or solids or fluids into the tracheobronchial passage.

Defining Risk Factors
- reduced level of consciousness
- depressed cough and gag reflexes (e.g., anesthesia, alcohol)
- presence of tracheostomy or endotrachial tube
- incomplete lower esophageal sphincter (e.g., preterm newborn)
- nasogastric tubes; gastrointestinal tubes; tube feedings
- medication administration
- situations hindering elevation of upper body
- increased intragastric pressure
- increased gastric residual (amount of feeding left in stomach from previous feeding when next feeding is due; more than 50–100 mL in an adult is excess residual volume but size of stomach must be considered)

- decreased gastrointestinal motility (signs and symptoms include faint, infrequent, or absent bowel sounds, abdominal distention, inability to pass gas, constipation)
- delayed gastric emptying (e.g., intestinal obstruction, anxiety, pain)
- impaired swallowing (e.g., myasthenia gravis, post-anesthesia)
- facial/oral/neck surgery or trauma
- wired jaws

Examples of Specific Nursing Diagnoses
1. High risk for aspiration related to wired jaws, decreased level of consciousness, depressed gag reflex secondary to fractured jaw surgery.
2. High risk for aspiration related to gavage tube feedings, presence of 10 mL of residual feeding, immature cough, gag reflex, small stomach capacity secondary to prematurity.
3. High risk for aspiration related to presence of tracheostomy tube, tube feedings, decreased level of consciousness, depressed gag reflex secondary to brain injury.

Examples of Specific Outcomes
1. Client's airway and lungs remain clear during recovery from surgery.
2. Client shows no aspiration of foods/fluids while jaws wired together.
3. Client shows no aspiration of tube feedings during this shift as evidenced by stable vital signs, clear breath sounds, no respiratory distress, no evidence of feeding in tracheal secretions.
4. Client shows no signs of coughing, gagging, respiratory distress during and after next tube feeding.

Examples of Specific Nursing Interventions
- Assess client and environment for risk factors.
- Eliminate or reduce risk factors whenever possible.
- Educate client and family to presence of current risk factors.
- Problem-solve with client/family ways to prevent aspiration when risk factors cannot be reduced or eliminated.

- Have suctioning equipment available when feeding clients with risk factors.
- Turn client on side if nausea develops or during high risk period (e.g., postanesthesia, postoperatively).
- Do not attempt to give food or fluids orally if level of consciousness is significantly decreased, respirations are very rapid, nausea present with wired jaws, possibility of surgery in near future, cough/gag reflex is absent or weak.
- Feed slowly watching for complete swallowing before continuing.
- Work with dietician and family for types and textures of food client will be most likely to swallow without choking.
- If tracheostomy present, inflate cuff before feeding and for 1 hour after feeding; suction pharynx before deflating cuff.
- Teach Heimlich maneuver to families of clients at risk.
- Remove any material from mouth and airway before emergency CPR; insert nasogastric tube during or after CPR to vent trapped air and decompress stomach.

For clients with tube feedings
- Assess for feeding tube placement, bowel sounds, abdominal girth, residual feeding volumes in stomach before administering each tube feeding; for continuous feeding assess every 4–8 hours.
- Hold tube feeding and check with physician if:
  capacity of stomach could be exceeded if this feeding given because of large residual remaining from last feeding (50–100 mL in an adult; as little as 5–10 mL in preterm infant).
  abdominal girth increased from baseline; tight-looking abdomen.
  uncertain of tube placement.
  absence of bowel sounds.
  nausea and/or vomiting.
- Place small amount of blue food coloring in tube feedings to detect presence in tracheal/respiratory secretions as evidence of aspiration.
- Elevate head of bed or have client sitting up for feedings; keep elevated for 30–60 minutes after feedings or continuously if feeding running continuously.

- Administer small feedings by gravity flow rather than large feedings under pressure to decrease risk of aspiration.
- Stop feeding or turn off tube feeding if any respiratory distress, choking, gagging, coughing develops.

Examples of Specific Evaluations for Outcomes 1 to 4

1. Outcome met. Airway and lungs clear during last 48 hours.
2. Outcome met. No aspiration of food/fluids during last 6 weeks while jaws wired shut.
3. Outcome partially met. Color became dusky, bluish during feeding with bradycardia; gavage tube removed and color and vital signs improved; clear breath sounds.
4. Outcome not met. Client began coughing and choking with feeding, traces of feeding suctioned from tracheostomy; respiratory distress present; breath sounds remain clear.

Key Index Words for Nursing Interventions

Look up these words in the index of fundamentals and medical-surgical nursing textbooks to find page references for additional nursing interventions and rationale for their selection:

- abdominal girth
- aspiration, high risk for
- cough, gag reflex
- gastric: aspirate, residual
- gavage feeding
- tube feedings
- tracheostomy, and feedings

HIGH RISK FOR SUFFOCATION

Definition

Accentuated risk of accidental suffocation (inadequate air available for inspiration).

Defining Risk Factors

- reduced olfactory sensation
- reduced motor abilities
- lack of safety education; lack of safety precautions
- cognitive or emotional difficulties
- disease or injury process
- pillow or propped bottle placed in an infant's crib
- vehicle warming in a closed garage

- children playing with plastic bags or inserting small objects into their mouths or noses
- discarded or unused refrigerators or freezers without removed doors
- children left unattended in bathtubs or pools
- household gas leaks
- smoking in bed
- use of fuel-burning heaters not vented to outside
- low-strung clothesline
- pacifier hung around infant's head
- persons who eat large mouthfuls of food

Examples of Specific Nursing Diagnoses
1. High risk for suffocation related to soft, pillow-like bedding around sides of portable infant bassinet.
2. High risk for suffocation related to forgetfulness, use of unvented gas space heater in house, decreased motor and sensory abilities.
3. High risk for suffocation related to young children playing in grandparent's home with unused refrigerator without door removed in basement.

Examples of Specific Outcomes
1. Infant's airway remains unobstructed by bedding.
2. Client eliminates risk of inadequate room oxygen by having gas heater vented within the next 2 weeks.
3. Grandparent prevents possible suffocation by turning refrigerator door to the wall, preventing opening before grandchild's next visit.

Examples of Specific Nursing Interventions
- Assess client and environment for risk factors.
- Eliminate or reduce risk factors whenever possible.
- Educate client and family to presence of current risk factors.
- Problem-solve with client/family ways to prevent suffocation when risk factors cannot be reduced or eliminated.
- Teach all new parents about risk factors and ways to make baby's environment safe, e.g., no pillows, no propped bottles, nothing tied around infant's neck; put to sleep on side or back rather than on stomach.
- Teach CPR and Heimlich maneuver to families of clients at risk.

Examples of Specific Evaluations for Outcomes 1 to 3

1. Outcome met. Parents returned bassinet to store and infants airway has remained unobstructed during first year of life.
2. Outcome not met. Client continues to use gas space heater without venting after 4 weeks.
3. Outcome partially met. Grandparents state refrigerator too heavy to move but are keeping basement door bolted.

Key Index Words for Nursing Interventions

Look up these words in the index of fundamentals and medical-surgical nursing textbooks to find page references for additional nursing interventions and rationale for their selection:

- aspiration
- carbon monoxide
- cardiopulmonary resuscitation (CPR)
- drowning
- Heimlich maneuver
- strangulation
- suffocation

IMPAIRED GAS EXCHANGE

Definition

A state in which an individual experiences a decreased passage of oxygen and/or carbon dioxide between the alveoli of the lungs and the vascular system.

Defining Characteristics

- confusion; somnolence; restlessness; irritability
- inability to move secretions out of lungs
- hypercapnia (excess carbon dioxide in the blood) e.g., arterial blood pCO_2 above 45 mmHg
- hypoxia (inadequate oxygenation of tissues) e.g., arterial blood pO_2 below 80 mmHg; oxygen saturation below 95%; elevated pulse, respirations and BP; dusky, cyanotic color

Related Factors

- reduced oxygen supply in inspired air
- reduced capacity for blood to carry oxygen (e.g., low hemoglobin in anemia; carbon monoxide in inspired air)
- ventilation perfusion imbalance
  adequate blood flow to pulmonary alveoli (perfusion) but inadequate movement of air in and out of lungs

(ventilation), e.g., pulmonary edema, pneumonia, atelectasis, mucus, tumor, chronic obstructive pulmonary disease (COPD)

adequate air movement in and out of lungs (ventilation) but inadequate blood flow to pulmonary alveoli (perfusion), e.g., pulmonary emboli, heart failure, hypovolemic shock

inadequate movement of gases in and out of lungs (ventilation) and inadequate blood flow to pulmonary alveoli (perfusion), e.g., pneumothorax (collapsed lung), adult respiratory distress syndrome (ARDS)

Examples of Specific Nursing Diagnoses

1. Impaired gas exchange related to inadequate ventilation of alveoli secondary to pulmonary edema.
   Impaired gas exchange related to inadequate ventilation of alveoli secondary to pulmonary edema as evidenced by crackles in all lobes, restlessness, elevated pCO_2 (48 mmHg), low pO_2 (60 mmHg). (PES format)
2. Impaired gas exchange related to inadequate perfusion of alveoli secondary to pulmonary emboli.
   Impaired gas exchange related to inadequate perfusion of alveoli secondary to pulmonary emboli as evidenced by anxiety, P 110, R 30, BP 120/60 mmHg, labored, difficult breathing, low pO_2 (48 mmHg), dusky blue skin color. (PES format)

Examples of Specific Outcomes

1. Client produces clear breath sounds in 48 hours.
2. Client is alert and oriented to time, place, person within 4 hours.
3. Client's pO_2 is above 50 mmHg within 1 hour.
4. pCO_2 is 35–45 mmHg in 2 hours.

Examples of Specific Nursing Interventions

- See General Respiratory/Breathing Nursing Interventions, page 179.
- Provide clear airway by positioning, chest physiotherapy, suctioning, maintaining oropharyngeal airway or tracheostomy tube in place.
- When repositioning, use side lying with clear, unaffected lung down to maximize blood flow to most effective lung for 1–2 hours.

- Remove any respiratory irritants, allergy-causing objects (e.g., smoke, hairspray, perfume, aftershave, cologne, flowers).
- Assess and maintain correctly functioning equipment during mechanical ventilation.
- Develop and document alternate methods of communicating with the client if intubated, on a ventilator, or with tracheostomy.
- Maintain closed chest drainage system; measure and record chest drainage (may be done every 1 hour initially; advancing to every 4–8 hours or every day as drainage decreases).
- Encourage maximum mobility by assisting with equipment when getting into chair or ambulating (e.g., IV, chest tubes and drainage system, Foley catheter).
- Administer nebulization treatments before meals to decrease risk of nausea and avoid fatigue common after eating; encourage coughing to clear secretions after treatments.
- In a client with COPD, administer oxygen carefully since hypoxia is the stimulus for breathing and raising flow rate of oxygen can cause apnea (cessation of breathing).
- Problem-solve with client and family ways to adapt activities of daily living to periods of improved respiratory functioning (e.g., COPD more disabling just after rising and after meals so that is a poor time for other activities).
- Encourage increasing activity but prevention of fatigue and dyspnea (difficult, labored breathing).
- Assist with planning daily fluid intake for fluid restriction.

Examples of Specific Evaluations for Outcomes 1 to 4

1. Outcome partially met. Upper lungs clear but crackles and wheezes still heard in lower left lobe.
2. Outcome met. Oriented to time, place, and person at 8 A.M.
3. Outcome met. pO_2 60 mmHg after 1 hour on oxygen at 3 L/min.
4. Outcome not met. pCO_2 remains elevated at 80 mmHg.

Key Index Words for Nursing Interventions

Look up these words in the index of fundamentals and medical-surgical nursing textbooks to find page references for additional nursing interventions and rationale for their selection:

- atelectasis
- blood gases, arterial
- breath sounds
- chest physiotherapy
- chronic obstructive pulmonary disease
- cystic fibrosis
- gas exchange, impaired
- hypoxemia
- hypoxia
- oxygen: administration of, saturation of (SaO_2), therapy
- partial pressure: carbon dioxide (pCO_2), oxygen (pO_2)
- pneumonia
- pneumothorax
- postural drainage
- pulmonary: edema, emboli, perfusion
- respiratory acidosis
- ventilation–perfusion imbalance
- ventilators, care of client

Case Management Example:
See Appendix for examples of a nursing diagnosis of Impaired Gas Exchange within clinical pathways for DRG 089, Pneumonia, page 460, and DRG 127, Congestive Heart Failure (CHF), page 466.

INABILITY TO SUSTAIN SPONTANEOUS VENTILATIONS

Definition
A state in which the response pattern of decreased energy reserves results in an individual's inability to maintain breathing adequate to support life.

Major Defining Characteristics
- dyspnea (labored, difficult breathing)
- increased metabolic rate

Minor Defining Characteristics
- increased restlessness, apprehension; decreased cooperation
- increased use of accessory muscles
- decreased tidal volume
- increased heart rate
- decreased pO_2; increased pCO_2; decreased SaO_2 (saturation)

Related Factors
- metabolic factors
- respiratory muscle fatigue

Examples of Specific Nursing Diagnoses
1. Inability to sustain spontaneous ventilations related to fatigue of respiratory muscles, increased metabolic needs secondary to sepsis (infection) and prematurity.

   Inability to sustain spontaneous ventilations related to fatigue of respiratory muscles, increased metabolic needs secondary to sepsis (infection) and prematurity as evidenced by T 101°F (38.3°C), P 188, R 86, retractions, nasal flaring, O_2 saturation of 88%, pCO_2 60 mmHg, pH 7.15. (PES format)

2. Inability to sustain spontaneous ventilations related to pneumonia, poor nutritional status, and chronic obstructive pulmonary disease (COPD).

   Inability to sustain spontaneous ventilations related to pneumonia, poor nutritional status, and COPD as evidenced by dyspnea, 38 breaths per minute, apprehension, pH 7.21, pO_2 48 mmHg on 60% oxygen. (PES format)

Examples of Specific Outcomes
1. Client maintains normal blood gases on 40% oxygen or less without use of ventilator and is gaining 0.25 oz/day in 14 days.
2. Client returns to baseline blood gas values and vital signs on spontaneous ventilations after 3 days on antibiotic therapy.
3. Client shows absence of dyspnea during spontaneous ventilations, clear breath sounds, and afebrile in 72 hours.

Examples of Specific Nursing Interventions
- See General Respiratory/Breathing Nursing Interventions, page 179.
- While on ventilator implement interventions to meet client's basic needs for hygiene, hydration, nutrition, mobility, pain relief, temperature maintenance, rest, and sleep.
- Initiate preventive interventions for complications caused by immobility until client ambulatory (see High Risk for Disuse Syndrome, page 106).

- Assess central venous pressure, pulmonary capillary wedge pressure, VS and urine output to evaluate adequacy of vascular blood volume and cardiac output.
- Assess client's psychosocial status and plan interventions to:

  promote communication while intubated.

  provide support, stay close to client to reduce fear/anxiety.

  increase client's knowledge and cooperation with all treatments, mechanical ventilation, and the weaning process.

  restore a sense of control by encouraging client participation in care and decision-making.

  encourage family and support people to touch, talk with, hold client and stay within visual field.
- Suction to remove increased secretions which occur with intubation and mechanical ventilation; develop and document suctioning protocol with physician and respiratory therapy to maximize clear airway and maintain client's oxygenation (e.g., hyperoxygenate and hyperventilate before and after suctioning).
- Assess equipment functioning; maintain ventilator at ordered settings; prevent pulling or twisting on endotracheal tube by ventilator tubing; monitor tracheostomy cuff pressure under 25 cm to prevent injury to trachea; remove water that accumulates in tubing; keep water levels adequate for humidifying oxygen.
- Have equipment available to manually ventilate if equipment malfunctions, client fights ventilator.
- Assess for development of complications related to mechanical ventilation: decreased venous return to heart, alveolar rupture, pneumothorax, pulmonary infection, fighting the ventilator.
- Provide oral hygiene every 8 hours and prn.
- Provide tracheostomy care at least every 8 hours and prn.
- Use good aseptic technique to prevent nosocomial infection.

Examples of Specific Evaluations for Outcomes 1 to 3
1. Outcome partially met. Newborn maintains blood gases in normal range on 36% oxygen with spontaneous

respirations of 60–76 per minute; some retractions and nasal flaring; no weight gain since weaned from ventilator.

2. Outcome met. Spontaneous ventilations for 8 hours; blood gases × 3 at acceptable levels; vital signs within client's normal range.
3. Outcome not met. Client remains febrile with crackles and wheezes in lower lobes of lung after 72 hours; continues on ventilator and IV antibiotic therapy.

Key Index Words for Nursing Interventions
Look up these words in the index of fundamentals and medical-surgical nursing textbooks to find page references for additional nursing interventions and rationale for their selection:

- mechanical ventilation: care of client, setting on, types of
- suctioning: use of hyperoxygenation, hyperinflation
- tracheostomy, care of
- ventilations, inability to sustain spontaneous
- ventilators
- ventilatory weaning

DYSFUNCTIONAL VENTILATORY WEANING RESPONSE (DVWR)

Definition
A state in which an individual cannot adjust to lowered levels of mechanical ventilator support, which interrupts and prolongs the weaning process.

Major Defining Characteristics
Responds to lowered levels of ventilator support with:

Mild DVWR
- respiratory rate slightly increased from baseline
- restlessness

Moderate DVWR
- respiratory rate increased by less than 5 breaths per minute
- heart rate increased by less than 20 beats per minute
- BP increased by less than 20 mmHg

Severe DVWR
- respiratory rate increased by 5 breaths per minute or more
- heart rate increased by 20 beats per minute or more
- BP increased by 20 mmHg or more
- deterioration in arterial blood gases from current baseline
- agitated

Minor Defining Characteristics
Responds to lowered levels of ventilator support with:

Mild DVWR
    expressed feelings of increased need for oxygen
    breathing discomfort
    fatigue
    warmth
    questioning possible machine malfunction
    increased concentration on breathing

Moderate DVWR
    hypervigilance to activities
    inability to respond to coaching
    inability to cooperate
    apprehension
    diaphoresis
    "wide-eyed look"
    decreased air entry on auscultation
    color becomes more pale, slightly cyanotic
    slight respiratory accessory muscle use

Severe DVWR
    profuse diaphoresis (sweating)
    full respiratory accessory muscle use
    shallow, gasping breaths
    paradoxical abdominal breathing
    discoordinated breathing with the ventilator
    decreased level of consciousness
    adventitious breath sounds
    audible airway secretions
    cyanosis

Related Factors
- physical: ineffective airway clearance; sleep pattern disturbance; inadequate nutrition; uncontrolled pain or discomfort

- psychological: knowledge deficit of the weaning process and client role; client perceived inability to wean; decreased motivation; decreased self-esteem; moderate/severe anxiety; fear; hopelessness; powerlessness; insufficient trust in nurse
- situational: uncontrolled episodic energy demands or problems; inappropriate pacing of diminished ventilator support; inadequate social support; adverse environment (e.g., noisy, active, negative events in room, low nurse-client ratio, extended nurse absence from bedside, unfamiliar nursing staff); history of ventilator dependence greater than 1 week; history of multiple unsuccessful weaning attempts

Examples of Specific Nursing Diagnoses

1. Severe DVWR related to 2 weeks on ventilator, severe anxiety about ability to breathe independently, inability to wean 3 days ago, lack of support/family.
   Severe DVWR related to 2 weeks on ventilator, severe anxiety about ability to breathe independently, inability to wean 3 days ago, lack of support/family as evidenced by physical agitation, P 110, R 46, BP 168/98 mmHg, pO_2 decreased to 52 mmHg from 80 mmHg; retractions and shallow gasping breaths. (PES format)
2. Mild DVWR related to anxiety from first experience with ventilators and weaning process, minimal knowledge, fatigue from inadequate sleep.
   Mild DVWR related to anxiety from first experience with ventilators and weaning process, minimal knowledge, fatigue from inadequate sleep as evidenced by slight restlessness and elevation of respirations from 16–20 to 18–25 breaths per minute; stating need for more air; attention focused on breathing. (PES format)

Examples of Specific Outcomes

1. Client is weaned from ventilator with no signs of respiratory distress within 5 days.
2. Client demonstrates no problems or only mild DVWR during next reduction in ventilatory weaning this morning.
3. Client's vital signs and blood gases remain within baseline values following planned termination of ventilatory support, by Friday.

Examples of Specific Nursing Interventions

- See General Respiratory/Breathing Nursing Interventions, page 179, and Specific Nursing Interventions for Inability to Sustain Spontaneous Ventilations, page 190.
- Develop weaning plan in collaboration with physicians, respiratory therapists, client, family and primary nurse.
- Maximize client's ability to wean from ventilator by eliminating related factors causing problems; time weaning process when client with trusted nurse, family available, client is rested and pain controlled, environment relaxed, secretions reduced, minimal energy demands anticipated, and when client feels ready (within a chosen time period).
- Wean from ventilator in small steps; assess client's physical and psychological response at each level; continue weaning, maintain current level of ventilator support or return to previous level based on overall client response.
- Stay with client, in visual field, breathe with client, demonstrate and encourage effective breathing pattern as weaning initiated.
- Assess for signs of inadequate oxygenation, ineffective breathing patterns, fear, and anxiety and intervene to correct or reduce when possible.
- Assess client, family, and home setting for possible home ventilator care if long-term mechanical ventilation is required.
- Teach home ventilator care for ventilator-dependent clients: client care, ventilator care and maintenance.

Examples of Specific Evaluations for Outcomes 1 to 3

1. Outcome not met. Client continues to show signs of mild to moderate DVWR with attempts to discontinue remaining ventilator support after 5 days.
2. Outcome met. Client's vital signs and breathing efforts were within normal limits following 8 A.M. reduction in ventilator support.
3. Outcome partially met. Prior to transfer out of ICU, client's blood gases were within normal baseline values 3 hours after termination of ventilator support but pulse and respirations were slightly increased; BP remained in normal range.

Key Index Words for Nursing Interventions
Look up these words in the index of fundamentals and medical-surgical nursing textbooks to find page references for additional nursing interventions and rationale for their selection:

- mechanical ventilation: care of client, setting on, types of
- suctioning: use of hyperoxygenation, hyperinflation

- tracheostomy, care of
- ventilators
- ventilatory weaning

INEFFECTIVE AIRWAY CLEARANCE

Definition
A state in which an individual is unable to clear secretions or obstructions from the respiratory tract to maintain airway patency.

Defining Characteristics
- abnormal breath sounds (rales/crackles or rhonchi/wheezes)
- changes in rate or depth of respirations; tachypnea (fast rate)
- cough which is effective or ineffective with or without sputum
- cyanosis
- dyspnea (difficult, labored breathing)

Related Factors
- decreased energy/fatigue
- tracheobronchial infection, obstruction, secretions
- perceptual/cognitive impairment
- trauma
- ineffective or suppressed cough reflex (e.g., intentional suppression to prevent pain; anesthesia; sedation)

Examples of Specific Nursing Diagnoses
1. Ineffective airway clearance related to weakness and decreased level of consciousness after surgery.
   Ineffective airway clearance related to weakness and

decreased level of consciousness after surgery as evidenced by ineffective cough, gurgling sound in trachea, dusky color, labored respirations 34 per minute, pulse 110. (PES format)
2. Ineffective airway clearance related to increased secretions and weakness secondary to pneumonia.
   Ineffective airway clearance related to pneumonia as evidenced by respiratory rate of 36 per minute, increased secretions, dyspnea and rales (crackles) in all lobes of lungs. (PES format)

Examples of Specific Outcomes
1. Client's breath sounds become increasingly clear during next 24 hours.
2. Client shows absence of gurgling sound in trachea and improved color within the next 30 minutes.
3. Client's respirations are 20 per minute or less with no dyspnea at rest after 24 hours on antibiotic therapy.
4. Client produces clear breath sounds in 48 hours.

Examples of Specific Nursing Interventions
■ See General Respiratory/Breathing Nursing Interventions, page 179.
■ Prevent, reduce, or eliminate physical obstructions to airway:

   Secretions: administer medications to reduce secretions and/or treat underlying condition (e.g., antibiotics); encourage coughing several times every hour until lungs clear.

   Oral structures: position with head elevated and with neck neither overflexed nor overextended; assess positioning of tongue for possible obstruction of airway.

   Food, objects: assess level of consciousness before feeding; hold feeding if choke, gag, swallowing reflexes impaired or if tachypnea present; position in high Fowler's if possible; encourage to eat slowly, chewing thoroughly; objects that could fit in mouth and become lodged in throat should be moved out of reach of children and clients who are confused or have decreased level of consciousness or cognition.

Edema/inflammation: provide humidified air or oxygen; elevate head; monitor for wheezing or stridor on inspiration; prevent trauma to tissues from airway, tubes, suctioning; prevent exposure to irritants, allergens.

Maintain correct placement of oral/tracheal airway.

- Maximize client's ability to clear own airway by effective pain management, chest physiotherapy, encouraging rest, promoting good nutrition and hydration.
- Assist in clearing airway by suctioning when needed rather than on set schedule (assess lung sounds, viscosity of secretions, and effectiveness of cough to help decide on need for suctioning); postural drainage; percussion and vibration.
- Teach Heimlich maneuver to new parents and to clients and family if risk of airway obstruction from food, objects is present.

Examples of Specific Evaluations for Outcomes 1 to 4

1. Outcome met. Lungs clearing at all assessments during last 24 hours following surgery; no crackles or wheezes now present.
2. Outcome partially met. No gurgling, clear breath sounds but color remains dusky.
3. Outcome not met. Continues to have tachypnea with rates between 35–48 per minute and dyspnea after 24 hours on antibiotics.
4. Outcome partially met. Upper lobes have cleared; fine crackles remain in left and right lower lobes.

Key Index Words for Nursing Interventions

Look up these words in the index of fundamentals and medical-surgical nursing textbooks to find page references for additional nursing interventions and rationale for their selection:

- airway: clearance, patency
- aspiration
- chest physiotherapy
- Heimlich maneuver
- postural drainage
- suctioning: bronchial, nasal, oral, tracheal
- vibration and percussion

INEFFECTIVE BREATHING PATTERN

Definition
A state in which an individual's inhalation and/or exhalation pattern does not enable adequate pulmonary inflation or emptying.

Defining Characteristics
- dyspnea (difficult, labored breathing); shortness of breath
- tachypnea (rapid rate)
- fremitus (vibration felt with palpation over chest in area of secretions)
- abnormal arterial blood gases
- cyanosis
- cough
- nasal flaring
- respiratory depth changes; shallow breathing; hyperventilation
- assumption of three-point position (sitting forward with hands on knees, bed, chair to elevate shoulders)
- pursed-lip breathing/prolonged expiratory phase
- increased anterior-posterior chest diameter
- use of accessory muscles to breathe
- altered chest excursion (e.g., reduced or asymmetrical chest movement)

Related Factors
- pain
- neuromuscular impairment (e.g., anesthesia, analgesia; brain or spinal cord injury, muscular dystrophy, poliomyelitis)
- musculoskeletal impairment (e.g., chest trauma, surgery)
- perceptual/cognitive impairment (e.g., drug overdose)
- impairment of airflow into and out of lungs (e.g., COPD such as chronic bronchitis, emphysema, asthma; pneumothorax; TB)
- anxiety
- decreased energy/fatigue

Examples of Specific Nursing Diagnoses
1. Ineffective breathing pattern related to postoperative pain.

Ineffective breathing pattern related to postoperative pain as evidenced by shallow respirations of 28 per minute, reduced breath sounds in lower lobes. (PES format)

2. Ineffective breathing pattern (hyperventilation) related to anxiety.

Ineffective breathing pattern related to anxiety as evidenced by very deep, rapid respirations of 40 per minute, feeling short of breath, tingling in fingers, dizziness. (PES format)

Examples of Specific Outcomes

1. Client respirations restored to normal rate and depth within 1 hour of analgesic administration.
2. Client's respirations are 30 per minute, normal depth within the next 20 minutes.
3. Client's blood gases within normal limits in 4 hours.
4. Client demonstrates pursed-lip, diaphragmatic breathing by discharge.

Examples of Specific Nursing Interventions

■ See General Respiratory/Breathing Nursing Interventions, page 179.
■ Assess for underlying physical or emotional factors contributing to client's ineffective breathing pattern and try to reduce or eliminate them.
■ Teach client/family breathing techniques to improve airflow.

Describe ineffective breathing pattern to client and family.

Explain why observed pattern is less effective.

Describe and demonstrate alternative breathing pattern (e.g., pursed-lip breathing, diaphragmatic breathing for COPD; sustained maximal inspirations for hyperventilation from anxiety).

Practice with positive reinforcement while at rest and during activity to prevent or reduce dyspnea.

■ Suggest and demonstrate relaxation techniques.

Examples of Specific Evaluations for Outcomes 1 to 4

1. Outcome met. After pain relief, client cooperated with deep breathing, coughing, position change; rate down to 20 per minute.

2. Outcome not met. Client remains very anxious and is unable to relax and slow breathing; continues to hyperventilate.
3. Outcome partially met. Blood gases returning to normal values but pH still slightly acidotic and pCO_2 elevated.
4. Outcome met. Client using pursed-lip and diaphragmatic breathing to reduce dyspnea by discharge.

Key Index Words for Nursing Interventions
Look up these words in the index of fundamentals and medical-surgical nursing textbooks to find page references for additional nursing interventions and rationale for their selection:

- apnea
- bradypnea
- breathing patterns, ineffective
- Cheyne-Stokes respirations
- dyspnea
- fremitus
- hyperpnea
- hyperventilation
- hypoventilation
- Kussmaul respirations
- oxygen administration
- tachypnea

Chapter 10

Rest/Sleep Problems

FOCUSED ASSESSMENT GUIDE

Complete this focused assessment if a general nursing assessment indicates a possible problem. Then turn to page 204 of this text for the Data ⇒ Diagnosis Matching Guide for rest/sleep problems to help you select the best nursing diagnosis to match a client's data.

ASK CLIENT

___ When did this sleep (or fatigue) problem begin? Tell me about it.
___ What do you think is causing or contributing to it?
___ What have you done about it?
___ What was your normal sleep pattern and energy level like before this?

TELL ME IF YOU ARE HAVING ANY OF THESE FEELINGS OR PROBLEMS

___ always feeling exhausted; not feeling well rested
___ having trouble getting through the day or maintaining routines
___ more physical discomfort or problems than usual
___ feeling irritable or very emotional
___ difficulty concentrating/performing activities; absent-minded
___ loss of interest in doing anything
___ becoming accident prone; falling
___ difficulty falling asleep
___ awakening earlier or later than desired
___ interrupted sleep

OBSERVE FOR

- actual sleep pattern (if sleeping at health care facility)
- nystagmus (rapid rhythmic movement of the eye), hand tremor, or ptosis (drooping of eyelid), expressionless face, dark circles under the eyes, frequent yawning, changes in posture
- thick speech with mispronunciation and incorrect words

NORMALS AND INFORMATION

- Sleep is unconsciousness from which the person can be aroused by sensory stimuli such as sound, light, touch, shaking
- Sleep has two stages: nonrapid eye movement (NREM) sleep with slow brain waves and REM (rapid eye movement) sleep when the brain is very active; the reason for two stages is not known
- The sleep center is located in the pons and medulla of the brain
- Most sleep at night is NREM sleep; it occurs when a person first falls asleep; it is deep restful sleep
- During NREM sleep:
  pulse and respirations drop by about 20–30%; BP decreases
  muscles relax, and skin vessels dilate (increasing heat loss)
  metabolic rate decreases by 10–30%, reducing caloric need
  body temperature decreases (decreased heat production)
- Episodes of REM sleep occur about every 90 minutes and last 5–30 minutes; REM sleep begins after about 90 minutes of sleep; it is associated with dreaming that is remembered
- During REM sleep:
  heart rate and respirations often become irregular
  metabolism increases and this increases temperature
- Need for sleep decreases with age: 14–18 hours/day as a newborn, 10 hours/day in school-age children, 7–9 hours/day as an adult, 6 hours/day in the elderly
- Sleep needs increase during illness

- Lack of sleep results in progressive deterioration in mental functioning, increased physical discomfort, feeling withdrawn
- Drugs and medications may interfere with sleep, often decreasing REM sleep (e.g., alcohol, amphetamines, sedatives, tranquilizers)

DATA ⇒ DIAGNOSIS MATCHING GUIDE

Compare your client data from the Rest/Sleep Focused Assessment to these related rest and sleep nursing diagnoses and abbreviated descriptions. Select the nursing diagnosis with the best match. Then turn to the page in this section with that specific diagnosis for help in planning care.

1. *Fatigue: page 205*
   - definition: overwhelming sustained sense of exhaustion and decreased capacity for physical and mental work
   - data: report of continual and overwhelming lack of energy; inability to maintain usual routines

2. *Sleep Pattern Disturbance: page 208*
   - definition: disruption of sleep time causing discomfort or interfering with desired lifestyle
   - data: verbal complaints of difficulty falling asleep, not feeling well rested; awakening earlier or later than desired; interrupted sleep

GENERAL OUTCOMES AND NURSING INTERVENTIONS
GENERAL REST/SLEEP OUTCOMES

- Client reports feeling well rested and having adequate energy.
- Client reestablishes normal sleeping pattern.
- Client meets sleep needs based on age and health status.

GENERAL REST/SLEEP NURSING INTERVENTIONS

- Identify and eliminate or reduce the related factors causing excess fatigue and/or altered sleep.

- Assess for medications/drugs that may be affecting sleep (e.g., drugs that decrease REM sleep, stimulants, poorly timed diuretics causing frequent voidings at night).
- Consolidate care, treatments, diagnostics to provide client with uninterrupted blocks of time for rest/sleep.
- Conserve the client's energy whenever possible.
- Provide rest before and after activities, treatments, diagnostic tests.
- Encourage client's usual bedtime routines that promote sleep.
- Manage the environment to promote sleep; sound, light, temperature adjusted for client comfort.
- Encourage good nutrition; bedtime snack of milk, protein foods.
- Encourage daily activity and exercise appropriate to health status.

RELATED NURSING DIAGNOSES

FATIGUE

Definition
An overwhelming sustained sense of exhaustion and decreased capacity for physical and mental work.

Major Defining Characteristics
- verbalization of an unremitting and overwhelming lack of energy
- inability to maintain usual routines

Minor Defining Characteristics
- perceived need for additional energy to accomplish routine tasks
- increase in physical complaints
- emotionally labile (unstable) or irritable
- impaired ability to concentrate
- decreased performance
- lethargy or listlessness
- disinterest in surroundings
- introspection (focus on own thoughts and feelings)
- decreased libido (decreased interest in sex)
- accident-prone

Related Factors
- decreased or increased metabolic energy production (e.g., pregnancy, periods of rapid growth in children, injury, fever, thyroid disease)
- overwhelming psychological or emotional demands
- increased energy requirements to perform activity of daily living (e.g., breast-feeding, pregnancy, using crutches, walking with a cast)
- excessive social and/or role demands (e.g., primary caregiver for ill family member, caring for child with disability, or chronic illness)
- states of discomfort (e.g., pain, cold, heat, hunger)
- altered body chemistry (e.g., medications, drug withdrawal, chemotherapy, radiation, renal or liver disease)

Other Related Factors
- sleep disorders; sleep disruptions; inadequate sleep
- acute and chronic illness (e.g., cancer, AIDS, rheumatoid arthritis, systemic lupus, multiple sclerosis, anemia)
- inadequate nutrition
- depression

Examples of Specific Nursing Diagnoses
1. Fatigue related to interrupted sleep at night, caring for new baby, breast-feeding.
   Fatigue related to interrupted sleep at night, caring for new baby, breast-feeding as evidenced by report of extreme exhaustion; unable to do anything but feed and care for baby. (PES format)
2. Fatigue related to poor nutrition, decreased exercise, reduced sleep time, and anxiety during final exam week at college.
   Fatigue related to poor nutrition, decreased exercise, reduced sleep time, and anxiety during final exam week at college as evidenced by report of total exhaustion after last final, feeling too tired to eat or fix appearance. (PES format)

Examples of Specific Outcomes
1. Client reports minimal fatigue level by 6-week postpartum checkup.

2. Client reports return of normal energy level 24 hours after last final.
3. Client reports ability to perform priority activities, roles without excessive fatigue by end of the week.
4. Client identifies ways to conserve energy and maximize ability to perform important activities by discharge.

Examples of Specific Nursing Interventions

- See General Rest/Sleep Nursing Interventions, page 204.
- Assess client and family understanding of health condition and treatments contributing to fatigue (when known) and provide information as needed.
- Assure clients that fatigue is experienced by many people with similar health problems and treatment; fatigue is real not just imagined or a sign of laziness.
- Explain to client/family that fighting fatigue and over-exertion may worsen health condition and cause physical damage.
- Help client to balance increased rest/sleep needs with important activities and family responsibilities.

    Assess daily activities, jobs, schedule; help client/family set priorities for where client should spend time and energy.

    Limit or eliminate low priority activities to conserve energy.

    Identify some tasks to go undone or be done less frequently.

    Organize priority activities to provide blocks of time for rest/sleep; explore ways to perform priority activities in more energy-efficient ways.

    Schedule daily rest/sleep periods.

    Encourage rest/sleep time before and after activities.

    Identify how others can help; encourage client to let others help (accepting help is often difficult and should be supported as crucial to client's health and ability to participate in priority activities).

    Explore option of hiring help for some tasks.

- Provide emotional support to minimize feelings of guilt and disappointment in self associated with inability to do all the things client wants to do and that others expect client to do.

Examples of Specific Evaluations for Outcomes 1 to 4

1. Outcome not met. Mother reporting continuing fatigue, exhaustion at 6-week postpartum checkup.
2. Outcome met. Student reports feeling full of energy after 14 hours of sleep and a large breakfast.
3. Outcome partially met. Reports energy level was good most of week and was able to participate in chosen activities; marital problems at the end of week left client exhausted, "too tired to talk".
4. Outcome partially met. Client identified ways to conserve energy and promote activity without causing exhaustion but is unaccepting of limits on activities and need for rest periods.

Key Index Words for Nursing Interventions

Look up these words in the index of fundamentals and medical-surgical nursing textbooks to find page references for additional nursing interventions and rationale for their selection:

- fatigue
- rest
- sleep

SLEEP PATTERN DISTURBANCE

Definition

Disruption of sleep time causes discomfort or interferes with desired lifestyle.

Critical Defining Characteristics

- verbal complaints of difficulty falling asleep
- not feeling well rested
- awakening earlier or later than desired
- interrupted sleep

Defining Characteristics

- changes in behavior and performance (increasing irritability, restlessness, disorientation, lethargy, listlessness)
- physical signs: mild fleeting nystagmus (involuntary rapid rhythmic movement of the eyeball), slight hand tremor, ptosis (drooping) of eyelid, expressionless face, dark circles under the eyes, frequent yawning, changes in posture
- thick speech with mispronunciation and incorrect words

Related Factors

- internal sensory alterations (illness, psychological stress): pain, needing to get up to the bathroom several times at night, snoring, sleep apnea (periods of no breathing between periods of snoring), night sweats, anorexia nervosa, alcoholism
- external sensory alterations (environmental changes, social cues): working different shift, crying baby, new sounds such as occur in the hospital, sleeping without usual partner

Examples of Specific Nursing Diagnoses

1. Sleep pattern disturbance related to knee replacement surgery, pain, immobility in continuous passive motion (CPM) machine, effects of anesthesia/analgesia, unfamiliar surroundings and nursing assessments every 2 hours during 11 P.M. to 7 A.M. shift.

   Sleep pattern disturbance related to knee replacement surgery, pain, immobility in CPM machine, effects of anesthesia and analgesia, unfamiliar surroundings and nursing assessments every 2 hours as evidenced by complaints of inability to fall asleep, interrupted sleep, feeling exhausted. (PES format)

2. Sleep pattern disturbance related to breast-feeding newborn every 2–4 hours during the night.

   Sleep pattern disturbance related to breast-feeding newborn every 2–4 hours during the night as evidenced by reports of interrupted sleep two or more times a night, feeling poorly rested all day. (PES format)

Examples of Specific Outcomes

1. Client returns to previous sleep pattern 3 weeks after joint replacement surgery.
2. Mother establishes a new sleep pattern by 6-week checkup to meet her sleep needs during next several months while night-feeding baby.
3. Client sleeps 6 hours or more during night by end of 2 weeks.
4. Client experiences five hours of uninterrupted sleep during 11 P.M. to 7 A.M. shift tonight.

Examples of Specific Nursing Interventions

■ See General Rest/Sleep Nursing Interventions, page 204.

■ Reduce or eliminate related factors causing sleep disturbance (e.g., administer analgesic before bedtime if in pain; reschedule diuretics to prevent increased urine output during sleep; offer to discuss concerns or worries with client; refer to social service for financial concerns).

■ Identify previous sleep routines when client was sleeping well and replicate as much as possible (e.g., toileting, hygiene, snacks, music, positioning, bedtime).

■ Alter environment to promote sleep.
>   Close door to block sound, light; turn on night-light
>   Use "Do not disturb" or "Check at nurses station" signs to provide periods of uninterrupted rest/sleep.
>   Adjust temperature to client's comfort level; provide adequate blankets.
>   For intermittent environmental noise, suggest a radio or tape for background sound.
>   Decrease or eliminate naps during the day.
>   Reduce coffee, caffeine, alcohol intake; eliminate them after supper; eliminate or reduce cigarette smoking.
>   Offer a cot/bed for family member to sleep in room.
>   Encourage use of favorite pillow, stuffed animal from home.
>   Provide clean dry bedding; straighten/retuck corners as needed.
>   Assist with good body alignment; position with pillows for support.
>   Private room, or roommate that will not interfere with sleep.

■ Suggest new activities to promote sleep.
>   Simple relaxation techniques
>   Backrub before bedtime
>   Milk or protein snack before bed
>   Quiet time before going to bed rather than having visitors, e.g., reading, watching TV
>   Use of fairly consistent bedtime and wake-up time

Examples of Specific Evaluations for Outcomes 1 to 4

1. Outcome met. Client reports no problem sleeping at night and feels well rested during follow-up nursing evaluation.

2. Outcome not met. Mother increasingly exhausted; reports almost no blocks of sleep during last 24 hours; feeding baby every 1–2 hours around-the-clock; baby crying frequently.
3. Outcome partially met. Client observed sleeping at least 6 hours/night but is reporting interrupted sleep, feeling tired.
4. Outcome met. Client observed sleeping 6 hours without interruptions following administration of pain medication, discontinuation of IV, and use of special neck pillow brought from home.

Key Index Words for Nursing Interventions
Look up these words in the index of fundamentals and medical-surgical nursing textbooks to find page references for additional nursing interventions and rationale for their selection:

- Circadian rhythm
- hypersomnia
- insomnia
- narcolepsy
- sleep: NREM, REM
- sleep apnea
- sleep deprivation
- sleep pattern disturbance
- sleep-wake patterns
- somnambulism

Chapter 11

Self-Care Problems

FOCUSED ASSESSMENT GUIDE: BATHING/HYGIENE/GROOMING/DRESSING/ FEEDING/TOILETING

Complete this focused assessment if the general assessment indicates a possible problem. Then turn to page 214 of this text for the Data ⇒ Diagnosis Matching Guide for self-care problems to help you select the best nursing diagnosis to match a client's data.

TELL ME WHAT KIND OF HELP YOU NEED WITH THE FOLLOWING ACTIVITIES

___ eating (e.g., opening containers, cutting meat, using regular or specialized silverware, extra time, getting dentures in)

___ drinking (e.g., use of straws or special cups)

___ bathing, showering, taking a tub bath, getting set up, brushing your teeth)

___ getting dressed or undressed, fastening buttons, getting shoes on, getting clothes out of suitcase (drawers or closet)

___ fixing hair, shaving

___ toileting (e.g., getting to the bathroom, getting on and off the toilet or commode, using bedpan or urinal)

OBSERVE FOR PROBLEMS WITH

___ cleanliness

___ grooming (nails cut, hair combed, shaved)
___ teeth or dentures brushed or cleaned; odor-free
___ dressing (getting clothes on and off, appropriate for environmental temperature; changing to clean clothes as needed)
___ feeding self (time taken to eat; fatigue, frustration occurring, ability to eat most of foods/fluids offered; chewing problems)
___ toileting (mobility or hygiene help needed; any dizziness)

NORMALS AND INFORMATION: BATHING/HYGIENE/GROOMING/DRESSING/FEEDING/TOILETING

- Loss of independence in self-care activities can result in feelings of embarrassment, loss of control, anger, depression, hopelessness, powerlessness, and loss of self-esteem
- Clients embarrassed or disgusted with themselves over loss of self-care ability may refuse to try to relearn these skills; they may become overly dependent on others rather than admit inability or perform self-care in a clumsy or inadequate way
- Clients may state they are not hungry or refuse to bathe and groom themselves if accepting help is difficult or unacceptable to their self-image
- Clients may need some time to grieve the loss of prior abilities and remain dependent on others before they are ready to relearn basic self-care skills and move toward independence
- Family members can retard or block client progress toward independent functioning by overprotective behavior
- Loss of self-care ability creates anxiety in clients who now must be partially or totally dependent on others for these basic, personal needs
- Caretakers, including health care professionals, will require patience, creativity, energy, and empathy to work with clients toward maximum independence; they will need time out to take care of themselves when they care for others on a continuing basis

DATA ⇒ DIAGNOSIS MATCHING GUIDE: BATHING/HYGIENE/GROOMING/DRESSING/ FEEDING/TOILETING

Compare your client data from the Self-Care Focused Assessment to these related nursing diagnoses and abbreviated descriptions. Select the nursing diagnosis with the best match. Then turn to the page in this section with that specific diagnosis for help in planning care.

SUGGESTED FUNCTIONAL LEVEL CLASSIFICATION

0 = Completely independent (no problem exists)

1 = Requires use of equipment or devices

2 = Requires help from another person, for assistance, supervision, or teaching

3 = Requires help from another person and equipment device

4 = Dependent, does not participate in activity

1. *Feeding Self-Care Deficit: page 222*
   - definition: an impaired ability to perform or complete feeding activities for oneself
   - data: inability to bring food from a receptacle to the mouth

2. *Bathing/Hygiene Self-Care Deficit: page 217*
   - definition: an impaired ability to perform or complete bathing and/or hygiene activities for oneself
   - data: inability to wash body parts; inability to obtain or get to water source; inability to regulate temperature or flow

3. *Dressing/Grooming Self-Care Deficit: page 220*
   - definition: an impaired ability to perform or complete dressing and grooming activities for oneself
   - data: impaired ability to put on or take off necessary items of clothing: impaired ability to obtain or replace articles of clothing; impaired ability to fasten clothing; inability to maintain appearance at a satisfactory level

4. *Toileting Self-Care Deficit: page 225*
   - definition: an impaired ability to perform or complete toileting activities for oneself
   - data: unable to get to toilet or commode; unable to sit on or rise from toilet or commode; unable to manipulate clothing for toileting; unable to carry out proper toilet hygiene

5. *Impaired Home Maintenance Management: page 395*
   - definition: inability to independently maintain a safe growth-promoting immediate environment (see Health Management Problems)

6. *Altered Health Maintenance: page 390*
   - definition: inability to identify, manage, and/or seek out help to maintain health (see Health Management Problems)

GENERAL OUTCOMES AND NURSING INTERVENTIONS: BATHING/HYGIENE/ GROOMING/DRESSING/FEEDING/TOILETING

GENERAL SELF-CARE OUTCOMES

- Client will perform self-care activities independently.
- Client will perform self-care activities at maximum level of independence possible.
- Client will participate in self-care activities.
- Client will maintain current level of ability in self-care activities.
- Client will adapt performance of self care activities to increase level of independence.

GENERAL SELF-CARE NURSING INTERVENTIONS

- Reduce or eliminate the related factors causing and/or contributing to the problem whenever possible.
  All self-care deficit diagnoses are related to:
  impaired transfer ability: intervene to promote transfer ability, e.g., install overbed trapeze.
  impaired mobility status: intervene to promote mobility (see General Mobility Nursing Interventions, page

96, and Specific Nursing Interventions for Impaired Physical Mobility, page 111).

intolerance to activity, decreased strength and endurance: intervene to increase activity tolerance, strength, and endurance (see General Mobility Nursing Interventions, page 96, and Specific Nursing Interventions for Activity Intolerance, page 100), e.g., encourage active and passive range of motion exercises, rest, good nutrition, isometric and isotonic exercises.

pain, discomfort: intervene to manage/prevent pain (see General Pain Nursing Interventions, page 131), e.g., give analgesic 1 hour before activities.

perceptual or cognitive impairment: intervene to promote cognitive/perceptual abilities (see General Communication, Thinking, and Knowledge Nursing Interventions, page 297, and Specific Nursing Interventions for Altered Thought Process, page 299, and Sensory/Perceptual Alterations, page 169), e.g., room calenders, use of glasses/hearing aids, repeated orientation to time, place, and person.

neuromuscular and/or musculoskeletal impairment: intervene to promote healing and treat underlying condition based on physician's orders, e.g., promote rest/sleep, good nutrition and hydration, exercise and activity as permitted, respiratory physiotherapy.

depression, severe anxiety: intervene to reduce anxiety, promote more positive outlook (see General Coping/ Adjustment Nursing Interventions, page 311, and Specific Nursing Interventions for Anxiety, page 313).

- Select self-care outcomes with client and family to prevent excessive caretaking and dependence; encourage independence.
- Problem-solve with client/family ways to accomplish self-care activities that enable the client's maximum independence (e.g., replace buttons with Velcro fasteners, pull-up sweats; write out daily grooming activities in a list for client to follow; provide finger foods).
- Set up environment to facilitate self-care (e.g., opening food packages, cutting meat, assisting to best eating position based on client's ability and physician-ordered movement restrictions, adequate lighting, adequate time

so client not rushed; railings in bathroom, raised toilet seat, walker at bedside).

■ Assist client into maximum functioning status (e.g., eyeglasses on, adaptive equipment on or within reach, pain control).

■ Teach self-care skills in ways that promote success.

Divide larger task into smaller simpler activities.

Be creative by suggesting different ways to do self-care skills based on client's current ability level.

Start with skills the client is likely to master fairly rapidly.

Support and praise efforts to relearn self-care skills; review progress over days, weeks, months.

Provide repeated opportunities for client to practice skills.

Develop a clear, detailed teaching plan to be used by all people working with client for consistency in what and how skills are retaught.

■ Provide rest before and after self-care activities and teaching.

■ Place call light/bell within reach and encourage client to use it for any needed help; answer promptly.

■ Encourage client's caretaker to take care of self, take time off and meet some of own needs to prevent fatigue and burnout.

■ Suggest support group for client and/or caretaker.

■ Refer to occupational therapy for adaptive devices to facilitate self-care, overcome physical limitations; social services for financial concerns, community and private resources for adult care, home care, therapy.

RELATED NURSING DIAGNOSES: BATHING/ HYGIENE/GROOMING/DRESSING/FEEDING/ TOILETING

BATHING/HYGIENE SELF-CARE DEFICIT

Definition

A state in which an individual experiences an impaired ability to perform or complete bathing/hygiene activities for oneself.

Critical Defining Characteristics
- inability to wash body parts

Defining Characteristics
- inability to obtain or get to water source
- inability to regulate temperature or flow

Related Factors
See General Self-Care Nursing Interventions, page 215.

Examples of Specific Nursing Diagnoses
1. Bathing/hygiene deficit level 2 related to confusion and disorientation secondary to Alzheimer's disease.
   Bathing/hygiene deficit level related to confusion and disorientation secondary to Alzheimer's disease as evidenced by inability to find or utilize shower, absence of dental hygiene and personal grooming without direct assistance and supervision. (PES format)
2. Bathing/hygiene deficit level 4 related to extreme muscle wasting, weakness, inability to get out of bed, and pain secondary to AIDS.
   Bathing/hygiene deficit level 4 related to extreme muscle wasting, weakness, inability to get out of bed, and pain secondary to AIDS as evidenced by inability to wash self other than face and hands. (PES format)

Examples of Specific Outcomes
1. Client maintains bathing/hygiene self-care level 2 for length of stay in nursing home.
2. Client washes own face and upper body this morning with supervision.
3. Client directs others in providing bathing/hygiene needs for duration of illness to promote sense of control.
4. Client returns to previous independent level of self-care 3 days following back surgery.

Examples of Specific Nursing Interventions
- See General Self-Care Nursing Interventions, page 215.
- Orient client to bathing options available in the health care facility based on current health status and physician-ordered limitations on activity; offer use of adaptive devices as appropriate based on client's strength and mobility.

■ Encourage the client to select the type of bathing and the timing whenever possible (consider other therapies, fatigue level, home routines, availability of preferred family members for help, availability of nursing staff to assist).

■ Assess the client's perception of needed help.

"How can I help you with your morning cleanup and bathing?"

"What kind of help do you need for your shower?"

"I'll wash your back off and rub in some lotion if you like."

Are there other areas you will need help washing?

■ Provide clean gown and towels, bath mat for bath/shower, lotion, soap, clean washbasin or clean tub/shower area.

■ Assemble within easy reach client's personal hygiene supplies such as toothbrush, denture cup, razor, comb/brush, deodorant.

■ Remove elastic stockings (unless contraindicated) and wash as needed; replace with clean pair in 30 minutes to let legs air-dry after bathing.

■ Provide warm clean water refills as needed when client doing bedbath.

■ Provide privacy.

■ Offer to assist with hair washing once a week or as needed.

■ Consider client safety and do not leave unattended in shower/tub if client is at risk (e.g., weak, confused, unsteady on feet).

■ Provide clean bed for client after bathing.

Examples of Specific Evaluations for Outcomes 1 to 4

1. Outcome met. Continues to bathe self with minimal assistance and supervision 1 year after admission.

2. Outcome partially met. Client began to wash face but was unable to complete task and needed assistance.

3. Outcome met. Client identifying what to do and how to do it during morning bathing.

4. Outcome not met. Client extremely anxious about moving and turning; being bathed by spouse; refuses to shower stating, "I did too much too soon with my last back surgery and it never did heal right."

Key Index Words for Nursing Interventions

Look up these words in the index of fundamentals and medical-surgical nursing textbooks to find page references for additional nursing interventions and rationale for their selection:

- bathing
- bedmaking: occupied, unoccupied
- dentures, care of
- foot care
- hygiene
- oral care (hygiene)
- perineal care
- self-care deficit, bathing/hygiene

DRESSING/GROOMING SELF-CARE DEFICIT

Definition

A state in which an individual experiences an impaired ability to perform or complete dressing and grooming activities for oneself.

Critical Defining Characteristics

- impaired ability to put on or take off necessary items of clothing

Defining Characteristics

- impaired ability to obtain or replace articles of clothing
- impaired ability to fasten clothing
- inability to maintain appearance at a satisfactory level

Related Factors

See General Self-Care Nursing Interventions, page 215.

Examples of Specific Diagnoses

1. Dressing self-care deficit level 1 related to bending restrictions secondary to hip replacement surgery.

   Dressing self-care deficit level 1 related to bending restrictions secondary to hip replacement surgery as evidenced by inability to get pants and shoes on without bending hip more than 90 degrees and needing continual reminders not to flex hip too much to prevent hip dislocation during dressing. (PES format)

2. Dressing and grooming self-care deficit level 2 related to depression and excessive sleeping.

   Dressing and grooming self-care deficit level 2 related to

depression and excessive sleeping as evidenced by no spontaneous dressing or grooming; client claims to be too tired to get dressed or fixed up. (PES format)

Examples of Specific Outcomes
1. Client returns to complete independence in dressing 4 months after hip replacement surgery.
2. Client performs own dressing and grooming without flexing hip more than 90 degrees before hospital discharge.
3. Client performs dressing and grooming every morning without supervision by end of 2 weeks.
4. Family to report at next doctor's visit that client is maintaining personal dressing and grooming after discharge.

Examples of Specific Nursing Interventions
■ See General Self-Care Nursing Interventions, page 215.
■ Offer to assist with hair washing at least once a week and as needed.
■ Identify dressing/grooming expectations; discuss with client what type of help will be needed for each activity, e.g., "For physical therapy you will need to have on loose-fitting pants, sweats, or pajama bottoms and shoes and socks. What kind of help do you think you will need?"
■ Arrange grooming equipment within client's reach; show client where electrical outlets are; plug in grooming tools for client if out of reach, unless client's cognitive ability makes this dangerous.
■ Ask for family's help in providing clothing; with familiar items, the client is more likely to dress and undress independently (base on client's current mobility, dexterity, and cognitive abilities), e.g., slip-on shoes and an over-the-head, casual dress for a client who must not bend at the hip more than 90 degrees.
■ If client seems physically able to dress and groom self but refuses or shows no interest in doing these activities, reflect your observations to the client and ask about other concerns, e.g., "You haven't shaved or combed your hair for the last 2 days. I'm worried that something is really getting you down and you're not taking care of yourself."

Examples of Specific Evaluations for Outcomes 1 to 4

1. Outcome met. No longer requires any help with dressing; has changed dressing technique to prevent overflexing hip.
2. Outcome not met. Continues to have trouble adapting dressing habits to prevent overflexing hip beyond 90 degrees.
3. Outcome met. After 13 days on antidepressant therapy, client is dressing and grooming spontaneously.
4. Outcome partially met. Client dressing without encouragement every day since discharge but family reporting interest in personal grooming is not as good as it used to be.

Key Index Words for Nursing Interventions

Look up these words in the index of fundamentals and medical-surgical nursing textbooks to find page references for additional nursing interventions and rationale for their selection:

- dressing, self-care deficit
- grooming, self-care deficit
- hair care
- nail care

FEEDING SELF-CARE DEFICIT

Definition

A state in which an individual experiences an impaired ability to perform or complete feeding activities for oneself.

Defining Characteristics

- inability to bring food from a receptacle to the mouth

Related Factors

See General Self-Care Nursing Interventions, page 215.

Examples of Specific Nursing Diagnoses

1. Feeding self-care deficit level 3 related to spinal cord injury and neuromuscular impairment in hands.
   Feeding self-care deficit level 3 related to spinal cord injury and neuromuscular impairment in hands as evidenced by inability to pick up and hold regular fork, open containers, cut meat, or pick up cup/glass. (PES format)

2. Feeding self-care deficit level 4 related to recent CVA cognitive impairment, and right-sided paralysis involving arm/hand.

   Feeding self-care deficit level 4 related to recent CVA, cognitive impairment, and right-sided paralysis involving arm/hand as evidenced by inability to follow directions to try to feed self and inability to use unaffected left hand to bring food to mouth. (PES format)

Examples of Specific Outcomes

1. Feeds self independently at all meals by end of week with use of adaptive silverware and tray setup.
2. Feeds self one-half of breakfast this morning using adaptive spoon.
3. Feeds self independently within 6 months of CVA.
4. Feeds self one mouthful of food with unaffected left hand during lunch today.

Examples of Specific Nursing Interventions

■ See General Self-Care Nursing Interventions, page 215.
■ Ask for the client's perception of needed eating help
   "How can I help you with this meal?"
   "What can you do yourself and what could you use some help with?"
■ Position for optimal feeding independence.
   In sitting position in bed or chair if possible to promote seeing the food, eating, swallowing and to decrease the risk of choking
   If unable to sit up, turn client on left side (if right-handed) and position tray on left side of bed level with mattress; if one-sided paralysis is present, position on affected side so functioning arm is up; place towel or waterproof pad between path from tray to client for spills.
■ Observe client's feeding activities and feeding help provided by family; make observations and suggestions to the client and family based on what you see, e.g., "You seem to be having some trouble getting the food to your mouth. Can I raise this bedside stand to bring your tray closer to you?"
■ Teach use of adaptive silverware, plates, cups, glasses provided by occupational therapy.

- Offer to reheat foods that become cool (self-feeding may take more time).
- Smaller meals with snacks in between may prevent client from becoming fatigued or discouraged when relearning feeding skills.
- Refer to dietician for foods the client can pick up (finger foods) if manipulating silverware is a problem.
- Explain to blind/visually impaired clients what food is on the tray and where it is located (e.g., baked potato located at 3 o'clock position on the plate, green beans at 9 o'clock).
- If clients become fatigued or discouraged or stop eating before consuming enough food to satisfy nutritional needs, assess for feelings of being too full or too nauseated to continue eating; if so, remove tray. If not nauseated or feeling too full to eat more:

    ask if you may help them to eat a little more.

    explain that they need the calories to maintain their strength and get better.

    praise their efforts at self-feeding.

    reassure them you have the time and this is important.

    ask them what food or drink they would like next.

    encourage clients to direct you as you feed them so they retain some feeling of control.

- Consider risk of choking based on observation of client; have suction equipment available; teach Heimlich maneuver to family before discharge.

Examples of Specific Evaluations for Outcomes 1 to 4

1. Outcome met. Client eating all meals independently with adaptive silverware and tray setup but does require extra time.
2. Outcome not met. Client became discouraged and refused to try after spilling food.
3. Outcome partially met. Client feeds self most of food on tray but becomes fatigued and needs help toward end of meals.
4. Outcome met. Client fed self three pieces of food using left hand at lunch today.

Key Index Words for Nursing Interventions
Look up these words in the index of fundamentals and medical-surgical nursing textbooks to find page references for additional nursing interventions and rationale for their selection:

- adaptive aids: silverware, plates, cups
- eating
- feeding, assisting with
- nutrition, self-care deficit
- silverware, adaptive

TOILETING SELF-CARE DEFICIT

Definition
A state in which an individual experiences an impaired ability to perform or complete toileting activities for oneself.

Critical Defining Characteristics
- unable to get to toilet or commode
- unable to sit on or rise from toilet or commode
- unable to manipulate clothing for toileting
- unable to carry out proper toilet hygiene

Defining Characteristics
- unable to flush toilet or commode

Related Factors
See General Self-Care Nursing Interventions, page 215.

Examples of Specific Nursing Diagnoses
1. Toileting self-care deficit level 2 related to continuous IV, two surgical drains, and pain with movement secondary to abdominal surgery.
   Toileting self-care deficit level 2 related to continuous IV, two surgical drains, and pain with movement secondary to abdominal surgery as evidenced by inability to get to bathroom without help, needing help to push IV stand and carry drains. (PES format)
2. Toileting self-care deficit level 2 related to bed rest restrictions.
   Toileting self-care deficit level 2 related to bed rest restrictions as evidenced by inability to obtain, position, or remove bedpan without help. (PES format)

Examples of Specific Outcomes
1. Client performs independent toileting in bathroom on third day post-op.
2. Client performs independent toileting when physician changes bed rest order to bathroom privileges.
3. Client uses toilet independently this shift, maintaining hip flexion no greater than 90 degrees using raised toilet seat.
4. Client walks to bathroom for voiding once this shift with use of walker.

Examples of Specific Nursing Interventions
- See General Self-Care Nursing Interventions, page 215.
- Assess client and family perception of the kind and amount of toileting help needed.
- Identify with family how client communicates toileting needs if client unable to communicate this information; record in chart.
- Record bowel and bladder patterns over several days; compare to expected normal patterns and client's previous patterns.
- Promote good fluid intake; fruits and vegetables.
- Develop a toileting schedule based on client's bowel/bladder patterns to promote independence.
    help client to void every few hours before bladder too full and urgency may cause incontinence; use urinal/bedpan if inadequate time to get to bathroom.
    provide extra time and privacy (as safety needs allow).
- Provide assistive devices based on assessment of mobility (e.g., walker at bedside, call light within reach in bed or bathroom, elevated toilet seat, handrails in bathroom, commode at bedside, urinal within reach, trapeze over bed, siderails down with bed in low position if safe for client).
- Encourage daily activity and exercise to promote strength and maintain range of motion of joints and mobility.
- Answer call light promptly.

Examples of Specific Evaluations for Outcomes 1 to 4
1. Outcome not met. Using commode; requires help out of

bed; fever for last 24 hours, IV antibiotic infusing; reports feeling very weak.

2. Outcome partially met. Client needs assistance walking to bathroom due to development of partial foot drop after 2 weeks on bed rest.
3. Outcome met. Client observed × 3 using elevated toilet seat without problems or excessive hip flexion.
4. Outcome met. Client voiding in bathroom; using walker correctly.

Key Index Words for Nursing Interventions

Look up these words in the index of fundamentals and medical-surgical nursing textbooks to find page references for additional nursing interventions and rationale for their selection:

- bedpan, types
- commode
- elimination
- incontinence
- toileting, self-care deficit
- urgency
- urinal

Chapter 12

Sex/Sexuality Problems

FOCUSED ASSESSMENT GUIDE

Complete this focused assessment if a general nursing assessment indicates a possible problem. Then turn to page 229 of this text for the Data ⇒ Diagnosis Matching Guide for sex/sexuality problems to help you select the best nursing diagnosis to match the client's data.

"TELL ME IF YOU OR YOUR PARTNER HAVE CONCERNS OR PROBLEMS IN ANY OF THESE AREAS:"

___ controlling your fertility; use of birth control
___ protecting yourself from sexually transmitted diseases
___ loss of interest or desire for sexual activity
___ decreased sexual satisfaction
___ changes in your usual sexual activity because of health problems, fatigue, pain, therapy, or other reasons
___ difficulty doing the things that are part of your role as a partner
___ conflicts about what you believe is right and wrong related to sexual feelings and behavior
___ feeling undesirable or unattractive
___ loss of interest in yourself and others
___ problems in relationships with people you love and care about

Assessment for problems in the area of sex and sexuality are often most appropriate during the recovery phase as part of discharge planning. Example questions to begin discussion are given below.

> "I have talked with you about your diet, medications, and resuming physical activity. Before going home, many people I work with like some information or have some questions about resuming sexual activity."

> "Many people I have worked with get a little anxious or have concerns about resuming sexual activity after a health problem. I am wondering if you or your partner have any concerns or questions in this area you would like to discuss with me or with your doctor."

NORMALS AND INFORMATION

- Clients may be heterosexual, bisexual, homosexual, or transsexual
- Many medications can reduce sexual desire and interfere with sexual functioning
- Alcohol consumption negatively affects erectile function
- Most clients consider sexual issues and concerns an appropriate area for nursing intervention
- Professional nursing organizations (American Nurses Association, Oncology Nursing Society, North American Nursing Diagnosis Association) believe it is part of nursing's role to promote a client's sexual health and functioning
- Many clients would prefer it to be the nurse who initiates discussion of sexual concerns
- The majority of clients are given inadequate opportunity to discuss sexual concerns with a nurse
- The majority of clients receive inadequate information related to the effect of their current health problem, injury and/or treatment on future sexual activity
- Loss of sexual functioning is not part of normal aging

DATA ⇒ DIAGNOSIS MATCHING GUIDE

Compare your client data from the Sex/Sexuality Focused Assessment to these related sex/sexuality nursing diagnoses and abbreviated descriptions. Select the nursing diagnosis with the best match. Then turn to the page in this section with that specific diagnosis for help in planning care.

1. *Altered Sexuality Patterns* (General Diagnosis): *page 232*
   - definition: expressed concern regarding own sexuality
   - data: reported difficulties, limitations, or changes in sexual behavior or activities

2. *Sexual Dysfunction* (More Specific Diagnosis): *page 234*
   - definition: a change in sexual functioning viewed as unsatisfying, unrewarding, or inadequate
   - data: client states there is a problem; changes in achieving perceived sex role; actual or perceived limitations imposed by disease and/or therapy; conflicts involving values; changes or inability to achieve sexual satisfaction; seeking confirmation of desirability; changes in relationship with significant other; change of interest in self and others

GENERAL OUTCOMES AND NURSING INTERVENTIONS

GENERAL SEX/SEXUALITY OUTCOMES

- Client will demonstrate ability to control own fertility.
- Client will participate in satisfying sexual relationship.
- Client will engage in behaviors to reduce or eliminate risk of infection.
- Client will achieve satisfying forms of sexual expression.
- Client will describe possible alterations, limitations in sexual functioning because of health condition and its treatment.
- Client will identify adaptations to promote optimum sexual functioning.
- Client will state comfort with own sexuality and sexual behavior.

GENERAL SEX/SEXUALITY NURSING INTERVENTIONS

- Increase professional knowledge base about sex/sexuality and high frequency health problems in your practice.

- Improve communication skills and personal comfort level in discussing sexual concerns with your clients. Ask at least one question to open up the topic during discharge planning.
- Use active listening; identify the fears and concerns as described by client and/or partner; be nonjudgemental.
- Give client permission to discuss sexual concerns and ask questions by introducing the topic during assessment and discharge planning regardless of age, marital status, or sex.
- Include information on sexual functioning in pamphlets about specific health problems designed for client education.
- Teach based on assessment of client's knowledge in areas of:
    growth and development; normal childhood sexual behavior.
    breast and/or testicular self-exam.
    reproduction and fertility control; preventing sexually transmitted diseases.
    possible effects of health problem and treatment on sexuality and sexual functioning.
    safe and unsafe forms of sexual expression based on current health status.
    specific suggestions for adapting sexual activity to client's physical health or medical condition; use of aids to optimize sexual functioning.
- Evaluate medications the client is taking or will be taking for possible negative effect on sexual desire and functioning.
- Offer client's partner an opportunity to be involved with physical care and grooming needs if desired by client.
- Demonstrate respect for client's sexuality by:
    providing privacy during physical care.
    asking about and providing for cycling needs of women clients.
    assisting with personal grooming needs as necessary to help client feel attractive and maintain self-esteem.
    providing privacy for clients when they are with loved ones so they may lay with, touch, hold, and engage in sexual activity that is safe for client's current level of heatlth.

excusing yourself and coming back later if you enter the client's room during sexual activity either with self or partner (if behaviors are not contraindicated by client's medical condition).

RELATED NURSING DIAGNOSES

ALTERED SEXUALITY PATTERNS

Definition
A state in which an individual expresses concern regarding own sexuality.

Major Defining Characteristics
- reported difficulties, limitations, or changes in sexual behavior or activities

Related Factors
- knowledge/skill deficit about alternative responses to health-related transitions, or altered body function or structure (illness or medical)
- lack of privacy (e.g., nursing home, living with large family)
- lack of significant other (e.g., death of spouse, isolated)
- ineffective or absent role models
- conflicts with sexual orientation or variant preferences
- fear of pregnancy or of getting a sexually transmitted disease
- impaired relationship with significant other

Examples of Specific Nursing Diagnoses
1. Altered sexuality patterns: abstinence related to lack of knowledge about safety and alternate positioning during pregnancy.
   Altered sexuality patterns: abstinence related to lack of knowledge about safety and alternate positioning during pregnancy as evidenced by report of abstaining from sex for last 2 months because husband was too heavy; afraid of hurting the baby. (PES format)
2. Altered sexuality patterns: belief that sexual functioning is no longer possible related to lack of knowledge about options for catheter during intercourse, anxiety related to erectile functioning secondary to spinal cord injury.

Altered sexuality patterns related to lack of knowledge about options for catheter during intercourse and anxiety related to erectile functioning secondary to spinal cord injury as evidenced by statements that client wouldn't ever have to worry about getting anyone pregnant; crying when talking about perceived loss of sexual function. (PES format)

Examples of Specific Outcomes

1. Client states confidence in ability to prevent unwanted pregnancy and infection by end of clinic visit.
2. Client identifies when resumption of sexual activity is safe post-MI (heart attack) and adaptations to reduce the workload on the heart before discharge.
3. By discharge, client identifies actual risk of repeat MI during sexual activity, sexual activities that may be risky or should be avoided, and what to do if chest pain develops.
4. Client states options for managing urinary function/catheter during sexual activity at the end of discharge planning.

Examples of Specific Nursing Interventions

- See General Sex/Sexuality Nursing Interventions, page 230.
- Reduce or eliminate specific related factors causing the problem whenever possible.
- Discuss pain management and suggest taking analgesics before sexual activity if this activity precipitates pain (unless contraindicated; does not apply to chest, cardiac, pain).
- Offer support groups for clients to discuss feelings, possible adaptations, alternative responses, and successful coping related to sexual issues and particular disease condition, injury, surgery, or treatment (e.g., diabetics, spinal cord injury, heart attack, joint/mobility diseases).

Examples of Specific Evaluations for Outcomes 1 to 4

1. Outcome not met. Client confused over measures to prevent pregnancy versus methods to prevent infection; client insists on use of condom during middle of menstrual cycle, but not at other times.

2. Outcome partially met. Client correctly restated information from physician on the timing for resumption of sexual activity but is confused about nitroglycerine use.
3. Outcome met. Client identified actual risk of causing repeat MI is low during sexual activity; listed avoidance of anal stimulation/anal receptive intercourse and to stop activity causing chest pain and take a nitroglycerine.
4. Outcome met. Client states he can fold catheter back under a condom or remove it and do self-cath after lovemaking.

Key Index Words for Nursing Interventions
Look up these words in the index of fundamentals and medical-surgical nursing textbooks to find page references for additional nursing interventions and rationale for their selection:

- sexual roles
- sexual dysfunction
- sexual functioning
- sexual response cycle
- sexuality

SEXUAL DYSFUNCTION

Definition
A state in which an individual experiences a change in sexual functioning that is viewed as unsatisfying, unrewarding, or inadequate.

Defining Characteristics
- verbalization of a problem (by client or partner)
- alterations in achieving perceived sex role
- actual or perceived limitations imposed by disease and/or therapy (e.g., pain with intercourse, fear of injury or repeat heart attack, indwelling catheter, activity restrictions)
- conflicts involving values
- alteration in achieving sexual satisfaction
  decreased or lost sexual desire (both sexes)
  arousal problems: dyspareunia (pain with intercourse) in women; impotence (erectile dysfunction) in men
  discharge problems: premature or retarded ejaculation in men; orgasmic dysfunction in women

- inability to achieve desired satisfaction
- seeking confirmation of desirability (may take form of seductive behavior, exposing, sexual harassment of nurses)
- alteration in relationship with significant other
- change of interest in self and others

Related Factors
- biopsychosocial alteration of sexuality
- ineffectual or absent role models
- physical abuse/psychosocial abuse (e.g., harmful relationships)
- vulnerability
- values conflict (e.g., belief that sexual activity is inappropriate for the elderly or mentally handicapped)
- lack of privacy
- lack of significant other
- altered body structure or function (e.g., pregnancy, vaginal dryness, ostomies, recent childbirth, drugs, surgery, anomalies, disease processes, sexually transmitted diseases, vaginal infections, trauma, radiation)
- lack of knowledge or misinformation

Other Related Factors
- erectile dysfunction associated with diabetes, multiple sclerosis, spinal cord injury, Parkinson's disease, post-MI or coronary bypass surgery, liver and kidney disease

Examples of Specific Nursing Diagnoses
1. Sexual dysfunction: loss of desire, dyspareunia related to recent childbirth, vaginal dryness, fatigue, and demands of newborn.
   Sexual dysfunction: loss of desire, dyspareunia related to recent childbirth, vaginal dryness, fatigue, and demands of newborn as evidenced by statement of pain with intercourse over last month; lack of interest in resuming sexual activity. (PES format)
2. Sexual dysfunction: erectile dysfunction related to anxiety, fear, perceived vulnerability of another MI (heart attack).
   Sexual dysfunction: erectile dysfunction related to anxiety, fear, perceived vulnerability of another MI (heart attack) as evidenced by client statements of impotence with sexual stimulation since heart attack; no previous sexual problems. (PES format)

Examples of Specific Outcomes

1. Client states return of sexual desire and absence of dyspareunia 3 months after delivery.
2. Client states return of normal erectile function 6 months following prostatectomy.
3. Client identifies options for managing bladder and catheter during sexual activity and intercourse by discharge.
4. Client states return of sexual desire within 2 weeks of change in medication for hypertension.

Examples of Specific Nursing Interventions

■ See General Sex/Sexuality Nursing Interventions, page 230.
■ Reduce or eliminate specific related factors causing a problem (e.g., suggest water-soluble lubrication for vaginal dryness; suggest analgesics for painful joints; administer medications for vaginal infections).
■ Increase your expertise in a particular area of practice by learning about the effects of specific health problems on sexual functioning and teach adaptations to promote optimum functioning. For example, for clients post-MI (heart attack):

suggest couple activities, such as walking, as client gradually increases activity level.

suggest maintaining physical closeness with less strenuous forms of sexual activity: touching, holding, kissing.

ask physician when it is medically safe for this client to resume sexual activity and include in discharge teaching; 3–4 months is average time post-MI.

discuss the fear most clients have related to repeat MI during sexual activity; provide actual risk information; workload on heart similar to climbing two flights of stairs.

inform client that some medications such as diuretics and antihypertensives may reduce sex drive and/or contribute to erectile problems and to notify the doctor if this becomes a problem for a dose or drug change.

rest before sexual activity; select time during day when more rested.

wait several hours after eating a large meal.

avoid alcohol consumption or smoking.

side-lying or client-below positions are less stressful on the heart.

sex with a familiar partner in familiar place is less stressful.

nitroglycerine 15–30 minutes before sex may be recommended by physician to prevent chest pain.

stop sexual activity if chest pain develops; use other less strenuous forms of pleasuring.

anal stimulation or anal receptive intercourse can cause a vagal response and slow the heart; avoid this form of sexual activity since it increases heart workload.

Examples of Specific Evaluations for Outcomes 1 to 4

1. Outcome met. Client states return of sexual activity and desire since baby began to sleep through the night at 3 months and no pain with the use of K-Y jelly for vaginal lubrication.

2. Outcome partially met. Client experiencing some erectile dysfunction (impotence) at 6 months but functioning seems to be improving each week. States confidence in continued recovery.

3. Outcome met. Client states she will either tape up catheter on abdomen and out of the way or will remove it prior to intercourse and do self-catheterization later.

4. Outcome met. Client states amazement that blood pressure drug was causing sex problems. Client states he is feeling previous level of interest in sex and new medication is working well to control blood pressure.

Key Index Words for Nursing Interventions

Look up these words in the index of fundamentals and medical-surgical nursing textbooks to find page references for additional nursing interventions and rationale for their selection:

- dyspareunia
- ejaculation, premature and retarded
- erectile dysfunction (impotence)
- intercourse, sexual
- orgasmic dysfunction
- sexual dysfunction
- sexual expression
- sexual response cycle
- vaginismus

Chapter 13

Skin/Mucous Membrane Problems

FOCUSED ASSESSMENT GUIDE

Complete this focused assessment if a general nursing assessment indicates a possible problem. Then turn to page 239 of this text for the Data ⇒ Diagnosis Matching Guide for skin/mucous membrane problems to help you select the best nursing diagnosis to match the client's data.

Provide privacy and assist the client into a hospital gown. Explain to the client that you will be examining the condition of the skin and mucous membrane of the mouth.

ASK THE CLIENT

___ Do you have any rashes or sores in your mouth? If yes, document the location, size, color, and how long the client has been aware of them.
___ Do you have any rashes or sores on your skin? If yes, document the location, size, color, and how long the client has been aware of them.
___ Are you able to control bowel movements?
___ Are you able to control urination or do you sometimes have accidents?
___ Are you able to change your position in bed or in a wheelchair unassisted?

EXAMINE

___ conjunctiva of eyes; note color and moisture
___ mucous membrane of mouth; note area under tongue, membrane moistness, pink color, tongue coating
___ condition of teeth, gums, dentures, breath
___ condition of scalp: dandruff, excessive oil, dryness
___ complete a head-to-toe inspection of skin, observing especially skin around bony prominences: wrists, elbows, coccyx, hips, ankles, heels, and around any areas of bowel/bladder incontinence
___ have client close eyes then assess for feeling on all extremities: touch the client with the blunt end of a closed safety pin and ask whether client can feel it: "Now? Now?"
___ document abnormal findings

If client has a prosthesis or uses crutches, examine the point of contact between the skin surface and the device. Document any skin discoloration, edema, blisters, or skin breakdown.

DATA ⇒ DIAGNOSIS MATCHING GUIDE

Compare your client data from the Skin/Mucous Membrane Focused Assessment to these related skin and mucous membrane nursing diagnoses and abbreviated descriptions. Select the nursing diagnosis which is the best match. Then turn to the page in this section with that specific diagnosis for help in planning care.

1. *Altered Oral Mucous Membrane: page 241*
   - definition: breaks in the tissues of the mouth
   - data: oral pain, coated tongue, dry mouth, sores in mouth, bad breath, infected or bleeding gums

2. *Impaired Skin Integrity: page 243*
   - definition: skin surface is adversely altered
   - data: break in skin surface; destruction of skin layers

3. *High Risk for Impaired Skin Integrity: page 246*
   - definition: skin is at risk of being adversely altered

- data: presence of risk factors such as immobility, incontinence, excessive heat or cold, poor nutritional status, lack of sensation

4. *Impaired Tissue Integrity: page 249*
   - definition: individual has damage to mucous membrane, corneal, integumentary, or subcutaneous tissue
   - data: damaged or destroyed tissue

GENERAL OUTCOMES AND NURSING INTERVENTIONS

GENERAL SKIN/MUCOUS MEMBRANE OUTCOMES

- Client's skin remains intact.
- Client's mucous membrane remains intact.
- Client's skin/mucous membrane is free of infection.
- Client's skin/mucous membrane has healed and is free of infection.
- Client states preventive skin care.
- Client or caregiver demonstrates skin care.
- Client demonstrates correct skin care/stump care for use of prosthesis/crutches.

GENERAL SKIN/MUCOUS MEMBRANE NURSING INTERVENTIONS

- Assess skin/mucous membrane condition on regular schedule.
- Plan and teach skin care routine.
- Teach oral hygiene: brushing, flossing.
- Complete nutritional intake assessment, evaluate and provide dietary teaching as indicated.
- Provide nutritional supplements as necessary to promote healing.
- Encourage fluids to 2000 mL/day unless contraindicated.
- Teach body positioning to avoid pressure over bones.
- Use assistive devices (egg crate mattresses, fluid beds) as indicated to prevent bedsores (decubitus ulcers).
- Assess for urinary/fecal incontinence. Clean skin promptly after soiling.

■ Use catheter if necessary.
■ Use skin barrier creams as necessary to protect skin.

RELATED NURSING DIAGNOSES

ALTERED ORAL MUCOUS MEMBRANE

Definition
A state in which an individual experiences disruptions in the tissue layers of the oral cavity.

Defining Characteristics
■ oral pain/discomfort
■ coated tongue
■ xerostomia (dry mouth)
■ stomatitis
■ oral lesions or ulcers
■ lack of or decreased salivation
■ leukoplakia (thickened white patches on mucous membranes)
■ edema
■ hyperemia (excess blood in an area; congestion)
■ oral plaque
■ desquamation (skin peeling off in scales)
■ vesicles
■ hemorrhagic gingivitis
■ carious teeth (tooth decay, cavities)
■ halitosis (bad breath)

Related Factors
■ pathological conditions: oral cavity (radiation to head or neck)
■ dehydration
■ trauma (chemical, e.g., acidic foods, drugs, noxious agents, alcohol; mechanical, e.g., ill-fitting dentures)
■ braces, tubes (endotracheal/nasogastric), surgery in oral cavity
■ NPO for more than 24 hours
■ ineffective oral hygiene
■ mouth breathing

- malnutrition
- infection
- lack of or decreased salivation
- medication

Examples of Specific Nursing Diagnoses
1. Altered oral mucous membrane related to mouth breathing caused by nasogastric tube.
   Altered oral mucous membrane related to mouth breathing caused by nasogastric tube as evidenced by dry, coated tongue, cracked lips, decreased salivation, and halitosis. (PES format)
2. Altered oral mucous membrane related to yeast infection.
   Altered oral mucous membrane related to yeast infection as evidenced by white, curd-like patches. (PES format)

Examples of Specific Outcomes
1. Client's mucous membrane and tongue will be pink, moist, and free of cracks or coatings within 48 hours.
2. Client will demonstrate effective oral hygiene routine before discharge.
3. Client will be free of oral pain and able to have oral dietary intake of 1600 cal/day.

Examples of Specific Nursing Interventions
- See General Skin/Mucous Membrane Nursing Interventions, page 240.
- Assess and document condition of mucous membrane and teeth. By wearing gloves and wrapping the tongue in a gauze, a nurse can view the oral cavity.
- Assess for fit of dentures, oral appliances, bridgework.
- Assess for pain, especially with oral intake.
- Assess the knowledge and ability of the client to do oral hygiene; if the client is unable to do own care, include a schedule for oral care in the written care plan.
- Provide teaching for client or caregiver if indicated.
- Assist with ordered mouthwashes (medicated for analgesia or infection), adhering to a schedule.
- Assist with or complete oral hygiene for clients unable to do own care. May use sponge or foam swabs in place of a toothbrush to provide more gentle cleansing.
- Apply lubricant to lips.

- Offer lozenges or hard candy to stimulate saliva secretion if not contraindicated.
- Assure adequate fluid intake (at least 1500 mL/day); set prescribed oral intake per waking hour (example, 100 mL per hour while awake).
- Provide dietician consultation to plan for nutritional intake; select foods that are mechanically soft, high in calories and protein (to promote healing); cool/frozen foods may increase comfort level.

Examples of Specific Evaluations for Outcome 1
1. Outcome not met. Client continues mouth breathing and oral mucous membrane is still cracked and dry.
2. Outcome partially met. Condition of mucous membrane is improved but problem not totally resolved.
3. Outcome met. Oral mucous membrane and tongue pink, moist, and free of cracks or coatings.

Key Index Words for Nursing Interventions
Look up these words in the index of fundamentals and medical-surgical nursing textbooks to find page references for additional nursing interventions and rationale for their selection:

- atrophy
- *Candida albicans* (thrush)
- gingivae
- *Herpes simplex*
- hyperplasia
- leukoplakia
- *Pseudomonas*
- stomatitis
- topical analgesics
- xerostomia

See additional nursing diagnoses:

- Impaired tissue integrity
- Impaired skin integrity
- High risk for impaired skin integrity

IMPAIRED SKIN INTEGRITY

Definition
A state in which an individual's skin is adversely altered.

Major Defining Characteristics
- disruption of skin surface
- destruction of skin layers
- invasion of body structures

Related Factors
External (Environmental)
- hyper- or hypothermia
- chemical substance
- mechanical factors (shearing forces, pressure, restraint)
- radiation
- physical immobilization
- humidity

Internal (Somatic)
- medication
- altered nutritional state (obesity, emaciation)
- altered metabolic state
- altered circulation
- altered sensation
- altered pigmentation
- skeletal prominence
- developmental factors
- immunological deficit
- alteration in turgor (change in elasticity)

Examples of Specific Nursing Diagnoses
1. Impaired skin integrity related to unrelieved pressure secondary to immobility.

   Impaired skin integrity related to unrelieved pressure secondary to immobility as evidenced by 4-in diameter, reddened circle with broken skin over coccyx. (PES format)

2. Impaired skin integrity related to impaired circulation secondary to diabetes.

   Impaired skin integrity related to impaired circulation secondary to diabetes as evidenced by foot ulcer approximately 2 in in diameter. (PES format)

Examples of Specific Nursing Outcomes
1. Client's skin will heal and be free of infection prior to discharge.
2. Client will demonstrate diabetic foot care prior to discharge.
3. Client/family caregiver will verbalize observations to be made and daily skin care needed to prevent skin breakdown.

Examples of Specific Nursing Interventions

- See General Skin/Mucous Membrane Nursing Interventions, page 240.
- Assess condition of skin at specified intervals, measure and document any abnormalities.
- Wash perianal area with mild soap and warm water, rinse well, and dry thoroughly after each episode of incontinence.
- Use products that wick moisture away from the client's skin and provide a dry surface in contact with the skin.
- Maintain room humidity to avoid drying the skin.
- Avoid massage over bony prominences.
- Position immobile client with the use of assistive pillows and devices, changing position at least every 2 hours. Document the condition of the skin as well as the new position.
- Use assistive devices to relieve pressure on heels, knees, and elbows.
- Assess the need for fluid, foam, alternating air, or water mattress.
- If using special type of bed/mattress, teach safety precautions to client and/or family caregiver.
- Teach wheelchair-bound client to shift weight every 15 minutes.
- Avoid use of plastic in contact with skin.
- Cleanse open wound using gloves and sterile technique.
- Apply barrier dressings as ordered.
- Maintain antibiotic therapy as ordered; assess and document response to therapy.

Examples of Specific Evaluations for Outcome 2

1. Outcome not met. Client refuses to participate in learning foot care.
2. Outcome partially met. Client attended diabetic foot care class but states, "I don't need to do that. I shower every day and that's good enough."
3. Outcome met. Client attended class and has completed a satisfactory return demonstration of diabetic foot care.

Key Index Words for Nursing Interventions

Look up these words in the index of fundamentals and medical-surgical nursing textbooks to find page references for additional nursing interventions and rationale for their selection:

- bony prominences
- debridement
- decubitus ulcer
- diabetes mellitus
- gangrene
- neuropathy
- paresthesia
- pressure sore
- wound healing

See additional nursing diagnoses:

- Impaired tissue integrity
- High risk for impaired skin integrity

Case Management Example
See Appendix for an example of a nursing diagnosis of Impaired Skin Integrity within a clinical pathway for DRG 209, Total Hip Replacement, page 474.

HIGH RISK FOR IMPAIRED SKIN INTEGRITY

Definition
A state in which an individual's skin is at risk of being adversely altered.

Defining Risk Factors
External (Environmental)
- hypo- or hyperthermia
- chemical substances
- mechanical factors (shearing forces, pressure, restraint)
- radiation
- physical immobilization
- excretions/secretions
- humidity

Internal (Somatic)
- medication
- alterations in nutritional state (obesity, emaciation)
- altered metabolic state
- altered circulation
- altered sensation
- altered pigmentation
- skeletal prominence
- developmental factors

- alterations in skin turgor (change in elasticity)
- psychogenic
- immunologic

Examples of Specific Nursing Diagnoses
1. High risk for impaired skin integrity related to physical immobility.
   High risk for impaired skin integrity related to physical immobility as evidenced by inability to shift position in wheelchair. (PES format)
2. High risk for impaired skin integrity related to fecal and urinary incontinence.
   High risk for impaired skin integrity related to fecal and urinary incontinence as evidenced by diarrhea stools in bed and urine in bed × 3. (PES format)

Examples of Specific Outcomes
1. Skin over client's coccyx will remain intact.
2. Client/family caregiver will verbalize observations that identify risk of skin breakdown before discharge.
3. Family caregiver will demonstrate skin care routine to prevent breakdown before discharge.

Examples of Specific Nursing Interventions
- Select interventions that decrease risk factors.
- See General Skin/Mucous Membrane Nursing Interventions, page 240.
- Assess condition of skin at specified intervals, noting any reddened areas, edema, blisters, tenderness. Document size and location of any abnormalities.
- Wash perianal area with mild soap and warm water, rinse well, and dry thoroughly after each episode of incontinence.
- Use products that wick moisture away from the client's skin and provide a dry surface in contact with the skin.
- Assess need for catheter, external or indwelling.
- Maintain room humidity to avoid drying the skin.
- Avoid massage over bony prominences.
- Position immobile client with the use of assistive pillows and devices, changing position at least every 2 hours. Document the condition of the skin as well as the new position.
- Use assistive devices to relieve pressure on heels, knees, and elbows.

- Assess the need for fluid, foam, alternating air, or water mattress.
- If using special type of bed/mattress, teach safety precautions to client and/or family caregiver.
- Teach wheelchair-bound client to shift weight every 15 minutes.
- Avoid use of plastic in contact with skin.
- Cleanse open wound using gloves and sterile technique.
- Apply barrier dressings as ordered.
- Maintain antibiotic therapy as ordered; assess and document response to therapy.
- Assess adequacy of nutritional intake: especially protein, calories, vitamin C, and zinc.
- Lift client, rather than dragging, during repositioning.
- Apply thin layer of cornstarch to client to reduce friction when moving in bed.
- Provide trapeze if client is able to assist in movement.
- Encourage caregiver to assist with active/passive range of motion exercises.

Examples of Specific Evaluations for Outcome 1

1. Outcome not met. Skin breakdown over coccyx with serous exudate.
2. Outcome partially met. Reddened area over coccyx but skin remains intact.
3. Outcome met. Skin intact over coccyx, no redness or edema noted.

Key Index Words for Nursing Interventions

Look up these words in the index of fundamentals and medical-surgical nursing textbooks to find page references for additional nursing interventions and rationale for their selection:

- bony prominences
- casts: body, leg orthopedic
- cerebral vascular accident (CVA)/stroke
- decubitus ulcer
- diabetes mellitus
- hemiplegia
- neuropathy
- paraplegia
- paresthesia
- quadriplegia
- shearing forces

See additional nursing diagnoses:
- Impaired tissue integrity
- Impaired skin integrity

IMPAIRED TISSUE INTEGRITY

Definition
A state in which an individual experiences damage to mucous membrane, corneal, integumentary, or subcutaneous tissue.

Major Defining Characteristics
■ damaged or destroyed tissue (cornea, mucous membrane, integumentary, or subcutaneous).

Related Factors
■ altered circulation
■ nutritional deficit/excess
■ fluid deficit/excess
■ knowledge deficit
■ impaired physical mobility
■ irritants, chemical (including body excretions, secretions, medications).
■ thermal (temperature extremes)
■ mechanical (pressure, shear, friction)
■ radiation (including therapeutic radiation)

Examples of Specific Nursing Diagnoses
1. Impaired tissue integrity related to accidental insertion of contact cleanser into eye.
   Impaired tissue integrity related to accidental insertion of contact cleanser into eye as evidenced by corneal pain, redness, edema, and abrasion. (PES format)
2. Impaired tissue integrity related to ingestion of lye.
   Impaired tissue integrity related to ingestion of lye as evidenced by burns in mouth and esophagus. (PES format)

Examples of Specific Outcomes
1. Cornea will heal without infection within 3 days.
2. Client will demonstrate safe procedure for cleaning contact lenses before the end of clinic visit.
3. Skin lesion will be completely healed within one month.
4. Damaged tissue will remain free of infection throughout hospitalization.

Examples of Specific Nursing Interventions
■ Select interventions that decrease risk factors.
■ See General Skin/Mucous Membrane Nursing Interventions, page 240.

- Assess the tissue damage and document condition at least every 8 hours. Observe and document the condition of the tissue adjacent to the wound.
- Document any drainage: amount, color, odor.
- Assess the cause of the tissue damage and determine whether client teaching is needed to prevent recurrence.
- Assess the client's pain and medicate as ordered.
- Teach alternative methods of pain control to enhance comfort.
- Protect client from infection: restrict visitors or personnel who may be ill; good handwashing; sterile dressing changes.
- Administer prophylactic antibiotics as ordered.
- Provide for cleanliness of affected area using sterile technique in treatments or dressing changes.
- Teach client and/or family caregivers the importance of aseptic technique and how to modify it for home care.
- Assess dietary intake and modify if necessary to assure adequate intake. Consider client preferences in nutritional planning.

Examples of Specific Evaluations for Outcome 1
1. Outcome not met. Eye is draining and irritated.
2. Outcome partially met. Corneal tissue is healing but still small amount of clear drainage.
3. Outcome met. Corneal tissue clear with no drainage or pain.

Key Index Words for Nursing Interventions
Look up these words in the index of fundamentals and medical-surgical nursing textbooks to find page references for additional nursing interventions and rationale for their selection:

- circulation
- edema
- epithelialization
- erythema
- exudate

- granulation tissue
- tissue induration
- tissue necrosis
- tissue regeneration
- wound assessment

See additional nursing diagnoses:
- Altered oral mucous membrane
- Impaired skin integrity
- High risk for impaired skin integrity

Chapter 14

Temperature Problems

FOCUSED ASSESSMENT GUIDE

Complete this focused assessment if a general nursing assessment indicates a possible problem. Then turn to page 253 of this text for the Data ⇒ Diagnosis Matching Guide for temperature problems to help you select the best nursing diagnosis to match the client's data.

ASSESS CLIENT AND CHART FOR

___ elevated body temperature during last 72 hours
___ lower than normal body temperature in last 72 hours
___ temperature fluctuating between normal and abnormal ranges during last 72 hours
___ flushed skin, warm to the touch
___ pale skin, cool to the touch
___ presence of risk factors
    ___ newborn, infant, child, elderly
    ___ overweight or underweight, emaciated
    ___ confused; decreased level of consciousness
    ___ dehydrated; unable to obtain fluids and drink independently
    ___ inactive or engaging in vigorous exercise
    ___ exposed to hot or cold environmental temperatures
    ___ inappropriately dressed for environmental temperature
    ___ lacking resources for adequately warmed/cooled housing
    ___ injury or illness affecting metabolism, hypothalamus in brain, or ability of body to vasoconstrict or

vasodilate blood vessels (e.g., burns, thyroid problems, brain tumors, spinal cord injury)
___ taking medications causing vasoconstriction or vasodilation

NORMALS AND INFORMATION

- The hypothalamus in the brain regulates temperature; it has a set point for temperature; if body temperature changes the hypothalamus initiates control mechanisms to return body temperature to its set point
- Pyrogens (produced by bacteria) can raise the hypothalamic set point; if this occurs, heat production increases and heat is conserved to raise body temperature; as infection resolves, the set point is returned to normal and heat production decreases and heat loss is increased to lower body temperature
- Internal "core" body temperature (rectal temperature) is maintained within $\pm 1°F$ ($0.6°C$) during health; skin temperature rises and falls with the environmental temperature
- Oral temperatures: average is 98–98.6°F (36.7–37°C); range 97–99.6°F (36.1–37.6°C); early morning may be 96–97°F (35.6–36.1°C); 99.6–101°F (37.6–38.3°C) with heavy exercise and in active children
- Rectal "core" temperatures: average is 99–99.6°F (37.3–37.6°C); range 97.6–100.2°F (36.4–37.9°C)
- Body temperature rises when heat production is greater than heat loss and decreases when heat production is less than heat loss
- Cellular metabolism produces body heat using oxygen (O_2) and glucose; as metabolism increases so does need for O_2 and glucose
- Thyroxin increases metabolism and consequently heat production
- Elevated body temperature causes increased cellular metabolism
- Shivering and muscle activity increase heat production
- Sympathetic nervous system stimulation:
  increases metabolic rate resulting in more heat

production
causes vasoconstriction to reduce heat loss to environment

- Heat is lost through radiation, conduction, convection, and evaporation of water (600 mL/day) from the skin and lungs
- Skin, subcutaneous tissue, and fat insulates the body conserving heat; excess fat overinsulates reducing normal heat loss; very thin people have inadequate insulation and have more heat loss
- Vasodilation of superficial blood vessels in the skin increases heat loss to the environment; vasoconstriction retains heat
- Sweat production can increase to 700 mL/hr to cool the body as long as hydration is adequate; people living in hot climates can increase sweat production as high as 2000 mL/hr to keep cool
- To reduce body temperature, the body initiates sweating and vasodilation, decreases heat production, and uses behavioral responses such as extended posturing, taking off extra clothing, and blankets, moving to cooler areas
- To raise body temperature, the body initiates vasoconstriction, piloerection (gooseflesh), shivering, increased heat production, and behavioral responses such as increased activity (stomping feet, pacing), closed body posture to decrease heat loss, putting on more clothing, blankets, moving to warmer areas

DATA ⇒ DIAGNOSIS MATCHING GUIDE

Compare your client data from the Temperature Focused Assessment to these related temperature nursing diagnoses and abbreviated descriptions. Select the nursing diagnosis with the best match. Then turn to the page in this section with that specific diagnosis for help in planning care.

1. *High Risk for Altered Body Temperature: page 255*
   - definition: at risk for failure to maintain body temperature within the normal range
   - risk factors: extremes of age or weight; cold/cool or warm/hot environments; dehydration; inactivity;

vigorous exercise; medications/drugs causing vasoconstriction or vasodilation; alcohol use; altered
metabolic rate; sedation or decreased level of consciousness; confusion; inappropriate clothing for
environmental temperature; inadequate housing; illness/
trauma affecting temperature regulation

2. *Hyperthermia: page 258*
   - definition: body temperature is elevated above normal
     range
   - data: body temperature above normal range; flushed
     skin

3. *Hypothermia: page 261*
   - definition: body temperature is reduced below normal
     range
   - data: body temperature below normal range; shivering;
     cool skin

4. *Ineffective Thermal Regulation: page 265*
   - definition: body temperature fluctuates between
     hypothermia and hyperthermia
   - data: fluctuations in body temperature above or below
     the normal range

GENERAL OUTCOMES AND NURSING INTERVENTIONS

GENERAL TEMPERATURE OUTCOMES

- Client will maintain body temperature within normal
  range.
- Client will return body temperature to normal range.
- Client will stabilize body temperature within normal
  range.
- Client will identify ways to promote normal body
  temperature.

GENERAL TEMPERATURE NURSING INTERVENTIONS

- Discuss identified risk factors with client and family; plan
  interventions together to reduce risk.

- Reduce or eliminate cold and/or heat stresses in client's environment.
- Adapt health treatments and procedures to better promote temperature maintenance, e.g., using caps to decrease heat loss, delaying bathing until body temperature back up to normal range.
- Assess vital signs more frequently for clients at risk (e.g., continuously, every 30–120 minutes); base frequency on status of client and potential cold/heat stress of treatment.
- Assess for data indicating a possible problem in thermal regulation: flushed or pale/blue skin color; cool or warm skin temperature, slow capillary refill (more than 3 seconds after compressing nail bed), decreased level of consciousness, client's report of temperature comfort/discomfort, presence of shivering, piloerection (gooseflesh) or sweating.
- Promote nutritional balance; increase nutritional intake to meet increased metabolic rate in both hypothermia and hyperthermia.
- Initiate I&O; maintain hydration.
- Place beds or cribs away from drafts and direct sunlight.

RELATED NURSING DIAGNOSES

HIGH RISK FOR ALTERED BODY TEMPERATURE

Definition
A state in which an individual is at risk for failure to maintain body temperature within the normal range.

Defining Characteristics
Presence of Risk Factors
- extremes of age (newborns, infants, children, and elderly)
- extremes of weight (thin/emaciated or overweight/obese)
- exposure to cold/cool or warm/hot environments
- dehydration (unable to sweat to cool self)
- inactivity or vigorous activity (reduced or excessive heat production)
- medications/drugs causing vasoconstriction (decreases ability to lose heat) or vasodilation (decreases ability to conserve heat)

- anesthesia (in genetically susceptable individuals malignant hyperthermia can result from anesthesia during surgery causing uncontrolled temperature elevation and possible death)
- alcohol consumption; alcoholic (causes vasodilation; "feel warm" and fails to act in ways to conserve heat)
- altered metabolic rate (reduced or excessive heat production)
- sedation; decreased level of consciousness; confusion
- inappropriate clothing for environmental temperature
- inadequate housing environment (e.g., homeless, no air-conditioning, unable to pay heating bill, inadequate heat in home; unable to control home temperature)
- illness or trauma affecting temperature regulation (e.g., surgery involving hypothalamus, infection, burns)

Examples of Specific Nursing Diagnoses

1. High risk for altered body temperature (hypothermia) related to birth in 70°F (21.1°C) room, being wet with amniotic fluid.
2. High risk for altered body temperature (hypothermia) related to living on the street in winter, poor nutritional status, alcohol consumption, lack of knowledge of community shelters.
3. High risk for altered body temperature (hyperthermia) related to planned 5-mile race in temperatures of 101°F (38.3°C), sunshine, age 12 years, no water stations along course.

Examples of Specific Outcomes

1. Newborn's rectal temperature will be above 98°F (36.7°C) when initially assessed after delivery.
2. Client will identify ways to stay warm, location of several shelters, and food shelves before end of clinic visit.
3. Temperature will be below 101°F (38.3°C) after running the race.

Examples of Specific Nursing Interventions

- See General Temperature Nursing Interventions, page 254.
- Reduce or eliminate risk factors whenever possible; prevent or reduce cold/heat stressors; treat infection with ordered antibiotics; keep client dry, hydrated, appropriately covered.

■ Assess client prior to surgery for any anesthesia-related complications in immediate family or with prior surgery; notify anesthesiologist immediately if history is positive.

■ Refer to social services as needed for financial or community help.

■ Promote maintenance of normal temperature/prevent chilling:

keep covered as much as possible for surgical experience, procedures, treatments, bathing.

delay bathing, or exposure until temperature stable.

when providing oxygen, use warmed, humidified oxygen for clients at risk of hypothermia (blowing room temperature oxygen over client's face is a cold stress, especially for infants).

provide extra blankets, warmed blankets, warm liquids, heat source during procedures that increase heat loss.

encourage movement and activity.

Examples of Specific Evaluations for Outcomes 1 to 3

1. Outcome met. Baby's rectal temperature was 98.2°F (36.8°C) on admission to the nursery.
2. Outcome partially met. Client correctly stated how to find two shelters and one food shelf but will not accept the risk of alcohol. Says it makes him "feel warmer."
3. Outcome not met. Child had febrile seizure at the end of the race with a body temperature of 105°F (40.6°C).

Key Index Words for Nursing Interventions

Look up these words in the index of fundamentals and medical-surgical nursing textbooks to find page references for additional nursing interventions and rationale for their selection:

■ body temperature
■ cold stress
■ hyperthermia, malignant hyperthermia
■ hypothermia
■ temperature: regulation of, maintenance of
■ vital signs, temperature

HYPERTHERMIA

Definition
A state in which an individual's body temperature is elevated above normal range.

Major Defining Characteristics
- increase in body temperature above normal range

Minor Defining Characteristics
- flushed skin
- skin feels warm to the touch
- increased respiratory rate
- increased heart rate; tachycardia (approximately 10 beats per minute for each 1°F rise and 18 beats per minute for each 1°C rise)
- seizures/convulsions (at high body temperatures, especially in children)

Other Characteristics
Temperature Rising: Chill Phase of Fever
When the hypothalamic set point has been raised (e.g., infection) the body tries to raise its temperature by increasing heat production and preventing heat loss.

- client reports having the "chills"
- client wants to put on more clothing, blankets
- piloerection (gooseflesh)
- shivering (to produce more heat)
- skin feels cool, looks pale (vasoconstriction to retain heat)
- temperature rises (reaches new set point over several hours)

Temperature Dropping: Crisis/Flush Phase of Fever
When the hypothalamic set point drops or returns to normal, the body tries to lower its temperature by decreasing heat production and increasing heat loss.

- client reports feeling hot
- client wants to remove blankets, extra clothing
- sweating (evaporation to lose heat)
- skin flushed; feels warm/hot (vasodilation to lose heat)
- temperature decreases ("fever breaks") over several hours

Severe Hyperthermia (Hyperpyrexia, Heat Stroke)
Hypothalamus loses ability to regulate temperature.

- temperature of 106°F (41.1°C) or higher
- decreased sweating
- dizziness
- abdominal pain
- delirium; loss of consciousness
- death

Related Factors
- exposure to hot, humid environment; hot tubs
- vigorous activity
- medications causing vasoconstriction or dehydration
- anesthesia (e.g., anesthesia can cause malignant hyperthermia and death in genetically susceptible individuals)
- inappropriate clothing (excess clothing prevents heat loss)
- increased metabolic rate (produces increased body heat)
- illness or trauma (e.g., brain tumors or surgery affecting the hypothalamus; bacterial infections, blood transfusion with contaminated blood)
- dehydration (decreases ability to sweat and lose heat)
- inability or decreased ability to perspire (e.g., infants, children, elderly, spinal cord injuries)

Examples of Specific Nursing Diagnoses
1. Hyperthermia related to overheating under warmer when skin sensor fell off newborn, inability to sweat.
   Hyperthermia related to overheating under warmer when skin sensor fell off newborn, inability to sweat as evidenced by T 102°F (38.9°C), P 178, R 88, flushed. (PES format)
2. Hyperthermia related to infection.
   Hyperthermia related to infection as evidenced by T 103°F (39.4°C), P 98, R 28; report of chills, pale skin. (PES format)

Examples of Specific Outcomes
1. Client's temperature to be down to 100°F (37.8°C) rectally or less within 1 hour.
2. Client's temperature to return to normal range within 24 hours of initiation of antibiotic therapy.

3. Client's temperature to drop to 102°F (38.9°C) in the next half hour.
4. Client's temperature in normal range by end of shift.

Examples of Specific Nursing Interventions

- See General Temperature Nursing Interventions, page 254.
- Reduce, eliminate, or treat factors causing the temperature elevation whenever possible.
- Report temperature elevation to physician for treatment orders; diagnostics and treatment usually begin at temperatures above 100.4–101°F (38.0–38.3°C) in adults.
- Assessments for severe hyperthermia may include continuous rectal temperature probe, cardiac monitor, blood gases, electrolytes; be alert for hyperthermia complications: cardiac arrhythmias, hypotension, shock, seizures.
- Administer antipyretics as ordered; request from physician if not ordered, except for heatstroke.
- Administer medications as ordered (e.g., antibiotics).
- Rehydrate as ordered with IV solutions (may be done slowly to prevent circulatory overload in clients at risk, elderly).
- Administer oxygen at ordered concentration; assess frequently.
- Change bedding or clothing to keep dry if sweating.
- Encourage minimal activity (to decrease heat production).
- Promote heat loss.
  Provide cool environment; turn down heat; use air-conditioning.
  Remove extra clothing or blankets to decrease insulation (the folk wisdom of putting on extra blankets to "sweat out the fever" is appropriate if client in chill phase and temperature is rising; it is contraindicated in crisis or flush phase when body is trying to lower temperature since it prevents heat loss).
  Expose skin surfaces to air.
  Provide air currents over client to increase evaporation.
  Encourage increased intake of cold fluids.
  Apply cool, wet cloth to face and neck; cool or tepid (not cold) baths/sponging to promote heat loss

through evaporation; ice baths or ice sponging may be ordered by physician but this technique often causes shivering, which increases heat production.
■ Apply and monitor hyperthermia blanket if ordered for continuous active cooling.

Examples of Specific Evaluations for Outcomes 1 to 4
1. Outcome met. Newborn's rectal temperature 99.8°F (36.7°C) after 1 hour in crib.
2. Outcome partially met. Temperature within normal range most of day but spiked to 101°F (38.3°C) in evening after 24 hours on ampicillin.
3. Outcome not met. Temperature dropped only 1°F (0.6°C) to 104°F (40.4°C).
4. Outcome met. Client reported feeling hot, sweating at 3 A.M. with temperature of 103°F (39.4°C); temperature 98.8°F (37.1°C) by 6 A.M.

Key Index Words for Nursing Interventions
Look up these words in the index of fundamentals and medical-surgical nursing textbooks to find page references for additional nursing interventions and rationale for their selection:

■ febrile seizures
■ fever
■ heat exhaustion
■ heat stroke
■ hyperprexia
■ hyperthermia

■ malignant hyperthermia
■ pyrexia
■ pyrogens
■ temperature: body, elevated

HYPOTHERMIA

Definition
A state in which an individual's body temperature is reduced below normal range.

Major Defining Characteristics
■ reduction in body temperature below normal range
■ shivering
■ cool, pale skin (due to vasoconstriction to conserve heat)

Minor Defining Characteristics

Signs and symptoms caused by body compensating for hypothermia by increasing metabolic rate to produce heat and vasoconstriction to conserve heat.

- slow capillary refill, cyanotic nail beds (vasoconstriction)
- hypertension (vasoconstriction; blood routed to core of body)
- tachycardia (increased metabolic rate, sympathetic stimulation)
- increased respiratory rate (increasing metabolic rate)
- piloerection (gooseflesh); sympathetic stimulation
- client reports feeling cold

Other Characteristics

Additional signs and symptoms develop as hypothermia worsens and body loses ability to compensate.

- apathy, sleepiness progressing to coma
- poor judgement; confused and disoriented
- poor muscle coordination; slurred speech; difficulty walking
- shivering ceases at body temperatures below 90°F (32.2°C)
- hypotension (as heart rate drops with continued hypothermia)
- slowed respirations (with continued hypothermia); apnea
- pupils dilate and stop reacting to light as hypothermia continues
- slow heart rate, bradycardia with body temperature below 90°F (32.2°C); in 60–70°F (15.6–21.1°C) range, rate may be only 2–3 beats per minute
- ventricular fibrillation, cardiac arrest, and death in severe hypothermia

Related Factors

- exposure to cool or cold environment; cold water submersion
- therapeutic induction of hypothermia (e.g., for cardiac and brain surgery, limb reattachment to decrease metabolism in cells thus decreasing need for oxygen; reduces tissue hypoxia)
- illness or trauma (e.g., spinal cord injuries, head trauma)
- damage to hypothalamus

- inability or decreased ability to shiver (e.g., spinal cord injuries, muscular dystrophy, emaciated, burns)
- anesthesia and surgery
- malnutrition; underweight for height (reduced insulation)
- inadequate clothing
- consumption of alcohol (causes vasodilation which increases heat loss; clouds judgement; decreases sensation of cold)
- medications causing vasodilation which increases heat loss
- evaporation from moist skin and body tissues (e.g., during surgery, birth, bathing, with burns)
- decreased metabolic rate which decreases heat production (e.g., hypothyroidism)
- inactivity; immobility (decreased heat production)
- elderly (decreased muscle mass, decreased shivering, decreased metabolic rate); infants and children (immature thermoregulation)

Examples of Specific Nursing Diagnoses

1. Hypothermia related to surgical experience, inactivity, exposure, evaporation, and anesthesia.

   Hypothermia related to surgical experience, inactivity, exposure, evaporation, and anesthesia as evidenced by rectal temperature of 97°F (36.1°C) in recovery room (PAR), shivering, report of being cold. (PES format)

2. Hypothermia related to birthing process, exposure while wet to cool room.

   Hypothermia related to birthing process, exposure while wet to cool room as evidenced by newborn's rectal temperature of 96.4°F (35.8°C), elevated respiratory rate (80 per minute), and elevated heart rate (174 per minute) on admission to the nursery. (PES format)

Examples of Specific Outcomes

1. Client reestablishes normal body temperature within 3 hours of surgery.
2. Client's rectal temperature up to 98°F (36.7°C) in 1 hour.
3. Client states causes and prevention of hypothermia before discharge.
4. Client exhibits reversal of present signs and symptoms of hypothermia after 12 hours of passive external rewarming.

Examples of Specific Nursing Interventions

■ See General Temperature Nursing Interventions, page 254.

■ Identify and eliminate or reduce the cold stress.

■ Assess temperature with thermometer capable of reading below 96°F (35.6°C).

■ Report decreasing urine output; output below 30 mL/h (decreased body temperature causes vasoconstriction; blood flow to kidney decreases resulting in inadequate perfusion and decreased urine production).

■ Hypothermia assessment may include continuous cardiac monitoring, indwelling urinary catheter, indwelling rectal temperature probe for continuous temperature monitoring, blood gases, electrolytes, and blood glucose levels.

■ Rewarm slowly to normal body temperature to avoid rewarming shock (drop in BP, cardiac arrhythmias, hypoxemia, acidosis). This may take many hours depending on severity and treatment.

    Passive external rewarming is for mild hypothermia when body can spontaneously generate enough heat to rewarm itself once cold stress has been removed. Dry the client if wet, place on dry bedding, remove any wet linen, raise environmental temperature if possible, warm blankets, hats, or head covers, encourage slow drinking of hot, calorie-containing liquids.

    Active external rewarming provides external heat. Use of hypo/hyperthermia blanket, overhead radiant warmers or isolettes for newborns and infants, warm (not hot) baths/soaks, warm packs, body-to-body contact (e.g., mother holding newborn against breasts with blankets over both).

    Active internal rewarming is used for severe hypothermia. Assist physician with techniques to rewarm. Rewarming of blood with cardiac bypass machines, gastric or colonic irrigation with warm solutions, giving warmed IV solutions, providing warmed humidified oxygen.

■ Delay any treatments or care that may increase heat loss such as bathing or weighing until body temperature back in normal range.

■ Administer IV fluids, oxygen, medications as ordered (e.g., warmed IV glucose solutions, antidysrhythmic drugs for cardiac arrhythmias, sodium bicarbonate for acidosis, warmed humidified oxygen).

■ Be prepared for emergency resuscitation measures if hypothermia is severe, if cardiac arrhythmias develop or if client arrests.

■ If hypothermia was accidental, review with client and family causes and prevention before discharge.

Examples of Specific Evaluations for Outcomes 1 to 4

1. Outcome met. Client's rectal temperature has returned to 99.2°F (37.3°C) and stabilized; no hypotension, cardiac arrhythmias, or respiratory distress noted.

2. Outcome not met. Newborn's temperature 97.4°F (36.3°C) after 1 hour under the radiant warmer.

3. Outcome partially met. Client blaming entire cause of hypothermia on outdoor temperature; refuses to acknowledge role of alcohol consumption and malnutrition.

4. Outcome partially met. Body temperature 98.6°F (37.0°C) orally and stable but still having occasional cardiac arrhythmias and shivering episodes.

Key Index Words for Nursing Interventions

Look up these words in the index of fundamentals and medical-surgical nursing textbooks to find page references for additional nursing interventions and rationale for their selection:

■ body temperature
■ heat: balance, application of, loss of, production of
■ hypothalamus, role in temperature regulation
■ hypothermia
■ metabolic rate, role in heat production
■ shivering
■ temperature, hypothermia
■ vasoconstriction: control of, role in heat conservation
■ vital signs, hypothermia

INEFFECTIVE THERMAL REGULATION

Definition

A state in which an individual's temperature fluctuates between hypothermia and hyperthermia.

Major Defining Characteristics
- fluctuations in body temperature above or below the normal range
- defining characteristics for Hyperthermia and Hypothermia

Related Factors
- trauma or illness (e.g., tumors or surgery to hypothalamus, spinal cord injury)
- immaturity (neonates, infants, children have a decreased ability to shiver, sweat, vasoconstrict, and vasodilate); elderly
- fluctuating environmental temperature

Examples of Specific Nursing Diagnoses
1. Ineffective thermal regulation related to newborn status.
   Ineffective thermal regulation related to newborn status as evidenced by inability to maintain normal temperature outside warmer; decrease in temperature to 97.4°F (36.3°C) rectally after 1 hour outside radiant warmer × 2. (PES format)
2. Ineffective thermal regulation related to spinal cord injury at C6 level.
   Ineffective thermal regulation related to spinal cord injury at C6 level as evidenced by loss of sensation of warm or cold over most of body; absence of shivering or sweating below level of injury; intermittent fever. (PES format)

Examples of Specific Outcomes
1. Client maintains body temperature above 98°F (36.7°C) rectally outside warmer after 2 hours in crib.
2. Client maintains body temperature between 97.6–99°F (36.4–37.2°C) during this shift.
3. Client identifies ways to maintain body temperature in normal range without sweating and shivering responses to environmental temperature.
4. Mother demonstrates activities to maintain newborn's body temperature while feeding, bathing, and caring for baby.

Examples of Specific Nursing Interventions
- See General Temperature Nursing Interventions, page 254, and Specific Nursing Interventions for Hypothermia, page 264, and Hyperthermia, page 260.

■ Reduce, eliminate, or compensate for client's specific risk factors.

Examples of Specific Evaluations for Outcomes 1 to 4

1. Outcome not met. Newborn's temperature was 97.6°F (36.4°C) after 2 hours in crib wrapped in two blankets.
2. Outcome met. Client had no febrile episodes this shift.
3. Outcome partially met. Client identified several interventions to maintain heat in cool environment but needs review in methods of heat loss for warm/hot environments.
4. Outcome met. Mother held baby skin-to-skin with blanket over both; used hat in cool room; delayed bathing until baby's temperature was warmer; kept extra layer on baby compared to layers for own comfort.

Key Index Words for Nursing Interventions

Look up these words in the index of fundamentals and medical-surgical nursing textbooks to find page references for additional nursing interventions and rationale for their selection:

■ children, temperature regulation
■ elderly: thermal regulation, temperature maintenance
■ fever, intermittent
■ infant, temperature maintenance (in maternal-child health text)
■ newborn, temperature maintenance (in maternal-child health text)
■ temperature, instability
■ vital signs, temperature

Chapter 15

Urinary/Voiding Problems

FOCUSED ASSESSMENT GUIDE

Complete this focused assessment if a general nursing assessment indicates a possible problem. Then turn to page 270 of this text for the Data ⇒ Diagnosis Matching Guide for urinary/voiding problems to help you select the best nursing diagnosis to match the client's data.

"TELL ME IF YOU ARE HAVING ANY OF THESE PROBLEMS:"

___ pain or difficulty urinating; trouble getting started or an interrupted stream
___ voiding in very small amounts (less than 100 mL) or very large amounts (more than 550 mL)
___ feeling like you have to urinate all the time
___ a full feeling in your bladder or like you're not emptying
___ voiding more often than every 2 hours or only 2–3 times a day
___ urinating two or more times a night or loss of urine while you sleep
___ loss of sensations related to emptying your bladder
___ health conditions or problems that you think are causing or are related to your urinary problem
___ urinary tract infections, burning, frequency, urgency
___ passing urine when you don't want to or before reaching a toilet; if yes:
    ___ Is there a strong urge to void before passing the urine or is client unaware of a need to void?

___ How long has it been going on?
___ Are there dry periods or a constant leaking?
___ Is client aware of passing urine at the time?
___ Is urine passed in small amounts and only with coughing, sneezing, laughing, or with exercise?
___ reasons for any previous urinary catheters
___ need help getting to the bathroom or on and off the toilet

OBSERVE FOR

___ abnormal I&O (pattern or amount) over last 24 hours
___ abnormal amounts and intervals for last 3–4 voidings
___ indwelling catheter or its removal in last few days
___ wetness under buttocks
___ distended bladder (if voiding small amounts frequently, no urination for last 5–6 hours, or report of feeling need to void but being unable to urinate)

ADULT NORMALS AND INFORMATION

- Normal voiding volume is 250–450 mL
- Voiding frequency is every 3–4 hours and 5–6 times/day (depending on fluid intake)
- Average urine output is 1500 mL/day; range 1000–2000 mL/day; more urine produced if fluid intake above average intake of 1300 mL
- Less urine is produced if client febrile (running a fever) and perspiring
- Fluids containing caffeine increase urine production
- Diuretics increase urine production
- Urine production is 40–80 mL/h; less than 30 mL/h is abnormal and should be reported to physician
- Adults usually sleep through the night without need to void (unless fluid intake is large before retiring); the need to void at night increases with aging
- Urine is sterile (no bacteria), clear, pale yellow, with no strong odor
- Urine is free of glucose, blood, ketones, and particulate matter

- Postvoiding residual urine (urine left in bladder after normal voiding) is minimal (approximately 5–10 mL); it is checked by inserting a catheter, draining out any remaining urine, and measuring the volume
- Activity and good muscle tone promote urinary function and control; immobility decreases bladder and sphincter tone and control
- Reflex for urination located in spinal cord at sacral level
- Any form of involuntary passage of urine (incontinence) is abnormal in adult
- Spinal/epidural anesthesia reduces or eliminates awareness of need to void and voluntary control of voiding

DATA ⇒ DIAGNOSIS MATCHING GUIDE

Compare your client data from the Urinary/Voiding Focused Assessment to these related urinary nursing diagnoses and abbreviated descriptions. Select the nursing diagnosis with the best match. Then turn to the page in this section with that specific diagnosis for help in planning care.

1. Altered Urinary Elimination (most general dx): page 274
- definition: a disturbance in urine elimination
- data: dysuria (painful or difficult urination); frequency (voiding more often than every 2 hours); hesitancy (difficulty or a delay in initiating voiding); incontinence (loss of control of urination); nocturia (excessive urination at night); retention (accumulation of urine in bladder because of inability to urinate or to empty bladder); urgency (feeling a strong and sudden need to void)

2. Stress Incontinence: page 281
- definition: a loss of urine less than 50 mL occurring with increased abdominal pressure
- data: loss of small dribble of urine occurs only with increased abdominal pressure (e.g., coughing, laughing, sneezing, strenuous exercise); nocturia (excessive urination at night) uncommon

3. *Reflex Incontinence: page 279*
   - definition: an involuntary loss of urine, occurring at somewhat predictable intervals when a specific bladder volume is reached
   - data: no awareness of bladder filling/full bladder; no urge to void; passes moderate amounts of urine at regular intervals; nocturia always present; increased postvoiding residual volumes; caused by spinal cord injuries/neurologic damage of nerve pathways to and from brain

4. *Urge Incontinence (most common in elderly): page 286*
   - definition: involuntary passage of urine occurring soon after a strong sense of urgency to void
   - data: client aware of very strong, sudden, unsuppressable need to void before passing urine; increased voiding frequency; nocturia present; minimal postvoiding residual volumes; associated with urinary tract infections, indwelling urinary catheters, bladder overfilling, alcohol, caffeine, and increased fluids

5. *Functional Incontinence: page 276*
   - definition: an involuntary, unpredictable passage of urine
   - data: client aware of urge to void; bladder contractions result in passage of urine before reaching a toilet; urinary system intact and functioning; incontinence caused by factors preventing client from reaching toilet/receptacle such as unfamiliar environment or sensory, cognitive and/or mobility deficits

6. *Total Incontinence (rare): page 284*
   - definition: continuous and unpredictable loss of urine
   - data: no strong urge to void; no awareness of bladder filling or emptying; constant flow of urine occurs day and night at unpredictable times; no bladder distention or increased postvoiding residual volumes; related to neurologic dysfunction or fistula (abnormal passageway for urine)

7. *Urinary Retention: page 289*
   - definition: incomplete emptying of the bladder

- data: inability to void; absence of urine output; bladder distention; small, frequent voidings (overflow voiding) with large amount of residual urine left in bladder because of inability to empty

8. *Toileting Self-Care Deficit: page 225 (in Self-Care Problem grouping)*
   - definition: an impaired ability to perform or complete toileting activities for oneself
   - data: unable to get to toilet/commode; unable to sit on or rise from toilet/commode; unable to manipulate clothing for toileting; unable to carry out needed toilet hygiene

GENERAL OUTCOMES AND NURSING INTERVENTIONS

GENERAL URINARY/VOIDING OUTCOMES

- Client will maintain normal urinary function and control.
- Client will regain normal urinary function and control.
- Client will regain previous level of urinary function and control.
- Client will stay free of urinary tract infections.
- Client will maintain urinary output of 1500 mL/day or more.
- Client will maintain urine output of 40 mL/h or more.
- Client will identify measures to promote normal urinary function.
- Client will empty bladder completely at regular intervals.
- Client will maintain postvoiding residual volumes below 50–100 mL.
- Client will state correct management of altered urinary function.
- Client will demonstrate correct use and care of any assistive devices needed to promote urinary function and control.

GENERAL URINARY/VOIDING NURSING INTERVENTIONS

- Demonstrate professionalism and understanding of client's situation to reduce embarrassment and/or stress; provide reassurance and support.

- Assess client's ability to get to the bathroom (use urinal, commode) and do own toileting hygiene; assist as needed.
- Assess client's voiding pattern over 48 hours and assist with toileting and bladder control based on voiding pattern.
- Assess client's knowledge and teach as needed related to tests, procedures, treatments, normal urinary functioning, promotion of optimum function, problem prevention, and new self-care skills such as self-catheterization or timed voidings.
- Measure and record intake and output (I&O); usually done every 4 hours, every shift and every 24 hours with totals starting and ending at 12:00 midnight.
- Observe urine color, odor, volume, and clarity every 2–4 hours.
- Report abnormal urinary and/or electrolyte data to charge nurse or physician.
- Assess client's medications for possible adverse reactions on urinary functioning; if present, discuss with physician.
- Increase fluid intake to >2000 mL/24 h unless contra-indicated.
- Encourage voiding every 3–4 hours.
- Prevent overdistention of bladder by promoting regular voiding or catheterizing if unable to void or empty (with physician's order).
- Administer antibiotics or other medications as ordered.
- Provide pain relief for urinary and other conditions.
- Provide privacy and adequate time to void (visitors out, curtains drawn, door shut, call light in reach).
- Encourage client to void in usual position whenever possible (male client standing, female client sitting on toilet/bedside commode).
- Raise the head of the bed for bedpan or urinal use.
- Keep client clean and dry; assess skin for signs of irritation and intervene to prevent damage/breakdown.
- Assist to turn, reposition, transfer to chair, and walk if urinary drainage system is in place to prevent backflow into bladder and/or interrupted urine drainage.
- Urinary incontinence may be treated with behavioral techniques such as bladder training, page 283, habit training (timed voiding), page 280, or pelvic muscle

exercise, page 283. Pharmacologic and surgical treatment may also be used.

- Assess postvoiding residual urine volume (physician's order) immediately after client voids.
- Condom catheters may be used for male incontinence to prevent skin breakdown or if bladder retraining is not successful.
- Irrigate catheter system to maintain patency if urine flow seems obstructed with clots or sediment (physician's order).
- Discontinue indwelling urinary catheters as soon as possible to reduce risk of infection and loss of bladder tone.

RELATED NURSING DIAGNOSES

ALTERED URINARY ELIMINATION

Definition
A state in which an individual experiences a disturbance in urine elimination.

Defining Characteristics
- dysuria (painful or difficult urination)
- frequency (voiding more often than every 2 hours)
- hesitancy (a delay or difficulty in initiating voiding)
- incontinence (loss of control of urination)
- nocturia (excessive urination at night)
- retention (accumulation of urine in the bladder because of inability to empty or inability to urinate)
- urgency (a strong, sudden need to void)

Other Characteristics
- increased or decreased force of stream
- change in amount, color, or odor of urine
- bladder distention

Related Factors
- anatomical obstruction (e.g., enlarged prostate; swelling)
- sensory/motor impairment
- urinary tract infection

Examples of Specific Nursing Diagnoses

1. Altered urinary elimination related to perineal swelling and loss of sensation secondary to episiotomy and epidural anesthesia.

   Altered urinary elimination related to perineal swelling and loss of sensation secondary to episiotomy and epidural anesthesia as evidenced by difficulty initiating voiding, bladder distention, no voiding for 6 hours. (PES format)

2. Altered urinary elimination related to urinary tract infection and increased fluid intake

   Altered urinary elimination related to urinary tract infection and increased fluid intake as evidenced by client's report of urgency, burning with urination, and frequent voiding pattern of every 1–2 hours. (PES format)

Examples of Specific Outcomes

1. Client to void at least 300 mL within 6 hours of surgery.
2. Client will report return of normal urinary elimination pattern 12 hours post-op.
3. Client to report absence of burning and urgency within 24 hours of initiation of antibiotic therapy.
4. Client completely empties bladder with next voiding as evidenced by postvoiding residual urine of less than 50 mL.

Examples of Specific Nursing Interventions

- See General Urinary/Voiding Nursing Interventions, page 272.
- Reduce or prevent anatomical obstruction (e.g., cold and heat to reduce/prevent swelling; positioning; removal of fecal impaction).
- Reduce or overcome sensory and mobility deficits (e.g., increased lighting, hearing aids, glasses; unobstructed path to bathroom, siderails down if safe, handrails, easily removed clothing, bed trapeze, urinal or bedside commode, offering assistance every 2–4 hours).
- Prevent or eliminate urinary tract infection (e.g., increase fluid intake to 2000–3000 mL; wipe front to back for females; give antibiotic therapy as ordered by physician; increase mobility to promote bladder tone; position

standing for males, sitting for females to promote complete emptying of bladder; encourage voiding every 2–4 hours).

Examples of Specific Evaluations for Outcomes 1 to 4
1. Outcome met. Client voided 450 mL five hours post-op.
2. Outcome partially met. Client voiding 250–400 mL of urine every 3–4 hours but still reports some difficulty initiating urination.
3. Outcome not met. Client continues to report burning and urgency after 24 hours on antibiotics.
4. Outcome met. Client catheterized for residual of 40 mL after voiding.

Key Index Words for Nursing Interventions
Look up these words in the index of fundamentals and medical-surgical nursing textbooks to find page references for additional nursing interventions and rationale for their selection:

- anuria
- catheter, urinary
- dysuria
- elimination, urinary
- micturition
- nocturia
- oliguria
- polyuria
- urination
- urinary frequency
- urinary hesitancy
- urinary incontinence
- urinary retention
- urinary urgency

Case Management Example:
See Appendix for an example of a nursing diagnosis of Altered Urinary Elimination within a clinical pathway, DRG 209, Total Hip Replacement, page 474.

FUNCTIONAL INCONTINENCE

Definition
A state in which an individual experiences an involuntary, unpredictable passage of urine.

Major Defining Characteristics
- urge to void or bladder contractions sufficiently strong to result in loss of urine before reaching an appropriate receptacle

Other Characteristics
- voiding in moderate to large amounts
- client aware of urge to void
- voiding at irregular intervals (no pattern to incontinence)
- nocturia (excessive urination at night) may be present

Related Factors
Causes of incontinence are factors that prevent client from reaching bathroom or appropriate receptacle rather than problems with the urinary system.
- altered environment (e.g., no access, long distance, poor lighting, call light out of reach, lack of available help, unanswered call light)
- sensory, cognitive, or mobility deficits (e.g., casts, drugs, or medications, head injury, confusion, paralysis, arthritis, restraints)

Examples of Specific Nursing Diagnoses
1. Functional incontinence related to mental confusion at night; difficulty using nurse call for help to bathroom.
   Functional incontinence related to mental confusion at night; difficulty using nurse call for help to bathroom as evidenced by bed wet with urine at every 4-hour assessment, calling out for help to find bathroom. (PES format)
2. Functional incontinence related to post-op anesthesia effects, decreased level of consciousness and impaired mobility secondary to hip replacement surgery.
   Functional incontinence related to post-op anesthesia effects, decreased level of consciousness and impaired mobility secondary to hip replacement surgery as evidenced by incontinence 2–3 times a shift since catheter removed, reports urge to void but "can't get to toilet." (PES format)

Examples of Specific Outcomes
1. Client experiences return of urinary continence on the third post-op day.
2. Client to remain continent during the night by discharge.
3. Client to use call light for help to the bathroom for voiding urge once this shift.
4. Client to use urinal for all voidings this shift.

Examples of Specific Nursing Interventions
- See General Urinary/Voiding Nursing Interventions, page 272.
- Alleviate the specific related factors preventing the client from reaching the toilet or appropriate receptacle.

    Adapt room and bathroom/toilet facilities to altered mobility needs (e.g., bed trapeze, urinal within reach, siderails down if safe, handrails, raised toilet seat).

    Leave bathroom light on at night; adequate room lighting.

    Call light in reach; prompt answering of all call lights.

    Prevent oversedation with pain medications/sleeping pills.

    Help client select clothing with simple fasteners; easily removable clothing to facilitate toileting.

- Encourage client to void every 2–3 hours; volunteer assistance at these intervals.
- Assess timing of bed-wetting and offer bedpan/urinal 30 minutes before that time (especially for nighttime wetting).
- Use of condom catheter to prevent wetness/skin breakdown.

Examples of Specific Evaluations for Outcomes 1 to 4
1. Outcome partially met. Client continent during day but incontinent at night, especially after pain medication.
2. Outcome met. Client continent all night using urinal when room light left on low and urinal placed on bedside stand.
3. Outcome not met. Client incontinent for all voidings this shift. Client remains confused and disoriented to time and place and unable to use call light.
4. Outcome met. Client left urinal in place and caught all voidings. Client able to call nurse to report two voidings.

Key Index Words for Nursing Interventions
Look up these words in the index of fundamentals and medical-surgical nursing textbooks to find page references for additional nursing interventions and rationale for their selection:

- catheter: condom, indwelling, intermittent
- incontinence, functional

REFLEX INCONTINENCE

Definition
A state in which an individual experiences an involuntary loss of urine, occurring at somewhat predictable intervals when a specific bladder volume is reached.

Major Defining Characteristics
- no awareness of bladder filling
- no urge to void or feelings of bladder fullness
- uninhibited bladder contractions/spasms at regular intervals

Other Characteristics
- moderate amount of urine passed
- nocturia (excessive urination at night) always present
- unaware of incontinence
- dry periods between voidings
- increased postvoiding residual urine volumes
- sympathetic response to full bladder before reflex voiding (e.g., perspiration, coldness in hands/feet, anxiety)

Related Factors
- neurological impairment (e.g., spinal cord lesion, tumors or degenerative changes above sacral region)

Examples of Specific Nursing Diagnoses
1. Reflex incontinence related to spinal cord injury.
   Reflex incontinence related to spinal cord injury as evidenced by involuntary passage of 250–400 mL of urine every 3–4 hours with no awareness of bladder filling, voiding urge, or urination. (PES format)
2. Reflex incontinence related to congenital spina bifida.
   Reflex incontinence related to congenital spina bifida as evidenced by involuntary passage of 100–250 mL of urine every 3–4 hours with no awareness of urination or need to void and no history of previous bladder control. (PES format)

Examples of Specific Outcomes
1. Client to remain continent by voiding every 4–6 hours in amounts no greater than 400 mL with postvoiding residual volumes less than 100 mL by discharge.

2. Client states signs and symptoms of a full bladder (when normal bladder sensation is absent) by discharge.
3. Client remains free of urinary tract infections during first 3 months of home management.
4. Client remains free of urinary stone formation for the next year.
5. Client correctly demonstrates self-catheterization using clean technique by the end of this week.

Examples of Specific Nursing Interventions

■ See General Urinary/Voiding Interventions, page 272.
■ Initiate habit training for voidings (timed voiding schedule).

> Keep voiding incontinence record for 72 hours to identify voiding frequency and timing related to fluid intake/meals.
> Teach techniques to elicit voiding reflex: stimulating skin in genital area; stroking inner thigh; digital stimulation of anal sphincter; assess effectiveness.
> Develop timed voiding schedule with client to match natural voiding pattern, fluid intake, and lifestyle; encourage client to void on this schedule.
> Instruct client not to resist urge or try to delay voidings (as in bladder training) since bladder overdistention is a common problem.
> Adapt timing of voidings to achieve volumes of no more than 400 mL at each voiding and no incontinence.
> Teach ways to promote complete emptying: sitting position, use of Valsalva maneuver; Crede's maneuver (check with physician first for client's safety).
> Assess effectiveness of bladder emptying by intermittent catheterization for postvoiding residual volume since incomplete emptying is a common problem.

■ Catheterize intermittently every 3–6 hours or use indwelling catheter to drain urine and prevent bladder distention (based on physician's order).
■ Encourage activity/mobility with early ambulation, tilt table, wheelchair.
■ Specify low calcium diet (to help prevent renal calculi/stones).

- Administer medications ordered by physician to increase contraction of bladder smooth muscle (e.g., urecholine).
- Teach client how to prevent bladder overdistention and risk of dysreflexia (see Dysreflexia, page 155).
- Teach self-catheterization skill using clean technique.
- Explain availability of absorbent products and incontinence underwear to manage incontinence.

Examples of Specific Evaluations for Outcomes 1 to 5

1. Outcome met. Client remaining continent and voiding 300–375 mL every 4–6 hours by applying pressure over bladder; less than 50 mL of residual urine after the last three voidings.
2. Outcome met. Client states perspiration, anxious feeling, and coldness of hands or feet as signs and symptoms of full bladder.
3. Outcome not met. Urinary tract infection developed and antibiotic therapy initiated.
4. Outcome partially met. No stones have formed after 6 months.
5. Outcome partially met. Successful at self-catheterizing most of the day but having trouble in the evening when fatigued.

Key Index Words for Nursing Interventions

Look up these words in the index of fundamentals and medical-surgical nursing textbooks to find page references for additional nursing interventions and rationale for their selection:

- automatic bladder
- bladder: flaccid, neurogenic, spastic, hypertonic
- bladder retraining program, habit training
- Crede's maneuver
- dysreflexia
- residual urine
- spinal cord injury, urinary problems and management

STRESS INCONTINENCE

Definition

A state in which an individual experiences a loss of urine less than 50 mL, occurring with increased abdominal pressure.

Major Defining Characteristics
- reported or observed dribbling with increased abdominal pressure (e.g., coughing, laughing, sneezing, exercise)

Minor Defining Characteristics
- urinary urgency (sudden with increased abdominal pressure)
- urinary frequency (more than every 2 hours)

Other Characteristics
- nocturia uncommon (excessive urination at night)
- aware of incontinence
- voiding habits normal with the exception of stress-induced incontinence
- postvoiding residual volume normal (minimal)

Related Factors
- degenerative changes in pelvic muscles and structural supports associated with increased age
- high intra-abdominal pressure (e.g., obesity, pregnancy)
- incompetent bladder outlet, unable to remain closed (e.g., prostate surgery, pelvic fracture, genitourinary surgery)
- overdistention (of bladder) between voidings
- weak pelvic muscles and structural supports

Other Related Factors
- estrogen deficiency
- multiple pregnancies; traumatic deliveries

Examples of Specific Nursing Diagnoses
1. Stress incontinence related to third trimester pregnancy. Stress incontinence related to third trimester pregnancy as evidenced by reports of urine leakage in the last month of pregnancy when laughing, coughing, or sneezing. (PES format)
2. Stress incontinence related to aging and generalized weakness. Stress incontinence related to aging and generalized weakness as evidenced by reports of increased passage of urine with laughing, sneezing, coughing over last 2 years beginning around age 78; emaciated appearance with reports of weight loss and weakness. (PES format)

Examples of Specific Outcomes
1. Stress incontinence resolved 6 weeks following birth of baby.
2. Client states ways to minimize passage of urine and ways to manage the incontinence by end of clinic visit.
3. Client regains complete bladder control within 6 months.
4. Client voids every 2 hours with no stress incontinence on first day of bladder training program.

Examples of Specific Nursing Interventions
■ See General Urinary/Voiding Nursing Interventions, page 272.
■ Teach and encourage use of pelvic muscle exercises (Kegels).
   Help client locate the muscle group by contracting muscles used to stop flow of urine without contracting abdomen, buttocks, or inner thigh.
   Contract the pelvic muscles for a period up to 10 seconds and relax for 10 seconds; repeat several times.
   Perform pelvic muscle exercises 30–80 times per day for at least 6 weeks; may need to continue indefinitely.
   Use exercises prior to and during situations where urine leaking may occur.

■ Discuss and initiate bladder training.
   Client voids on a set schedule, every 2–3 hours initially rather than waiting for urge to void.
   Voiding interval is gradually increased.
   Client encouraged to delay voiding and resist urge.
■ Explain and administer medications ordered to prevent/improve stress incontinence (e.g., phenylpropanolamine, estrogen replacement therapy, imipramine).
■ Use preoperative teaching and postoperative management if surgical repair is done.
■ Discuss use of absorbent shields or undergarments to manage urine for high risk times (e.g., when client has a cold, during exercise, or out socially).
■ Encourage to avoid long periods of standing.
■ Encourage walking and general body conditioning.
■ Discuss and implement weight loss program if obese.

Examples of Specific Evaluations for Outcomes 1 to 4
1. Outcome met. Client states complete return of bladder control at 6-week follow-up visit.
2. Outcome met. Client identified ways to reduce pressure on bladder when coughing, sneezing, and laughing and states she will wear minipad when she is out in case of incontinence.
3. Outcome partially met. Client states incontinence episodes less frequent with less urine released but still a problem.
4. Outcome not met. Client voiding every 2 hours but had two incontinent episodes when coughing in a standing position.

Key Index Words for Nursing Interventions
Look up these words in the index of fundamentals and medical-surgical nursing textbooks to find page references for additional nursing interventions and rationale for their selection:

- bladder training; retraining
- Kegel exercises
- incontinence, stress
- pelvic muscle exercises (pubococcygeus muscle)
- stress incontinence
- urinary incontinence

TOTAL INCONTINENCE

Definition
A state in which an individual experiences a continuous and unpredictable loss of urine. (rare)

Major Defining Characteristics
- constant (or near constant) flow of urine
- urine passed at unpredictable times without distention or uninhibited bladder contractions/spasms
- unsuccessful incontinence treatments
- nocturia present (excessive urination at night)

Minor Defining Characteristics
- lack of perineal or bladder-filling awareness
- unaware of incontinence

Other Characteristics
- no awareness of urge to void
- no dry periods
- little or no postvoiding residual urine volumes

Related Factors
- neuropathy (nerve damage) preventing transmission of reflex indicating bladder fullness (e.g., prostate surgery, perineal surgery, trauma, radiation, spinal cord tumors)
- neurological dysfunction causing triggering of micturition (voiding) at unpredictable times (e.g., multiple sclerosis)
- independent contraction of detrusor (bladder) reflex
- trauma or disease affecting spinal cord nerves
- anatomic (e.g., urinary fistula, which is an abnormal passage or opening from the urinary tract; congenital defects)

Examples of Specific Nursing Diagnoses
1. Total incontinence related to prostate surgery.
   Total incontinence related to prostate surgery as evidenced by client's report of post-op development of continuous uncontrollable dribbling of urine. (PES format)
2. Total incontinence related to fistula, urethral lacerations secondary to assisted obstetrical delivery of 12-lb baby.
   Total incontinence related to fistula, urethral lacerations secondary to assisted obstetrical delivery of 12-lb baby as evidenced by involuntary passage of urine with massage of uterus, urine mixed with vaginal blood on Kotex pad at every assessment; no urge to void or sense of bladder filling. (PES format)

Examples of Specific Outcomes
1. Client states understanding of cause of post-op urinary incontinence and identifies ways to reduce and manage the dribbling by end of shift.
2. Client experiences return of complete continence by discharge following repair of urinary fistula.
3. Client experiences return of normal bladder control by 6 months post-op.
4. Client maintains maximum dryness without skin breakdown or use of indwelling catheter for remainder of stay in nursing home.

Examples of Specific Nursing Interventions

- See General Urinary/Voiding Nursing Interventions, page 272.
- Assess every 2 hours for wetness and encourage voiding attempt.
- Teach pelvic muscle exercises (Kegels): tighten muscles as if to stop urine stream and hold for 10 seconds; relax for 10 seconds and repeat several times; repeat 30–80 times a day for 6 weeks or indefinitely.
- Use incontinence pads and underwear to control wetness.
- Use condom catheter to control wetness.
- Provide postoperative care for fistula repair; urinary surgery.
- Assess skin every 4 hours; use good skin care to prevent breakdown (see Specific Nursing Interventions for High Risk for Impaired Skin Integrity, page 247).

Examples of Specific Evaluations for Outcomes 1 to 3

1. Outcome partially met. Client states understanding of cause but is very upset and angry; refusing to consider ways to manage dribbling at this point in time.
2. Outcome met. Post-op fistula repaired; client is voiding every 2–3 hours, small to moderate amounts of urine with no periods of incontinence.
3. Outcome partially met. Six months post-op, client reports no dribbling urine except when laughing or coughing.

Key Index Words for Nursing Interventions

Look up these words in the index of fundamentals and medical-surgical nursing textbooks to find page references for additional nursing interventions and rationale for their selection:

- incontinence, total
- Kegel exercises
- pelvic muscle exercises
- prostate surgery: TURP, prostatectomy

URGE INCONTINENCE

Definition

A state in which an individual experiences involuntary passage of urine occurring soon after a strong sense of urgency to void. (most common form of incontinence in elderly)

Major Defining Characteristics
- urinary urgency (very sudden, strong need to void)
- frequency (voiding more often than every 2 hours)
- bladder contractions/spasms (results in urine flow client cannot stop)

Minor Defining Characteristics
- nocturia common (excessive urination at night)
- voiding in small amounts (less than 100 mL) or in large amounts (more than 550 mL)
- inability to reach toilet in time

Other Characteristics
- client aware of full bladder and incontinence
- loss of urine in any position (lying, sitting, standing)
- minimal postvoiding residual volumes

Related Factors
- decreased bladder capacity (e.g., history of PID, abdominal surgeries, bladder tumors, indwelling urinary catheters; fecal impaction)
- irritation of bladder stretch receptors causing spasm (e.g., bladder infection, concentrated urine)
- alcohol; caffeine; increased fluids
- overdistention of bladder (from diuretics, increased intake and/or decreased frequency of voiding)

Other Related Factors
- neurologic disorders (e.g., Alzheimer's disease, Parkinson's disease, stroke, multiple sclerosis, brain tumor)

Examples of Specific Nursing Diagnoses
1. Urge incontinence related to discontinuation of indwelling catheter, increased fluid intake, and large coffee intake.
   Urge incontinence related to discontinuation of indwelling catheter, increased fluid intake, and large coffee intake as evidenced by report of sense of urgency with involuntary passage of 75–100 mL of urine every hour. (PES format)
2. Urge incontinence related to urinary tract infection.
   Urge incontinence related to urinary tract infection as evidenced by report of urgency followed by passage of small amounts of urine every 1–2 hours. (PES format)

Examples of Specific Outcomes
1. Client delays voiding until places urinal once this shift.
2. Client delays all voidings until reaches toilet by discharge.
3. Client voids 250–400 mL every 2–5 hours in toilet by discharge with no incontinence.
4. Client experiences return of normal voiding pattern 48 hours after initiation of antibiotic therapy for urinary tract infection.

Examples of Specific Nursing Interventions
■ See General Urinary/Voiding Nursing Interventions, page 272.
■ Select interventions to reduce or eliminate the related factors causing the incontinence whenever possible.
    Discuss ways to prevent urinary tract infections.
    Discuss ways to prevent concentrated urine by increasing fluid intake to >2000 mL/day.
    Administer ordered antibiotic therapy.
    Manage fecal impaction; prevent recurrence by promoting normal bowel function.
    Before discontinuing an indwelling catheter, clamp for 1–3 hours and release; repeat several times to help restore bladder tone and increase bladder capacity.
    Prevent bladder overdistention by catheterizing client as needed (physician's order).
■ Administer medications ordered to improve urge incontinence (e.g., propantheline, oxybutynin, tricyclic antidepressants, terodiline).
■ Use of a condom catheter continuously or at night to prevent wetness or skin breakdown.
■ Place urinal within reach of male client or between the legs with penis inside urinal.
■ Discuss and initiate bladder training.
    Client voids on a set schedule, every 1–2 hours initially rather than waiting for urge to void.
    Voiding interval gradually increased as bladder capacity increases and ability to delay urge improves.
    Client encouraged to delay voiding and resist urge.
■ Teach and encourage pelvic muscle exercises, Kegels, page 283.
■ Decrease fluid consumption prior to bedtime.
■ Encourage client to limit use of caffeine and alcohol.

Examples of Specific Evaluations for Outcomes 1 to 4

1. Outcome not met. Client unable to position urinal before passing urine for both voidings this shift.
2. Outcome partially met. Client able to void in bathroom during day but requires urinal at night to prevent incontinence.
3. Outcome met. Client voiding normal volumes every 2–4 hours in bathroom with no incontinence at discharge.
4. Outcome met. Client reports no burning, frequency, or small voidings this shift on second day of antibiotic therapy.

Key Index Words for Nursing Interventions

Look up these words in the index of fundamentals and medical-surgical nursing textbooks to find page references for additional nursing interventions and rationale for their selection:

- bladder: training, retraining
- catheter, condom or condom catheter
- incontinence, urge or urge incontinence
- pelvic muscle exercises (Kegels)
- unstable bladder

URINARY RETENTION

Definition

A state in which an individual experiences incomplete emptying of the bladder. (common postoperatively or postdelivery of newborn)

Major Defining Characteristics

- bladder distention
- small, frequent voidings or absence of urine output

Minor Defining Characteristics

- sensation of full bladder
- dribbling
- large postvoiding residual urine volume (100–150 mL or more measured by catheterization after client voids)
- dysuria (reports difficulty starting, interrupted stream, or decreased force of stream)

- overflow incontinence (involuntary loss of urine related to overdistention of bladder from urinary retention; client has continuous or intermittent leakage of urine)

Other Characteristics
- any decrease in urine output (or output less than intake)
- restless, diaphoretic (sweaty)

Related Factors
- high urethral pressure caused by weak detrusor (smooth muscles of bladder responsible for emptying)
- inhibition of reflex arc (e.g., anxiety, stress, pain, general/spinal anesthesia, surgery, medications)
- strong sphincter
- blockage (e.g., enlarged prostate, fecal impaction, swelling of urinary meatus, hemorrhoids, pressure from baby's head during labor)

Other Related Factors
- spinal cord injury
- multiple sclerosis
- herniated disks
- alcoholism

Examples of Specific Nursing Diagnoses
1. Urinary retention related to surgical anesthesia, absence of voiding urge, and no sensations of full bladder.
   Urinary retention related to surgical anesthesia, absence of voiding urge, and no sensations of full bladder as evidenced by no voiding for 6 hours, distended bladder. (PES format)
2. Urinary retention related to urethral swelling and bladder overdistention.
   Urinary retention related to urethral swelling and bladder overdistention as evidenced by inability to void for 5 hours, continuous sensation of full bladder with bladder distention for last hour. (PES format)

Examples of Specific Outcomes
1. Client to void at least 300 mL within the next 4 hours.
2. Residual urine to be less than 100 mL following next voiding.
3. Resolution of bladder distention by end of shift.
4. Output of 1500 mL without catheterization by 2/21.

Examples of Specific Nursing Interventions
- See General Urinary/Voiding Nursing Interventions, page 272.
- Nurse-initiated I&O when retention suspected.
- Relieve pain and anxiety that can inhibit voiding reflex.
- Administer medications to correct retention (e.g., urecholine may be ordered on prn basis for high risk clients).
- Run water in bathroom; soak hand in warm water during voiding attempt; instruct client to deep breathe and relax with an exhale and allow voiding to occur.
- Have client try to void in warm sitz bath/bathtub/shower.
- Pour warm water over perineum and let it drain into toilet (bedpan, commode) as client trys to void.
- Warm bedpan by running warm water over it before offering to client (cold can inhibit voiding).
- Encourage client to apply gentle pressure over lower abdomen during voiding attempt (Crede's maneuver) if no obstruction present that is preventing flow of urine.
- Have client try Valsalva maneuver while attempting to void (if discussed and approved by physician).
- Have client try to double-void (after passing urine, continue to sit on toilet while relaxing and try to void again).
- Insert indwelling catheter if unable to void (physician's order); catheterize before bladder overdistended.
- Catheterize to assess postvoiding residual urine volume; if greater than 100–150 mL physician may direct nurse to leave catheter in for 24 hours or a specific time period.

Examples of Specific Evaluations for Outcomes 1 to 4
1. Outcome met. Client voided 500 mL in an interrupted flow pattern over 5 minutes on toilet.
2. Outcome not met. Client catheterized for residual of 400 mL after last voiding.
3. Outcome partially met. Bladder distention is less after voiding of 250 mL but still palpable; with external pressure over bladder area client reports urge to void.
4. Outcome not met. Client unable to void and indwelling catheter inserted for 24 hours; 24-hour output of 1800 mL.

Key Index Words for Nursing Interventions

Look up these words in the index of fundamentals and medical-surgical nursing textbooks to find page references for additional nursing interventions and rationale for their selection:

- dysuria
- micturition
- overflow incontinence (outflow incontinence or overflow)
- residual urine
- retention, urinary
- urinary retention
- urecholine (bethanechol chloride)

PART 2

PSYCHOSOCIAL PROBLEMS

Chapter 16

Communication, Thinking, and Knowledge Problems

FOCUSED ASSESSMENT GUIDE

Complete this focused assessment if a general nursing assessment indicates a possible problem. Then turn to page 296 of this text for the Data ⇒ Diagnosis Matching Guide for Communication, Thinking, and Knowledge related problems to help you select the best nursing diagnosis to match the client's data.

FROM YOUR CONVERSATION WITH THE CLIENT NOTE IF ANY OF THE FOLLOWING ARE PRESENT

____ unable to speak English (or dominant language in health care facility)
____ speaks with difficulty
____ great effort to speak
____ speech accompanied by facial confusion
____ words unclear
____ inappropriate response to questions
____ stuttering or slurring of words
____ repetition of same word, e.g., "I, I…" or "No, no, no!" with increasing frustration
____ hallucinations
____ delusions (fixed false belief)

___ memory problems

    As a test for intermediate memory ask, "What did you have for dinner last night?"

    As a test for short term memory, "Repeat the following: 6-9-2-1-8-4, 2-1-9-7-1-3."

___ client unusually distracted by events/persons outside the immediate conversation, for example, client's eyes follow someone walking past the door or client focuses on roommate's television despite being asked a direct question.

___ client asks questions about health problem or treatment

___ client unable to perform self-care procedures

___ inaccurate statement of health problem cause and/or treatment

___ inaccurate or unsafe performance of self-care procedure

DATA ⇒ DIAGNOSIS MATCHING GUIDE

Compare your client data from the Communication, Thinking, and Knowledge Focused Assessment to these related diagnoses and abbreviated descriptions. Select the nursing diagnosis which is the best match. Then turn to the page in this section with that specific diagnosis for help in planning care.

1. *Altered Thought Processes: page 298*
   - definition: client experiences difficulty in interpreting and making sense out of stimuli in the environment; may hallucinate (see things that are not there), may be easily distracted
   - data: inaccurate interpretation of environment; cognitive dissonance (conflicting beliefs and attitudes); distractibility; memory deficit problems; egocentricity (self-centered), hyper/hypovigilance (alertness)

2. *Knowledge/Skill Deficit* (Specify): page 300*
   - definition: to be developed by NANDA
   - data: client statement, behavior, or skill demonstration indicates a lack of knowledge or skill necessary for self-care or coping with health problem

---

*Note that the present authors include skill deficit in this diagnosis.

3. Impaired Verbal Communication: page 303
  - definition: decreased or absent ability to speak or understand language
  - data: problems speaking or understanding

GENERAL OUTCOMES AND NURSING INTERVENTIONS

GENERAL COMMUNICATION, THINKING, AND KNOWLEDGE OUTCOMES

- Client is safe and unharmed within health care environment.
- Client is able to communicate needs either verbally or using alternative methods without frustration.
- Client is oriented to time, person, and place.
- Client requests (or accepts) health care information necessary for self-care or informed decision-making.
- Client practices/demonstrates skills necessary for self-care under the supervision of the registered nurse.
- Client will accurately interpret stimuli (visual, auditory, tactile) within the environment.

GENERAL COMMUNICATION, THINKING, AND KNOWLEDGE NURSING INTERVENTIONS

- Maintain client in safe environment. The first responsibility of the nurse is to provide for this most basic need. For some clients, this may mean the use of restraints, tranquilizing medications, a room with decreased stimulation, and careful evaluation of all items that might be harmful to the client such as shoelaces, razor blades, and electrical appliances.
- Frequent reorientation to reality: time, date, place, person. ("This is Tuesday at 8 o'clock in the morning. You are in the hospital and I am your nurse, Ms. Smith.") Use of calendars, open shades, dressed if appropriate to setting.
- Assess client current level of understanding to determine beginning point for further teaching.
- Assess cultural implications for planning care and teaching the client.

- Plan and implement teaching plan.
- Consider and select various teaching modalities: videos, pamphlets, written instructions, demonstration/return demonstration.

RELATED NURSING DIAGNOSES

ALTERED THOUGHT PROCESSES

Definition
A state in which an individual experiences a disruption in cognitive operations and activities.

Defining Characteristics
- inaccurate interpretation of environment
- cognitive dissonance
- distractibility
- memory deficit/problems
- egocentricity
- hyper- or hypovigilance

Other Possible Characteristics
- Inappropriate nonreality-based thinking

Related Factors
- To be developed by NANDA

Examples of Specific Nursing Diagnoses
1. Altered thought process related to Alzheimer's disease.
   Altered thought process related to Alzheimer's disease as manifested by absentmindedness, neglectful appearance, loss of memory. (PES format)
2. Altered thought process related to schizophrenia.
   Altered though process related to schizophrenia as manifested by auditory and visual hallucinations. (PES format)

Examples of Specific Outcomes
1. Client will remain safe from harm throughout hospitalization.
2. Client will perform activities of daily living (ADLs) with supervision by discharge.

3. Client will be able to accurately interpret environmental stimuli, (i.e., client will not experience auditory or visual hallucinations) by discharge.
4. Client will be able to watch a 30-minute television show of choice, and comment appropriately on the content, by discharge.

Examples of Specific Nursing Interventions

■ See General Communication, Thinking, and Knowledge Nursing Interventions, page 297.
■ Provide permanent identification and emergency information in the form of identity band on the client.
■ Assess and remove from the environment objects that could be potentially dangerous to the client, for example, shade or blind cords, razor blades, electric appliances, glass or hard plastic objects, pens/pencils, scissors, bathrobe belts, silverware.
■ Place a sign on the door (JIM'S ROOM) in large clear letters (if appropriate).
■ Decrease any excess stimulation in the environment, for example, one visitor at a time, television, printed instructions or rules.
■ Limit choices/decision-making to "this or that" (e.g., apple or orange).
■ Assist/supervise client in activities of daily living (bathing, brushing teeth, eating, toileting, exercise).
■ Provide consistent caregiver.
■ Speak slowly with simple sentences; do not speak louder!
■ Avoid use of touch as intervention (this could be very frightening to the client who is misinterpreting environmental stimuli) unless client is in contact with reality.
■ Establish a routine for sleep hygiene; client may shower, have a snack, a medication, read in bed for 30 minutes, then turn off lights and provide quiet.
■ Provide "picture" directions if reading or following verbal instructions is difficult, for example, a picture of handwashing in the bathroom.
■ Reorient to reality prn, "This is Tuesday morning and you are in the hospital. I am Ms. Jones, your nurse."

Examples of Specific Evaluations for Outcomes 1 to 4

1. Outcome met. Client remained safe throughout hospitalization.

2. Outcome partially met. Client can bathe self but needs assistance with hair washing and toileting.

3. Outcome met. Client does not report any incidence of hallucinations.

4. Outcome partially met. Client able to remain seated to watch TV for 30 minutes but cannot comment on content of program.

Key Index Words for Nursing Interventions

Look up these words in the index of fundamentals and medical-surgical nursing textbooks to find page references for additional nursing interventions and rationale for their selection:

- Alzheimer's disease
- delusion
- hallucinations, auditory
- hallucinations, visual
- organic brain syndrome
- safety (physical need)
- schizophrenia
- senile dementia
- substance abuse
- suicide

KNOWLEDGE/SKILL DEFICIT (SPECIFY)

Definition

To be developed (NANDA). (Defined by present authors.) A state in which the client or significant others does not have sufficient information or understanding of the health problem needed to make informed decisions about health care and treatment. Or the client or significant others lack the skills necessary to provide self-care for a specific health problem.

Defining Characteristics

- verbalization of problem
- inaccurate follow-through of instructions
- inaccurate performance on test
- inappropriate or exaggerated behaviors (e.g., hysterical, hostile, agitated, or apathetic)

Related Factors

- lack of exposure
- information misinterpretation
- cognitive limitation (low IQ)

■ lack of interest in learning
■ unfamiliarity with information sources
■ lack of recall

Examples of Specific Nursing Diagnoses
1. Knowledge deficit (low fat diet) related to lack of correct information.
   Knowledge deficit (low fat diet) related to lack of correct information as evidenced by client statement, "That is something I really am confused about and I want to try to eat a healthier diet." (PES format)
2. Skill deficit (self-administration of insulin) related to new diagnosis.
   Skill deficit (self-administration of insulin) related to new diagnosis as evidenced by client statement, "I will have to learn to give my own insulin if I want to be able to continue to travel for my job." (PES format)

Examples of Specific Outcomes
1. Client will plan 7 days of menus which meet the requirements for a low fat diet within 72 hours using menu selector pamphlet.
2. Client will demonstrate self-administration of insulin using sterile technique by 3/23.
3. Client will demonstrate all available sites for insulin injection and describe site rotation procedure by discharge.

Examples of Specific Nursing Interventions
■ See General Communication, Thinking, and Knowledge Nursing Interventions, page 297.
■ Assess client's current level of knowledge or skill. This is always the place to begin a teaching plan and will assist the nurse in determining an appropriate starting point. The nurse might ask the following questions of a client newly diagnosed with diabetes:

> How has diabetes affected you?
> What have you had to do to take care of yourself since you got diabetes?
> What do you notice when you begin to have an insulin reaction?
> Could you show me how you give yourself your insulin?

What do you look for on your body when you shower/bathe?

- Assess the cognitive abilities (ability to learn) of the client. Do not equate formal education with ability to learn or to master motor skills. Include an assessment of cultural factors which may require adaptation of teaching process.
- Assess readiness of the client to learn. If clients refuse to acknowledge their disease, they may be unwilling to learn to cope with it.
- Assess anxiety level of the client; some anxiety interferes with learning.
- Provide client with an opportunity to verbalize anxiety and deal with it before attempting to teach. "Can you tell me what bothers you about having to take insulin?"
- Ask what the client would like to learn about health care while in the hospital.
- Determine if significant others/family members want/need to be included in the teaching plan.
- Determine what the client needs to learn (scope) and in what order (sequence).
- Prioritize learning needs. First, what does the client need to maintain physical safety? Next, what does the client need to enhance quality of life?
- Divide content of instruction into logical groupings or classes. The client may be able to tolerate only brief instructions due to physical limitations.
- Match method of instruction to content and client preference: audiotapes, videotapes, one-to-one instruction, demonstrations, books or pamphlets, etc.
- Schedule teaching sessions with client and family or significant others. Select a time when client is rested, free from pain, and distractions are minimized.
- If teaching a skill, plan the steps in the procedure and demonstrate to the client in stages (not beginning to end but rather four or five steps at a time). Provide the opportunity for the client to practice each stage before proceeding to the next stage.
- Provide the client with support and honest praise during the instruction. Be specific about what the client does well.
- Provide opportunities for the client to ask questions in an accepting and nonjudgmental environment.

■ Evaluate the learning by asking questions or by having the client provide a return demonstration.

Examples of Specific Evaluations for Outcomes 1 to 2

1. Outcome met. Client able to plan a week's menus which meet the requirements for a low fat diet.
2. Outcome partially met. Client able to correctly draw up insulin using sterile technique but is unable to give it to self.
3. Outcome not met. Client refuses to learn self-administration of insulin and says, "My wife will give it to me. I can't give myself a shot."

Key Index Words for Nursing Interventions

Look up these words in the index of fundamentals and medical-surgical nursing textbooks to find page references for additional nursing interventions and rationale for their selection:

■ cognitive ability
■ developmental disability
■ Pattern 8: Knowing
■ psychomotor skills
■ teaching/learning process

Case Management Example

See Appendix for examples of a nursing diagnosis of Knowledge/Skill Deficit within a clinical pathway for the medical diagnoses:

■ DRG 89, Pneumonia with Complications, page 460
■ DRG 127, Congestive Heart Failure, page 466
■ DRG 209, Total Hip Replacement, page 474

IMPAIRED VERBAL COMMUNICATION

Definition

A state in which an individual experiences a decreased or absent ability to use or understand language in human interaction.

*Major Defining Characteristics**

■ unable to speak dominant language

*The first three items are critical.

- speaks or verbalizes with difficulty
- does not or cannot speak
- stuttering, slurring
- difficulty forming words or sentences
- difficulty expressing thought verbally
- inappropriate verbalization
- dyspnea
- disorientation

Related Factors
- decrease in circulation to the brain
- brain tumor
- physical barrier (tracheostomy, intubation)
- anatomical defect (cleft palate)
- psychological barriers (psychosis, lack of stimuli)
- cultural differences
- developmental or age-related

Examples of Specific Nursing Diagnoses
1. Impaired verbal communication related to cerebrovascular accident/stroke (CVA).
   Impaired verbal communication related to CVA as manifested by client making sounds but not speech pattern; signs of frustration. (PES format)
2. Impaired verbal communication related to inability to speak English.
   Impaired verbal communication related to inability to speak English as manifested by Spanish conversation, statement from daughter, "Mom can understand a bit of English but only speaks Spanish." (PES format)

Examples of Specific Outcomes
1. Client will use communication board or written communication to meet needs within 48 hours.
2. Client will meet with hospital interpreter and establish activities of daily living (ADL) schedule and instruction for postoperative care within 24 hours.
3. Client and daughter, who serves as interpreter, will establish schedule for teaching preoperative tests and procedures and postoperative care within 24 hours.

Examples of Specific Nursing Interventions

■ See General Communication, Thinking, and Knowledge Nursing Interventions, page 297.

■ Do gross assessment for hearing and document any abnormalities. This can be done by whispering a number with your hand covering your mouth and asking the client to hold up the corresponding number of fingers. This is a gross screening and if any difficulties are noted, the nurse documents and reports to the physician.

■ Establish unhurried environment with minimal interruptions and noise.

■ Provide all instructions in simple sentences; use visual aids if available.

■ Provide client with pencil/paper for communication if appropriate.

■ Sit when speaking to client to provide clear view of your face and to convey unhurried attitude to decrease stress on client.

■ Provide client with communication board (pictures of activities of daily living, e.g., use of toilet) for use at bedside.

■ Provide interpreter and establish a schedule (to be kept at bedside and nursing station) that coincides with tests/procedures.

■ Establish a schedule of availability of family members (or hospital interpreting service) for interpretation.

■ Use touch to reassure and comfort client.

■ Provide clock with large numerals and indicate time of next nursing visit.

■ Instruct in the use of the call light/intercom system using interpreter if necessary. Demonstrate and practice until client is able to return demonstration. Be aware that intercom will probably not be useful and reassure client that when nurses note the signal, they will come to the room rather than talk over the system.

■ Request consultation from speech pathologist.

■ Assign same nurse to client each shift as much as possible.

Examples of Specific Evaluations for Outcomes 1 to 3

1. Outcome met. Client able to use communication board to request food, bath, toilet, grooming needs, telephone.

2. Outcome partially met. Client met with hospital

interpreter who will return at 7 A.M. to talk with physician and do preop instruction interpretation.
3. Outcome not met. Daughter not available. Daughter will come in at 6 P.M. tomorrow (3/20) to work with Nurse D. Armis to interpret preop teaching.

Key Index Words for Nursing Interventions
Look up these words in the index of fundamentals and medical-surgical nursing textbooks to find page references for additional nursing interventions and rationale for their selection:

- aphasia
- cerebrovascular accident
- developmental disability
- hearing deficit

- Pattern 2: Communicating
- safety and security needs
- tracheostomy

Chapter 17

Coping/Adjustment Problems

FOCUSED ASSESSMENT GUIDE

Complete this focused assessment if a general nursing assessment indicates a possible problem. Then turn to page 308 of this text for the Data ⇒ Diagnosis Matching Guide for coping/adjustment problems to help you select the best nursing diagnosis to match the client's data.

Assess for presence of:
___ tension, apprehension, scared, jittery (unspecific causes)
___ trembling, increased pulse rate, restless, pupil dilation, insomnia, increased perspiration
___ able to identify object of fear
___ unable to accept change in health status or to participate in problem solving
___ lack of progress toward independence
___ passivity, decreased speech, "I can't"
___ lack of initiative, decreased response to stimuli
___ statements of having no ability to control or influence the situation or self-care; apathy
___ denial of obvious problems; projection of blame
___ superior attitude, difficulty establishing relationships
___ lack of follow-through or participation in treatment or therapy
___ inability to make a decision or feelings of distress while attempting to make a decision
___ verbalizes inability to cope or to ask for help
___ inability to solve problems
___ delays seeking health care or refuses health care

___ self-treatment of symptoms and/or minimizes symptoms
___ change in environment or location
___ statements about willingness to move with or without
   sleep disturbances, change in eating habits, sad affect
___ anticipated loss of loved object
___ denial, guilt, anger, verbal expression of distress at loss
   to excessive degree
___ questioning meaning of life/death/suffering/diety
___ accident-prone, high illness rate

NORMALS AND INFORMATION

Table 17.1

Anxiety Level	Effect
Mild	Helps one to deal with stress Heightens perceptions and awareness Example: student taking exam
Moderate	Narrows perceptual field, intense focus Example: preoperative patient

Severe	Decreased sensory reception
	Increased BP, pulse, respiration, vasoconstriction
	   Example: client having visual hallucinations of harmful
	      creatures

Panic	Completely disrupted perceptual field; intense terror Example: survivors of plane crash at the scene

Adapted from *Psychiatric Nursing*, H. S. Wilson, C. R. Kneisl, Addison-Wesley, 1992, pp. 86–87.

DATA ⇒ DIAGNOSIS MATCHING GUIDE

Compare your client data from the Coping/Adjustment Focused Assessment to these related coping/adjustment nursing diagnoses and abbreviated descriptions. Select the nursing diagnosis which is the best match. Then turn to the page in this section with that specific diagnosis for help in planning care.

1. Anxiety: page 312
   ■ definition: vague, uneasy feeling whose source is often
   unknown

■ data:
subjective: tension, apprehension, fearful, scared
objective: increased pulse rate, dilated pupils, tremors,
increased perspiration, insomnia, quivering voice

2. *Defensive Coping: page 315*
   ■ definition: individual projects falsely positive self-
   evaluation that protects against threats to self-esteem
   ■ data: denial of obvious problems, projection of blame
   and responsibility, rationalizes failures, superior attitude,
   difficulty establishing relationships

3. *Ineffective Individual Coping: page 318*
   ■ definition: diminished ability to adapt and solve
   problems
   ■ data: statements of inability to cope or ask for help;
   inability to solve problems; high illness or accident rate

4. *Decisional Conflict: page 321*
   ■ definition: inability to make a decision
   ■ data: statements of uncertainty about choices; vacillation
   between alternatives

5. *Fear: page 323*
   ■ definition: feelings of dread from identified source
   ■ data: ability to identify object of fear

6. *Anticipatory Grieving: page 326*
   ■ definition: future loss of loved person or significant
   object
   ■ data: statements of loss; guilt, anger, sorrow

7. *Dysfunctional Grieving: page 328*
   ■ definition: prolonged, excessive, or extreme grief
   response to a degree that interferes with life functioning
   ■ data: statements of distress at loss; crying, anger;
   changes in sleeping/eating patterns

8. *Hopelessness: page 331*
   ■ definition: state in which individual sees few or no
   choices and is unable to take initiative on own behalf
   ■ data: passive, decreased affect, lack of initiative,
   decreased appetite and sleep, lack of involvement in
   care

9. *Impaired Adjustment: page 334*
   - definition: state in which the individual is unable to make changes in lifestyle to change health status
   - data: statements indicating nonacceptance of health status; lack of participation or unsuccessful participation in problem solving; lack of progress toward independence

10. *Ineffective Denial: page 336*
    - definition: conscious or unconscious attempt to reject the meaning of a situation in order to reduce anxiety
    - data: delays seeking help or refuses treatment for health problem; self-treatment; minimizes symptoms

11. *Powerlessness: page 339*
    - definition: belief that one's actions will not affect an outcome; perceived lack of control over situation
    - data: statements of having no control or influence over situation or self-care; apathy

12. *Relocation Stress Syndrome: page 342*
    - definition: physical and psychosocial problems as a result of moving from one environment to another
    - data: change in location; loneliness, apprehension, sleep/appetite/GI disturbances

13. *Spiritual Distress: page 346*
    - definition: state in which individual questions belief/value system which has been a comfort or source of strength in the past
    - data: expresses concern about meaning of life/death/suffering; anger towards God; crying, withdrawal, anxiety

GENERAL OUTCOMES AND NURSING INTERVENTIONS

GENERAL COPING/ADJUSTMENT OUTCOMES

- Client is able to establish therapeutic, trusting relationship with nurse.
- Client is able to accurately assess own capabilities and limitations in meeting demands of health situation.

- Client is able to identify resources available to assist in times of crisis and how to access these resources.
- Client is able to validate the source of fear.
- Client verbalizes statements of decreased fear/anxiety.
- Client accurately describes alternative treatment options and their pros/cons.
- Client is able to assess for effectiveness of self-care routine.
- Client describes self-care regimen to be followed after discharge.
- Client verbalizes realistic description of diagnosis and recommended treatment.
- Client evidences reduced physiological indicators of stress: decreased pulse rate, blood pressure, diaphoresis (sweating), tremors, pupils normal, color normal for the client.

GENERAL COPING/ADJUSTMENT NURSING INTERVENTIONS

- Establish a therapeutic, trusting relationship with the client. All these nursing diagnoses involve a client with a fragile sense of self-esteem. While this may be true of many or all clients, it is accentuated here.
- Use a nonjudgmental approach; accept clients as they present themselves.
- Avoid false reassurances or statements which lessen the problems of the client.

    "You have lots to live for, I don't know why you're feeling this way."

    "That's not so bad, I know lots of people who are worse off than you."

- Offer praise of client accomplishments citing specific examples of what was well done.
- Assist the client in step-by-step problem solving; write out the process (the steps of the nursing process can be the basis for this approach: assess, identify the problems, determine goals, set up a plan, evaluate, and revise as necessary).
- Use communication techniques: reflection, summarizing, clarification.

- Use nonverbal communication: touch, staying within the client's frame of reference.
- Seek to gain an understanding of the client's perception of the problem before planning intervention.

RELATED NURSING DIAGNOSES

ANXIETY

Definition
A vague uneasy feeling whose source is often nonspecific or unknown to the individual.

Defining Characteristics
Subjective
- increased tension
- uncertainty
- scared
- worried
- overexcited
- jittery
- painful and persistent increased helplessness
- feelings of inadequacy
- fear of unspecific consequences
- expressed concerns about changes in life events
- apprehension
- fearful
- regretful
- anxious
- jittery
- shakiness

Objective
- *Sympathetic stimulation/cardiovascular excitation, superficial vasoconstriction, pupil dilation
- restlessness
- glancing about
- trembling/hand tremors
- voice quivering
- increased wariness

*Critical.

- extraneous movement (foot shuffling, hand/arm movements)
- insomnia
- poor eye contact
- facial tension
- focus on self
- increased perspiration

Related Factors
- unconscious conflict about essential values/goals of life
- threat to self-concept
- threat to or change in health status
- threat to or change in role functioning
- threat to or change in environment
- threat to or change in interaction patterns
- situational/maturational crises
- interpersonal transmission/contagion
- unmet meeds

Examples of Specific Nursing Diagnoses
1. Moderate anxiety related to change in health status.
   Moderate anxiety related to change in health status as evidenced by statement, "I have never been in a hospital before. You have to be *really serious* to be hospitalized." (PES format)
2. Severe anxiety related to staging procedure for Hodgkin's disease (cancer of the lymphatic system).
   Severe anxiety related to staging procedure as evidenced by inability to sleep, shaking hands, elevated blood pressure, and statement "This is terrifying—I can't think of anything else." (PES format)

Examples of Specific Outcomes
1. Client will state he feels less anxious and make an accurate statement of the reason for hospitalization by hour of sleep (hs).
2. Client will demonstrate reduced anxiety within 24 hours by decreased blood pressure, sleeping for at least 4 hours, and absence of shakiness in hands.

Examples of Specific Nursing Interventions
- See General Coping/Adjustment Nursing Interventions, page 311.

- Speak in short sentences; clear, calm voice facing the client.
- Decrease sensory stimulation: turn off television, limit number of visitors, decrease noise in hallway.
- Provide for the client's basic needs: warmth, food, elimination, privacy, telephone contact with significant others.
- Assess what the client knows about condition.
    "What brought you to the hospital?"
    "What has your doctor told you about Hodgkin's disease (or any other condition)? What does this mean to you?"
    "Have you ever known anyone else who has had Hodgkin's (or any other condition)?"
- Provide consistency of caregiver in order to develop a trusting relationship.
- Carefully consider the use of touch; this is easily misinterpreted by an anxious client.
- Assess client's coping skills: "What do you do at home when you cannot sleep or when you are worried?"
- Encourage use of coping skills which were successful in the past and which are appropriate to the present situation.
- Provide factual, relevant information to the client in amounts and at levels the client can understand.
- Communicate client status to physician; client may require medication to reduce anxiety and/or to facilitate sleep.
- Use stress reduction techniques: guided imagery or muscle relaxation.

Examples of Specific Evaluations for Outcomes 1 and 2
1. Outcome met. Client states, "So far I can handle this. After the test tomorrow I will have a better sense of what is going on."
2. Outcome partially met. Client understands hospital environment but states, "I am still a wreck with worry."
3. Outcome not met. Client unable to sleep and pacing at the nurses' station at 2 A.M.

Key Index Words for Nursing Interventions
Look up these words in the index of fundamentals and medical-surgical nursing textbooks to find page

references for additional nursing interventions and rationale for their selection:

- adult respiratory distress syndrome
- anger, guilt, depression
- anxiety disorders
- anxiolytic medications
- fear
- "fight or flight" response
- myocardial infarction
- panic
- stress

Case Management Example
See Appendix for an example of a diagnosis of Anxiety within a clinical pathway for the medical diagnosis DRG 89, Pneumonia with Complications, page 460.

DEFENSIVE COPING

Definition
A state in which an individual repeatedly projects falsely positive self-evaluations based on a self-protection pattern that defends against underlying perceived threats to positive self-regard.

Major Defining Characteristics
- denial of obvious problems/weaknesses
- projection of blame/responsibility
- rationalized failures
- hypersensitive to slight criticism
- grandiosity

Minor Defining Characteristics
- superior attitude towards others
- difficulty establishing/maintaining relationships
- hostile laughter or ridicule of others
- difficulty in reality testing perceptions
- lack of follow-through or participation in treatment or therapy

Examples of Specific Nursing Diagnoses

1. Defensive coping related to diagnosis of Alzheimer's disease.

   Defensive coping related to diagnosis of Alzheimer's disease as evidenced by client statement, "Lot's of people forget things, it's just normal aging, and now you tell me I have Alzheimer's. No way!" (PES format)

2. Defensive coping related to being denied a promotion.

   Defensive coping related to being denied a promotion as evidenced by client statement, "They had to hire a woman for the job or I would have gotten it". (PES format)

Examples of Specific Outcomes

1. Client will make accurate statement of the perceived threat during hospitalization.
2. Client will make statement of feelings associated with the threat before discharge.
3. Assisted by nurse, client will identify three alternative coping strategies by discharge.

Examples of Specific Nursing Interventions

- See General Coping/Adjustment Nursing Interventions, page 311.
- Establishment of trusting relationship, nonjudgmental, consistency of caregiver.
- Elicit the client's perspective of the stressful event.
- Do not attempt to alter or correct the perception of the stressor or to confront the incongruities of the client's perception.
- Assist the client to identify coping methods that have been successful in the past.

  "Have you had to resolve other difficult problems in the past?"

  "And what things did you do to cope with that?"

  "What was helpful in that situation?"

- Assist the client to identify similarities between the stressful situations and the coping strategies that provided relief.
- Provide information about support groups and if client agrees, make initial contact for client.

- Provide accurate information for the client, in alternative forms: videotapes, pamphlets, audiotapes, books.
- Assist the client to maintain supportive relationships: provide privacy for visiting, guest meals; include family in teaching/problem solving if client agrees.
- Spend time with client when physical care is not being given in order to sit and encourage expression of fears/worries.
- Share observations of client behavior in general: "I have cared for several other persons who have been diagnosed as having Alzheimer's disease. They were really afraid and thought that their world had ended. I wonder if you are feeling some of these same things."
- Assist the client to set realistic goals and develop plans to achieve them. This may include something as simple as seeing a movie with a friend, physical exercise, or trying a new hobby.

Examples of Specific Evaluations for Outcomes 1 and 2
1. Outcome not met. Client states, "I may as well commit suicide now and spare my family all the misery of the next years."
2. Outcome partially met. Client willing to talk with physician and learn about Alzheimer's disease but refuses contact with support group or other clients.
3. Outcome met. Client states, "I understand the progress of the disease but I am going to make the most of all the time I have left..... ..beginning now".

Key Index Words for Nursing Interventions
Look up these words in the index of fundamentals and medical-surgical nursing textbooks to find page references for additional nursing interventions and rationale for their selection:

- death/dying
- defense mechanisms
- denial
- ego-integrity
- group therapy
- hypersensitivity
- paranoid
- reality testing
- self-esteem
- suspiciousness
- terminal illness

INEFFECTIVE INDIVIDUAL COPING

Definition
Impairment of adaptive behaviors and problem-solving abilities of a person in meeting life's demands and roles.

Defining Characteristics
- *verbalization of inability to cope or inability to ask for help
- inability to meet role expectations
- inability to meet basic needs
- *inability to problem solve
- alterations in societal participation
- destructive behavior toward self or others
- inappropriate use of defense mechanisms
- change in usual communications patterns
- verbal manipulation
- high illness rate
- high rate of accidents

Related Factors
- situational crisis
- maturational crisis
- personal vulnerability

Examples of Specific Nursing Diagnoses
1. Ineffective individual coping related to inadequate financial/insurance resources.
   Ineffective individual coping related to inadequate financial/insurance resources as manifested by client statement, "I will be in debt forever. I can't pay for any of this; it is all I think about". (PES format)
2. Ineffective individual coping related to diagnosis of terminal cancer.
   Ineffective individual coping related to diagnosis of terminal cancer as evidenced by client statement, "I just want to throw in the towel, hang it up. There is nothing to be done." Client remains in bed and refuses to eat, bathe, or maintain hygiene. (PES format)

*Critical.

Examples of Specific Outcomes
1. Client will agree to meet with hospital financial counselor/social worker to resolve financial issues within 24 hours.
2. Client will talk with spouse and physician to choose treatment plan within 3 days.
3. Client will verbalize feelings related to diagnosis within 48 hours.

Examples of Specific Nursing Interventions
- Match interventions to related factors causing ineffective coping.
- See General Coping/Adjustment Nursing Interventions, page 311.
- Assist the client to verbalize own perception of the stressor: "This seems like a very difficult time for you. Can you talk about what this illness means to you?"
- Review interventions for nursing diagnosis of Self-esteem Disturbance, page 424. Clients who perceive themselves as unable to pay for their care may be experiencing shame or guilt.
- Assess for any self-harm or suicidal thoughts, plans, gestures.
    "Have you ever thought of harming yourself?"
    "Have you a plan?"
    "How would you do it?"
    If positive data for suicide/self-harm is present seek assistance from a mental health clinician (psychologist, clinical nurse specialist, psychiatrist).
- Offer hospital financial aid resources: "Many people, no matter how well insured, have concerns about their hospital bills. Would you like to meet with a financial counselor here at the hospital? They can often find help for these problems".
- Assist client in maintaining physical hygiene. It may be necessary to do complete care of the client or to merely put articles within the client's reach. The nurse will assess the level of dependency and intervene as needed.
- Assess client's previous coping strategies: "When you've had major problems in the past, what has helped you in dealing with them?"

- Assist client in identifying similarities between problems now and those in the past.
    "Have you ever had to deal with crises in the past?"
    "Can you describe that time in your life?"
    "How did you feel then?"
    "Were there people that were especially helpful at that time?"
- Assist the client to identify and try out new coping strategies: "Some patients I have cared for have told me that physical exercise is very helpful in learning to relax. Would you like to try an exercise plan to help you?"
- Offer assurance that many clients have similar feelings in this situation.
- Teach the client a problem-solving process: gather facts, analyze, name the problems, identify possible solutions, choose a best solution, try out solutions one at a time, evaluate, and try again as necessary. Assist the client in using the process.
- Assist the client to maintain supportive relationships with significant others: plan nursing care to avoid interruptions during visiting hours, provide guest meal trays, assist with grooming prior to visits.
- Provide information on alternative forms of stress reduction and assist client in use if requested: biofeedback, imagery, hypnosis, relaxation, massage, meditation.

Examples of Specific Evaluations for Outcome 1
1. Outcome not met. Client refuses to meet with financial counselor stating in angry voice, "I'm no charity case. What do you take me for?"
2. Outcome partially met. Client states he made a decision to take out a second mortgage to pay for hospital expenses. Client refuses further discussion with a hospital financial counselor.
3. Outcome met. Client met with financial counselor and worked out payment schedule stating. "Wow, that's a load off my mind. I bet I sleep tonight."

Key Index Words for Nursing Interventions
Look up these words in the index of fundamentals and medical-surgical nursing textbooks to find page references for additional nursing interventions and rationale

for their selection:

- activities of daily living (ADLs)
- biofeedback
- depression
- ego
- ego integrity
- hypnosis
- imagery
- lethality assessment
- massage
- perception
- reality testing
- self-esteem
- self-hypnosis
- stress/stress management
- suicide

DECISIONAL CONFLICT (SPECIFY)

Definition
A state of uncertainty about course of action to be taken when choice among competing actions involves risk, loss, or challenge to personal life values.

Major Defining Characteristics
- verbalized uncertainty about choices
- verbalization of undesired consequences of alternative actions being considered
- vacillation between alternative choices
- delayed decision-making

Minor Defining Characteristics
- verbalized feelings of distress while attempting a decision
- self-focusing
- physical signs of distress or tension (increased heart rate, increased muscle tension, restlessness, etc.)
- questioning personal values and beliefs while attempting a decision

Related Factors
- unclear personal values/beliefs
- perceived threat to value system
- lack of relevant information
- support system deficit
- multiple or divergent sources of information

Examples of Specific Nursing Diagnoses
1. Decisional conflict (ostomy surgery versus continued symptoms of chronic ulcerative colitis) related to two perceived negative choices.

Decisional conflict related to ostomy surgery as evidenced by verbalized uncertainty and stress, "I don't know which is worse, the ostomy or life with 20 stools a day, but the indecision is making me worse". (PES format)
2. Decisional conflict (medical versus surgical treatment of myocardial infarction) related to lack of knowledge of alternatives.
   Decisional conflict (medical versus surgical treatment of myocardial infarction) related to lack of knowledge about alternatives as evidenced by client statement, "So is the surgery like when I had my appendix out?" (PES format)

Examples of Specific Outcomes
1. Client will verbalize the positive and negative aspects of each alternative and make decision within 1 week.
2. Client will verbalize accurate knowledge of alternative choices prior to decision-making.
3. Client will verbalize decreased anxiety once decision has been made.
4. Client will have decreased muscle tension and improved sleep and appetite after decision has been made.

Examples of Specific Nursing Interventions
- See General Coping/Adjustment Nursing Interventions, page 311.
- Attempt to be present with the client when the physician explains the treatment alternatives. This is helpful since the client is under stress and may not be able to focus on the explanation at the time. Reinforce/repeat/clarify the physician's explanation; this is different from gaining informed consent for procedures. Gaining informed consent is the responsibility of a physician and should not be delegated to a nurse.
- Intervene appropriately to request physician to repeat explanations to client.
- Assess client's level of understanding to determine beginning point for teaching.
- Provide accurate information in a variety of learning modalities such as audiotapes, pamphlets, videos, magazines, supportive persons with the same diagnosis.
- Assist client to identify positive and negative aspects of

each alternative; it often helps to encourage the client to make a written list.

■ Encourage physical activity if the client is able; this may assist in stress reduction.

■ Assist in sleep hygiene: bathing, quiet, food if helpful, massage, relaxation tapes, medication if ordered.

■ Support the decision the client has made.

■ Offer to assist client in communicating choice to family and/or significant others.

Examples of Specific Evaluations for Outcome 1

1. Outcome not met. Client refuses to participate in discussion and repeats, "Just tell me what to do."

2. Outcome partially met. Client understands surgery but does not understand that ostomy surgery will be permanent, "When it heals, they can close the hole with more surgery."

3. Outcome met. Client is able to accurately state the positive and negative aspects of surgery versus medical treatment regimen.

Key Index Words for Nursing Interventions

Look up these words in the index of fundamentals and medical-surgical nursing textbooks to find page references for additional nursing interventions and rationale for their selection:

■ anxiety
■ informed consent
■ patient rights

■ relaxation techniques
■ stress
■ value clarification

FEAR

Definition

Feeling of dread related to an identifiable source which the person validates.

Defining Characteristics

NANDA: ability to identify object of fear

Present authors: irritability, nervousness, pacing; inability to process or comprehend information; difficulty sleeping; eating patterns may change to excessive eating or decreased appetite; may have nausea or vomiting, constipation or diarrhea; increased pulse, diaphoresis, increased blood pressure

Related Factors
To be developed by NANDA.

Examples of Specific Nursing Diagnoses
1. Fear related to diagnosis of breast cancer.
   Fear related to diagnosis of breast cancer as evidenced by client statement, "I'm afraid that I will lose the whole breast." (PES format)
2. Fear related to pain of terminal illness.
   Fear related to pain of terminal illness as evidenced by client statement, "I've always been afraid that when I die I would be alone and screaming in pain." (PES format)

Examples of Specific Outcomes
1. Client will identify the object of fear, verbalize own understanding of it, and two methods for dealing with it during hospitalization.
2. Client will state willingness to accept help in dealing with fear within 48 hours.
3. Client reports reduced fear level within 24 hours.

Examples of Specific Nursing Interventions
- See General Coping/Adjustment Nursing Interventions, page 311.
- Initiate establishment of therapeutic trusting relationship: introduce self, state purpose of interaction with client, express concern about client's comfort before proceeding. "I am Ms. Jones and I will be completing your admission. This may take about 30 minutes. Are you comfortable, can I get you anything before beginning?"
- Share your observations with the client in order to provide the opportunity for the client to express fears. "I often care for clients admitted for this type of surgery. They often tell me how afraid they are when they are hospitalized. I wonder if you might be afraid too?"
- Assist the client to identify the source of fear. "Can you tell me more about what it is that makes you afraid now?"
- Accept the client's perception of the fear without minimizing its significance. Offer information and teaching to correct misinformation.

■ Assist the client to identify strategies to reduce the fear.
  "Would it be helpful to understand what will happen tomorrow during the procedure?"
  "There are many things we can do to help make you comfortable. Would you like to learn about some of them?"
■ Teach the client stress reduction/comfort measures such as the use of distraction, muscle relaxation, guided imagery.
■ Limit sensory stimulation if the client indicates that this is irritating or annoying. This might include television noise, frequent interruptions by caregivers, or hallway noise.
■ Encourage presence of significant others as appropriate and offer them support.
■ Assess fear level at least daily.
■ Offer to remain with the client for a time, especially at night when the client is alone.
■ Assist the client to communicate fears to physician.

Examples of Specific Evaluations for Outcomes 1 and 3
1. Outcome met. Client identified fear of disfigurement from loss of breast; viewed filmstrip about surgery and requested visit from American Cancer Society volunteer.
2. Outcome partially met. Client able to verbalize fear but stated, "I just can't handle any information at this time. I just need to be alone".
3. Outcome not met. Client stated, "The report from the CAT scan just made it worse. Now there is no denying it. It's real and there is nothing I can do about it."

Key Index Words for Nursing Interventions
Look up these words in the index of fundamentals and medical-surgical nursing textbooks to find page references for additional nursing interventions and rationale for their selection:

■ anxiety
■ body image
■ fight or flight response
■ sympathetic stimulation
■ terminal cancer

ANTICIPATORY GRIEVING

Definition
Future loss of loved person or significant object. (Defined by present authors. Note that this can be a healthy reponse requiring no nursing intervention other than support/empathy.)

Defining Characteristics
- potential loss of significant object
- expression of distress at potential loss
- denial of potential loss
- guilt, anger, sorrow, choked feelings
- change in eating habits
- alteration in sleep patterns
- alteration in activity level
- altered libido
- altered communication pattern

Examples of Specific Nursing Diagnoses
1. Anticipatory grief related to planned mastecomy.
   Anticipatory grief related to planned mastectomy as evidenced by client statement, "I will feel so damaged, so mutilated; how can I wear my clothes?" (PES format)
2. Anticipatory grief related to diagnosis of cancer with liver/bone metastasis.
   Anticipatory grief related to diagnosis of cancer with liver/bone metastasis as evidenced by statement, "Why me? What did I do to deserve this? This means I won't be around for my kids!" (PES format)

Examples of Specific Outcomes
1. Client will verbalize own perception of the mastectomy and express own feelings related to it before surgery.
2. Client will maintain maximum control possible over life and health care throughout hospitalization.
3. Client will express feelings to family members and share meaning of relationship before death.
4. Client will participate in life review before death assisted by pastor or person of choice.

Examples of Specific Nursing Interventions
- See General Coping/Adjustment Nursing Interventions, page 311.

- Establish trusting, therapeutic relationship.
- Consistency of caregiver.
- Assess the meaning of the illness/death within the culture of the client.
  "How is it in your family at a time like this?"
  "What does your family do when someone is very ill?"
  "What has been helpful in your family during times of crisis?"
- Spend time with client when not giving physical care. At this time it may be helpful to sit at the client's bedside.
- Plan care to accommodate visits by significant others.
- Establish a relationship with significant others; offer comfort measures to them as they stay with client (pillows, blankets, beverages, meal trays).
- Provide broad opening questions to client.
  "How is it going for you?"
  "What can I do that would be helpful to you?"
  "What is it that worries you most?"
- Work with client to establish a plan for pain control. Begin by assessing the current level of pain and the effectiveness of the current treatments for it. If the current plan is effective, document the status of the client. If the current regimen is not effective in controlling pain, communicate concern to client and offer to work with client until a solution is found that is satisfactory to the client. Explain that client is the only one to know about pain levels and the client's assessment contains factual data needed by staff see Specific Nursing Interventions for Pain.
- Offer client as many choices as possible regarding care and treatment: timing of care and treatments, self-medication, dietary choices, visiting times, care plan.
- Assist client/family to identify resources available to them: church, legal/financial aid, support groups, community organizations. Take care over establishment of any new relationships; at this time they may require excessive energy expenditure by the client/family.
- Assist client to identify coping strategies that have been useful in the past and to apply them to the present situation.
- Offer client the opportunity to be visited by a person who has experienced a similar health problem.

- Accept client's right to refuse offers of nursing intervention, conversation, problem solving; clients will be at different levels of grief process and nurses will need to respect the rights of clients even when they are not choosing what the nurse would define as health-promoting behavior.
- Assist the client in the life review process, formally or informally. This is a value-laden choice and may not be selected by all clients, but the nurse can provide the opportunity.

Examples of Specific Evaluations for Outcome 1

1. Outcome not met. Client in bed, facing wall, and refuses to talk.
2. Outcome partially met. Client states, "The surgeons can give me some hope, but I don't want my hopes up only to crash again. It's easier just to block it all out."
3. Outcome met. Client states, "I've done all my thinking. The surgery is my best hope and there are lots of cosmetic options. I can live with these choices."

Key Index Words for Nursing Interventions

Look up these words in the index of nursing fundamentals and medical-surgical nursing textbooks to find page references for additional nursing interventions and rationale for their selection:

- AIDS
- amputation
- bereavement
- body image
- cancer
- grief and loss

- life review
- loneliness
- metastasis
- ostomy
- support group

DYSFUNCTIONAL GRIEVING

Definition

Prolonged, excessive, or extreme grief response to a degree that interferes with life functioning. (Defined by present authors.)

Defining Characteristics

- verbal expressions of distress at loss

- denial of loss
- expression of guilt
- expression of unresolved issues
- anger
- sadness
- crying
- difficulty in expressing loss
- alteration in eating habits, sleep patterns, dream patterns, activity level or libido
- idealization of lost object
- reliving of past experiences
- interference with life functioning
- developmental regression; labile (changing, unstable) affect
- alteration in concentration and/or pursuit of tasks

Related Factors
- actual or perceived loss (in the broadest sense)
- objects may include people, possessions, jobs, status, home, ideals, and parts and processes of the body

Examples of Specific Nursing Diagnoses
1. Dysfunctional grieving related to loss of spouse 5 years ago.
   Dysfunctional grieving related to loss of spouse 5 years ago as evidenced by daily visits to graveside and extreme distress when unable to do so; refusing all activities that interfere with this ritual. (PES format)
2. Dysfunctional grieving related to below-the-knee (BK) amputation.
   Dysfunctional grieving related to BK amputation as evidenced by refusal to participate in physical therapy stating "I am a cripple and nothing will change that. Everyone just pities me." (PES format)

Examples of Specific Outcomes
1. Client will make one statement indicative of progress in grieving or hope within 1 week.
2. Within 1 month, client will resume one activity enjoyed before death of spouse.
3. Within 1 month, client will decrease graveside visits to 1–3 per week at times when it does not interfere with recreational activities.

4. Client will agree to participate in physical therapy within 1 week.
5. Client will perform activities of daily living (ADLs) unassisted within 1 week.

Examples of Specific Nursing Interventions

- See General Coping/Adjustment Nursing Interventions, page 311.
- Assess feelings of client related to loss; begin with a broad opening statement such as, "Tell me how it has been for you since your partner died?"
- Assess client's perception of present situation and effectiveness of coping strategies:
    "And how are you doing now?"
    "What has helped you to cope with this difficult loss?"
    "And has that been effective for you?"
    "What has worked and what has not helped?"
- Assess client's willingness to learn new coping strategies: "Do you think that you would like to work to learn other ways to cope?"
- Spend time with client when no physical care is necessary. Sit at bedside and make offer of intervention: "I am concerned about how much you are grieving the loss of your husband. I would like to help to make things better for you."
- Share observations about client's behavior that cause concern: "You told me you visit the graveside daily. I wonder if this interferes with other activities that might be of interest to you. How would you feel if you were not able to go one day? What do you think about that?"
- Assure client of normalcy of feelings when appropriate, especially when client expresses negative feelings. Guilt and anger are a normal part of the grieving process.
- Explore client's activities prior to loss and assist in planning gradual resumption of one.
- Assist client in identifying community resources: support groups, social groups, spiritual support, peer counselors.
- Encourage maximum independence in ADLs.
- Point out capacities and abilities unaffected by loss (e.g., amputation, mastectomy, spinal cord injury).
- Assist client in learning modifications necessary to

continued participation in activities enjoyed before loss.
■ Provide contact with support person who has had similar loss, if agreeable to client.

Examples of Specific Evaluations for Outcomes 1 and 3

1. Outcome not met. Client states, "I just have to visit the grave every day. It is the only contact I can have with him now."
2. Outcome partially met. Client states, "Maybe I could miss on Thursdays so I could go to the Senior Center."
3. Outcome met. Client planning 2-week vacation to visit daughter over Christmas.

Key Index Words for Nursing Interventions

Look up these words in the index of fundamentals and medical-surgical nursing textbooks to find page references for additional nursing interventions and rationale for their selection:

■ amputation
■ anger/guilt
■ anticipatory grieving
■ body image disturbance
■ death/dying
■ depression

■ fixated/regression
■ hope
■ loneliness
■ self-esteem
■ suicide assessment
■ terminal illness

HOPELESSNESS

Definition

A subjective state in which an individual sees limited or no alternatives or personal choices available and is unable to mobilize energy on own behalf.

Major Defining Characteristics

■ passivity, decreased verbalization
■ decreased affect
■ verbal cues (despondent content, "I can't," sighing)

Minor Defining Characteristics

■ lack of initiative
■ decreased response to stimuli

- decreased affect
- turning away from speaker
- closing eyes
- shrugging in response to speaker
- decreased appetite
- increased/decreased sleep
- lack of involvement in care/passivity in allowing care

Related Factors
- prolonged activity restriction creating isolation
- failing or deteriorating physiological condition
- long-term stress; abandonment
- lost belief in transcendent values/God

Examples of Specific Nursing Diagnoses
1. Hopelessness related to diagnosis of brain tumor.
   Hopelessness related to diagnosis of brain tumor as evidenced by client statements, "I always knew that I would die young. I just can't handle this." (PES format)
2. Hopelessness related to diagnosis of breast cancer.
   Hopelessness related to diagnosis of breast cancer as evidenced by client statement, "I knew that I would get it. My mother and sister both had to have mastectomies for cancer. It was just a matter of time. No one can help me." (PES format)

Examples of Specific Outcomes
1. Client will make one positive statement related to ability to handle this illness before discharge.
2. Client will remain physically safe throughout hospitalization (absence of self-injurious behavior and suicide ideas or attempts).
3. Client will verbalize three future goals within 48 hours.
4. Client will identify one meaningful interpersonal relationship within 24 hours.

Examples of Specific Nursing Interventions
- See General Coping/Adjustment Nursing Interventions, page 311.
- Provide opportunities for client to express feelings. One way is to spend 5–10 minutes with client in addition to physical care; sit and listen using active communication skills.

- Provide consistency of caregiver.
- Assess level of self-care and assistance necessary.
- Direct client in personal hygiene/grooming activities: provide supplies and assist as necessary.
- Organize care to provide for uninterrupted visits by significant others.
- Assess for suicide potential: ask clients about thoughts of self-harm and if present, have they plans.
- Observe, document, and report any sudden change in mood or behavior. This could be indication of a decision made to commit suicide.
- Provide opportunities for client to make decisions about care and treatment regimen.
- Verbalize observations of positive response to treatment.
- Reinforce information from physician to client about treatments for breast cancer and the choices client may make. When possible, provide teaching in multiple learning modalities: pamphlets, videos, books, visits from support person. Materials the client can take home are especially useful.
- Offer referral to religious counselor if client indicates this is acceptable.
- Assist client in identification of goals: "What do you want to accomplish in the next week, month, year?" This could be as simple as seeing a movie or a particular TV show. After client identifies a goal, work on strategies to achieve it.
- Provide physical environment which promotes hope: light, windows, furniture (to encourage client out of bed).
- Offer option of company at mealtimes; could be significant others or other clients in the area.
- Provide meals to client out of bed.

Examples of Specific Evaluations for Outcome 1

1. Outcome not met. Client unwilling to talk; remains in dark room with covers over head.
2. Outcome partially met. Client states, "You always hear about miracles, but then I have never believed in that stuff."
3. Outcome met. Client states, "My doctor explained three alternative treatments. Things may be looking up."

Key Index Words for Nursing Interventions
Look up these words in the index of fundamentals and medical-surgical nursing textbooks to find page references for additional nursing interventions and rationale for their selection:

- activities of daily living
- AIDS
- alcoholism
- death/dying
- depression
- lethality assessment
- self-esteem
- stress
- suicidal ideation
- terminal illness

IMPAIRED ADJUSTMENT

Definition
A state in which an individual is unable to modify lifestyle/behavior in a manner consistent with a change in health status.

Major Defining Characteristics
- verbalization of nonacceptance of health status change
- nonexistent or unsuccessful ability to be involved in problem solving or goal setting

Minor Defining Characteristics
- lack of movement towards independence
- extended period of shock, disbelief, or anger regarding health status change
- lack of future-oriented thinking

Related Factors
- disability requiring change in lifestyle
- inadequate support systems
- impaired cognition
- sensory overload
- assault to self-esteem
- altered locus of control
- incomplete grieving

Examples of Specific Nursing Diagnoses
1. Impaired adjustment related to changing food intake to follow diabetic diet.
   Impaired adjustment related to changing food intake to

follow diabetic diet as evidenced by client statement, "I've been OK for 35 years eating whatever I want. I'm not going to change now." (PES format)

2. Impaired adjustment related to visual changes of multiple sclerosis.

Impaired adjustment related to visual changes of multiple sclerosis as evidenced by client statement, "It's time to die if I can't see. How will I ever take care of myself?" (PES format)

Examples of Specific Outcomes

1. Client verbalizes rationale for diabetic diet within 24 hours.
2. Client will state own particular benefits of following diabetic diet within 48 hours.
3. Client will work with nurse to plan a week of menus which follow the diabetic diet plan and include own favorite foods by discharge.
4. Client will make statement of ability to complete ADLs using assistive devices for blindness within 1 week.

Examples of Specific Nursing Interventions

- See General Coping/Adjustment Nursing Interventions, page 311.
- Convey acceptance of client at the present level of adjustment, and encourage client to continue to express feeling and perception of the disease process. Some helpful statements might include:

    "This seems difficult for you."

    "Is this the first time you have been ill?"

    "How might having diabetes affect your life?"

    "I guess I might be angry too if all of a sudden I had to make some major changes in the foods I enjoy."

- Provide opportunities for client to make choices and exercise control. Illness involves a loss of control over one's body, so provide opportunities for control in other areas. Bear in mind the client is a consumer and is not required to accept health care. This may be especially difficult when clients make choices that do not promote health.
- Include family or significant others in teaching as client permits.

- Identify likely outcomes if client chooses not to modify lifestyle/behavior.
- Provide client with realistic, factual alternatives from which to choose.
- Provide instruction in multiple modalities: pamphlets, videotapes, audiotapes, one-to-one instruction classes. Materials the client can take home are especially useful.
- Offer support group information and suggest visit from member of group.
- Assess client capabilities and limitations as impacted by illness; identify modifications and/or assistive devices as necessary to enhance capabilities.
- Identify community resources which can be used post-discharge and initiate contact while client is hospitalized.

Examples of Specific Evaluations for Outcomes 1 and 4
1. Outcome met. Client able to discuss reason for diabetic diet in controlling symptoms of diabetes.
2. Outcome partially met. Client willing to plan 4 days of menus using a diabetic diet but refuses to limit intake of ice cream, beer, and chocolate.
3. Outcome not met. Client remains in bed and refuses to attempt self-care.

Key Index Words for Nursing Interventions
Look up these words in fundamentals and medical-surgical nursing textbooks to find page references for additional nursing interventions and rationale for their use:

- amputation
- depression
- hemiplegia
- loss of function
- occupational therapy
- quadriplegia
- rehabilitation
- specific disease process
- trauma

INEFFECTIVE DENIAL

Definition
A conscious or unconscious attempt to disavow the knowledge or meaning of an event to reduce anxiety/fear to the detriment of health.

Major Defining Characteristics
- delays seeking or refuses health care attention to the detriment of health
- does not perceive personal relevance of symptoms or danger

Minor Defining Characteristics
- uses home remedies (self-treatment) to relieve symptoms
- does not admit fear of death or invalidism
- minimizes symptoms
- displaces source of symptoms to other organs
- unable to admit impact of disease on life pattern
- makes dismissive gestures or comments when speaking of distressing events
- displaces fear of impact of the condition
- displays inappropriate affect

Examples of Specific Nursing Diagnoses
1. Ineffective denial related to myocardial infarction.
   Ineffective denial related to myocardial infarction as evidenced by client statement, "This is just indigestion; the hot salsa is really too much for my system. All this fuss is not necessary." (PES format)
2. Ineffective denial related to loss of hearing.
   Ineffective denial related to loss of hearing as evidenced by client denial of hearing loss, inability to follow conversation, smiling at inappropriate times, lack of appropriate participation in conversation. (PES format)

Examples of Specific Outcomes
1. Client will immediately report all symptoms of chest pain to nurse throughout hospitalization
2. Client will exhibit only symptoms of mild anxiety; will be able to focus on learning about diagnosis of myocardial infarction before discharge
3. Client will be able to give explanation of cause of symptoms of myocardial infarction before discharge
4. Client will acknowledge difficulty hearing and make a decision whether or not to accept evaluation and treatment.

Examples of Specific Nursing Interventions
Denial may be a useful response in dealing with anxiety. It becomes a nursing diagnosis when it interferes with

health-seeking behavior. Because denial is a coping device used by the client to deal with anxiety, most interventions will focus on anxiety. Review Specific Nursing Interventions for Anxiety.

- See General Coping/Adjustment Nursing Interventions, page 311.
- Assess the level of anxiety the client is demonstrating. Is the client able to focus on conversation? Are there physical symptoms of anxiety: increased pulse rate, hand tremors, elevated blood pressure, increased respiratory rate?
- Assess client's understanding of disease and symptoms.
    "What does a heart attack mean to you?"
    "How do you think it will affect your life?"
    "What changes, if any, do you think you will need to make in your life?"
- Provide accurate information about disease and treatment options which have been presented by physician.
- Offer to leave printed information with client, "just in case you may want to read it later." This provides client with opportunity to read the information in private when ready.
- Offer group instruction with other clients. This provides opportunity for client to observe other client's responses and to question/challenge/discuss in a safe environment.
- Maintain nonjudgmental attitude, remembering that denial is an ego-protective device needed by client at the time.
- Provide opportunities for client to meet another client with the same disease; facilitate a conversation that may include:
    "What was it like for you when you found out you had a heart attack?"
    "What do you remember about that time?"
    "What did your family or nurses do that was helpful?"
- Provide referral to appropriate community resources.

Examples of Specific Evaluations for Outcome 1

1. Outcome not met. Client denies any symptoms and complains, "This is a lot of fuss about nothing. I want to go home!"

2. Outcome partially met. Client states, "Yes, I'll let you know if it gets really bad."
3. Outcome met. Client reported mild chest pain to nurse twice during last 24 hours and at present reports no pain at all.

Key Index Words for Nursing Interventions

Look up these words in the index of fundamentals and medical-surgical nursing textbooks to find page references for additional nursing interventions and rationale for their selection:

- anxiety
- coping techniques
- defense mechanisms
- ego integrity
- group therapy as treatment modality or teaching method
- reality testing
- safety/security (as basic human need)
- stress/stress management

POWERLESSNESS

Definition

Perception that one's own actions will not significantly affect an outcome; perceived lack of control over current situation or immediate happening.

Defining Characteristics

Severe
- verbal expressions of having no control or influence over situation
- verbal expression of having no control or influence over outcome
- verbal expression of having no control over self-care
- depression over physical deterioration which occurs despite patient compliance with regimens
- apathy

Moderate
- nonparticipation in care or decision-making when opportunities are provided

- expression of dissatisfaction and frustration over inability to perform previous tasks and/or activities
- does not monitor progress
- expression of doubt regarding role performance
- reluctance to express true feelings, fearing alienation from caregivers
- passivity
- inability to seek information regarding care
- dependence on others that may result in irritability, resentment, anger, and guilt
- lack of defense of self-care practices when challenged

Low
- expression of uncertainty about fluctuating energy levels
- passivity

Related Factors
- health care environment
- interpersonal interactions
- illness-related regimen
- lifestyle of helplessness

Examples of Specific Nursing Diagnoses
1. Powerlessness related to diagnosis of multiple sclerosis.
   Powerlessness related to diagnosis of multiple sclerosis as evidenced by client statement, "I understand how this disease progresses and how I will end up. Nothing I do will make a difference." (PES format)
2. Powerlessness related to history of alcoholism.
   Powerlessness related to history of alcoholism as evidenced by client statement, "I can go without a drink for a few days, even made it a few months once, but I always go back to drinking and that makes my life miserable." (PES format)

Examples of Specific Outcomes
1. Client will identify situations of powerlessness within next 2 days.
2. Client will identify areas of life within control within 48 hours.
3. Client will participate in decision-making regarding care with support of nurse before discharge.

Examples of Specific Nursing Interventions

■ See General Coping/Adjustment Nursing Interventions, page 311.
■ Encourage client to express feelings by spending time with client when there is no need for specific physical care, use of communication techniques, reflection of observations to client, "You seem a bit down tonight."
■ Provide client with accurate information about disease process and treatment regimen.
■ Identify alternative treatments and positive and negative aspects of each.
■ Provide choices for client to make about care, daily routine, rest/activity/nutrition alternatives.
■ Ask about client's home routine and if possible, adapt the hospital routine to the home schedule, recording it in the care plan.
■ Ask client's preference for bathing, dressing, etc., and include them in the care plan.
■ Provide opportunities for family members/significant others to learn about disease process and treatment alternatives with the permission of the client.
■ Provide opportunities for family members/significant other to participate in care, with the permission of the client.
■ Consult with physical therapist or rehabilitation therapist to assess and provide assistive devices that maximize the client's independence. This might include a tripod cane, adapted eating utensils, motorized wheelchairs, electric page turner for books.
■ Provide information about support groups.
■ Offer to make contact with a support group if client agrees (often clients do not have the emotional energy to seek this contact even if it is perceived as helpful).

Examples of Specific Evaluations for Outcome 1

1. Outcome not met. Client remains in bed with covers over head and refuses to talk.
2. Outcome partially met. Client states, "What will be will be," and asks to be left alone.
3. Outcome met. Client states he can not even control his bowel movements and this makes him feel like a child.

Client states he is no longer able to drive "and I did that when I was 16."

Key Index Words for Nursing Interventions

Look up these words in the index of fundamentals and medical-surgical nursing textbooks to find page references for additional nursing interventions and rationale for their selection:

- activities of daily living (ADLs)
- AIDS
- alcoholism
- Alzheimer's disease
- cancer
- chronic illness
- dependency

- depression
- hemiplegia
- hope
- paraplegia
- quadriplegia
- rehabilitation
- substance abuse

RELOCATION STRESS SYNDROME

Definition

Psychological and/or psychosocial disturbances as a result of transfer from one environment to another.

Major Defining Characteristics

- change in environment/location
- anxiety
- apprehension
- increased confusion (elderly population)
- depression
- loneliness

Minor Defining Characteristics

- verbalization of unwillingness to relocate
- sleep disturbance
- change in eating habits, weight change
- dependency
- gastrointestinal disturbances
- increased verbalization of needs
- insecurity
- lack of trust
- restlessness

- sad affect
- unfavorable comparison of post/pretransfer staff
- verbalization of being concerned/upset about transfer
- vigilance; withdrawal

Related Factors
- past, concurrent, and recent losses
- losses involved with decisions to move
- feeling of powerlessness
- lack of adequate support system
- little or no preparation for the impending move
- moderate to high degree of environmental change
- history and types of previous transfers
- impaired psychosocial health status
- decreased physical health status

Examples of Specific Nursing Diagnoses
1. Relocation stress syndrome related to move from own home to nursing home.
   Relocation stress syndrome related to move from own home to nursing home as evidenced by depression, sleep disturbance, lack of appetite. (PES format)
2. Relocation stress syndrome related to out-of-state move.
   Relocation stress syndrome related to out-of-state move as evidenced by change in eating habits, frequent crying jags, weight gain of 10 lb in 1 month, and frequent complaints about new city. (PES format)

Examples of Specific Outcomes
For Nursing Home Client
1. Client will participate in one scheduled activity of choice at nursing home within 1 week.
2. Client will make one positive statement about nursing home within 1 week of admission.

For Client with Out-of-State Move
1. Client will make one positive statement about new community within 1 week.
2. Client will attend one community activity of choice within 1 week.

Examples of Specific Nursing Interventions
- See General Coping/Adjustment Nursing Interventions, page 311.

- Nurse maintains nonjudgmental attitude and does not attempt to refute client's negative evaluations of new environment.
- Acknowledgement of client's feelings, "This must really be a difficult time for you. Can you tell me more about it?"
- Avoid use of false reassurance or platitudes.
    "In a couple of months you'll just love it here."
    "All the residents felt like you do on their first days here."
    "C. is a great place to live."
    "It was rated number six in the country by *Money* magazine."
- Orient to new environment; provide guide if possible, perhaps another client in the nursing home might volunteer.
- Encourage client to retain comfortable, familiar objects and furniture, a photograph display may be especially helpful.
- Provide privacy for family visits, provide refreshments to make home-like atmosphere.
- "Repeople" the interpersonal environment; provide introductions to other clients; provide information about community groups that might be of interest; if possible, have a member of an interest group call client with invitation to join.
- Assist client to identify means to maintain relationships in the previous environment: telephone, letters, subscription to familiar newspaper, planned visit.
- Encourage participation in communal meals.
- Identify form of physical exercise that client likes and provide information about that activity within the new community.
- If requested by client, provide information about weight-control and support groups.
- Assist client to maintain personal hygiene and grooming habits.
- Assist client to set an achievable personal goal daily; this may be as simple as
    "I will smile and say good morning to three persons before 10 A.M."
    "I will shower and be at breakfast by 8 A.M. tomorrow."
    "I will watch the news at 6 P.M. in the lounge today."

Examples of Specific Evaluations for Outcomes
Outcome 1 for Nursing Home Client

1. Outcome not met. Client refuses to leave room.
2. Outcome partially met. Client walks in hall but declines invitation to join activity.
3. Outcome met. Client attended choir performance in the dining room after dinner.

Outcome 2 for Client with Out-of-State Move

1. Outcome not met. Client refuses to consider community activities saying, "Those are for senior citizens; I wouldn't fit in."
2. Outcome partially met. Client reading city magazine and discussing activities which are of interest but declines to go alone to anything.
3. Outcome met. Client attended Book and Brunch session at the library and states, "I met a woman who said she will call this week. She is going to loan me a book by the same author as the one we discussed today. I almost felt alive again!"

Key Index Words for Nursing Interventions
Look up these words in the index of fundamentals and medical-surgical nursing textbooks to find page references for additional nursing interventions and rationale for their selection:

- adaptation
- aging process
- altered nutrition: less than body requirements
- altered nutrition: more than body requirements
- dependency
- depression
- interpersonal relationships
- life review
- loneliness
- love and belonging as a basic human need
- psychological safety as a basic human need

SPIRITUAL DISTRESS

Definition
Disruption in the life principle which pervades a person's entire being and which integrates and transcends one's biological and psychosocial nature.

Defining Characteristics
- *expresses concern with the meaning of life/death and/or belief systems
- anger towards God
- questions meaning of suffering
- verbalizes inner conflict about beliefs
- verbalizes concern about relationship with deity
- questions meaning of own existence
- inability to participate in usual religious practices
- seeks spiritual assistance
- questions moral/ethical implications of therapeutic regimen
- gallows humor
- displacement of anger towards religious representatives
- description of nightmare/sleep disturbances
- alteration in behavior/mood evidenced by anger, crying, withdrawal, preoccupation, anxiety, hostility, apathy, and so forth

Related Factors
- separation from religious/cultural ties
- challenged belief and value system (e.g., due to moral/ethical implications of therapy, due to intense suffering)

Examples of Specific Nursing Diagnoses
1. Spiritual distress related to metastasis of cancer and threat of death.
   Spiritual distress related to metastasis of cancer and threat of death as evidenced by client statement, "Why is God punishing me like this? My family still needs me!" (PES format)
2. Spiritual distress related to chronic pain.
   Spiritual distress related to chronic pain as evidenced by

*Critical.

client statement, "Why does God let people suffer so? There is no good in this." (PES format)

3. Spiritual distress related to separation/nonparticipation in church.

Spiritual distress related to separation/nonparticipation in church as evidenced by statement, "I used to be a Catholic but I haven't been to church for years. I hate to go back to God only when I need help but it would be such a comfort now." (PES format)

Examples of Specific Outcomes

1. Client will express understanding that illness is not a punishment.
2. Client will express anger at God and reestablish previous comforting relationship with God.
3. Client will reestablish relationship with church group.

Match Interventions to Related Factors Causing Distress

- See General Coping/Adjustment Nursing Interventions, page 311.
- As a first intervention, nurses need to understand their own belief/value system with the understanding that all human beings have the right to their own belief/value system and that their beliefs are to be respected.
- Establish therapeutic relationship with consistency of caregiver.
- Spend time listening to the client when no physical care is necessary.
- Offer to assist clients in practicing their faith: "How can I help you to practice your faith?"
- Offer to contact the chaplain/minister for a hospital visit.
- If the nurse is comfortable with prayer and if the client has given some indication that this is appropriate, the nurse may offer to pray with the client, to read from the Bible, or to read other spiritual texts.
- Support the expression of feelings by active listening techniques: "Can you tell me more about that? And how did that make you feel?"
- Use silence as a communication technique to promote the expression of feelings. Some nurses are uncomfortable with silence and attempt to "fill in the blanks" in conversation but if the nurse can tell the client, "I'd like

to just sit here and be with you for a while" it provides an invitation to the client to talk as well as an offer of support.

■ Offer to assist the client to reconnect with church group perhaps by saying, "Many persons that I have cared for find that during hospitalization it is a time in their lives to rethink church membership and they choose to make contact with their church again. I wonder if you are thinking about this?"

■ Some clients find it helpful to talk to God and need reassurance that God understands the expression of anger and doubt.

■ While many spiritual practices are specific to a religious denomination or cultural group, many persons are comforted by the reading of the 23rd psalm: "The Lord is my Shepherd..." The nurse may offer to read this with the client or to leave it for the client to read.

■ Provide privacy and minimize interruption during spiritual practices.

Examples of Specific Evaluations for Outcome 1

1. Outcome not met. Client continues to search life for deeds deserving of punishment.
2. Outcome partially met. Client states, "I know in my head that God is not punishing me with this but I can't believe it in my heart."
3. Outcome met. Client states, "I still don't understand God's plan for me but I know that God is a loving being and that my cancer is not a punishment".

Key Index Words for Nursing Interventions

Look up these words in the index of fundamentals and medical-surgical nursing textbooks to find page references for additional nursing interventions and rationale for their selection:

■ active listening
■ alienation
■ belief system
■ death/dying
■ egocentrism
■ ethnocentrism
■ guilt

■ life review
■ reconciliation
■ spirituality
■ suffering
■ terminal illness
■ value clarification

Chapter 18

Family and Growth/ Development Problems

FOCUSED ASSESSMENT GUIDE

Complete this focused assessment if a general nursing assessment indicates a possible problem. Then turn to page 350 of this text for the Data ⇒ Diagnosis Matching Guide for family and growth/development problems to help you select the best nursing diagnosis to match the client's data.

____ Is client able to respond to questions at age-appropriate level.

____ Is client able to perform skills at age-appropriate level.

____ Who is caring for client at home?

____ Approximately how many hours of care per day is required?

____ What care is required by client at home?

____ Who is available to relieve the caregiver?

____ Is the family pulling together at present time to meet all members needs?

____ Is the family asking for information or assistance in coping with family member's health problem?

____ Are you getting the help or support you want/need from spouse or those closest to you?

____ How has your illness affected being a parent? What parental jobs or tasks are difficult to accomplish?

____ Who is caring for your children while you are in the hospital?

____ Is the arrangement for child care satisfactory to you?

DATA ⇒ DIAGNOSIS MATCHING GUIDE

Compare your data from the Family and Growth/
Development Focused Assessment to these related family
and growth/development nursing diagnoses and abbreviated
descriptions. Select the nursing diagnosis which is the best
match. Then turn to the page in this section with that specific
diagnosis for help in planning care.

1. *Altered Family Processes: page 353*
   - definition: normally functioning family experiences dysfunction
   - data: family system unable to meet needs of its members

2. *Altered Growth and Development: page 356*
   - definition: deviations from what is normal for age-group
   - data: delay in verbal or motor skills or physical growth

3. *Altered Parenting: page 359*
   - definition: parent unable to meet needs of infant/child
   - data: history of abuse or abandonment by primary caregiver; inattention to infant/child needs; inappropriate caretaking behavior

4. *High Risk for Altered Parenting: page 363*
   - definition: parent is at risk for being unable to meet needs of infant/child
   - data: presence of risk factors such as history of abuse or abandonment by primary caregiver, inattention to infant/child needs, inappropriate caretaking behavior

5. *Caregiver Role Strain: page 366*
   - definition: caregiver's felt difficulty in performing the family caregiver role
   - data: caregivers report lack of resources to provide care, difficulties in providing care, family conflict over care issues, own depression, stress, nervousness

6. *High Risk for Caregiver Role Strain: page 371*
   - definition: caregiver is susceptible to experiencing difficulty in caregiver role

■ data: physical status of care receiver; caregiver not ready to assume responsibility of role; marginal relationship with care receiver prior to illness; situational stressors affecting ability to give care such as poverty, history of abuse, lack of recreation for caregiver, inexperience, inadequate physical environment

7. *Family Coping: Potential for Growth: page 374*
   ■ definition: effective management of adapting to illness; family member shows signs of desire and readiness to enhance health for self and client
   ■ data: family members describe growth impact of illness; family member(s) seeking health-promoting lifestyle

8. *Ineffective Family Coping: Compromised: page 377*
   ■ definition: insufficient or ineffective support from family or close friend
   ■ data: client verbalizes concern about family response to health problem or family member/significant other verbalizes lack of knowledge which interferes with effective ability to support client; family member or significant other displays behaviors which are not effective in supporting client

9. *Ineffective Family Coping: Disabling: page 380*
   ■ definition: behavior of family member or significant other which destroys own or client's ability to deal with health problem
   ■ data: neglect or abandonment of client; neglectful care of client's basic human needs; distortion of reality/denial about client health status

10. *Parental Role Conflict: page 383*
    ■ definition: parent experiences confusion/conflict in response to crisis
    ■ data: parent expresses concerns about ability to provide for child's needs during hospitalization or at home; concerns about changes in parental role, family function

GENERAL OUTCOMES AND NURSING INTERVENTIONS

GENERAL FAMILY AND GROWTH/DEVELOPMENT OUTCOMES

- Client is able to perform tasks appropriate to developmental level.
- Client is able to communicate at appropriate developmental level.
- Client maintains/attains maximum level of health possible.
- Family caregiver maintains intact self/personality while providing or delegating care of family member.
- Family members interact in ways that are mutually supportive and satisfying.
- Family members acknowledge existence of problems and identify when assistance is needed.
- Family members engage in constructive problem solving to meet each member's needs.
- Parents accurately assess parenting skills.
- Parents seek assistance in learning new parenting skills.

GENERAL FAMILY AND GROWTH/DEVELOPMENT NURSING INTERVENTIONS

- Review own biases about what family "should" look like or how family "should" function in order to become aware of cultural or class stereotypes, possible prejudices.
- Assess family from perspective of "Is this a functional/satisfying arrangement for meeting members' needs?"
- Assess client and family members/significant others comparing data to appropriate developmental norms.
- Observe client interaction with family group and consider impact on health status.
- Assess strengths and limitations of family group in assisting client.
- Provide for health teaching for both client and family members.
- Assist family to identify sources of support or assistance within own community.
- Assist client and family to learn and practice problem-solving skills.

RELATED NURSING DIAGNOSES

ALTERED FAMILY PROCESSES

Definition
A state in which a family that normally functions effectively experiences dysfunction.

Defining Characteristics
- family system unable to meet physical needs of its members
- family system unable to meet emotional needs of its members
- family system unable to meet spiritual needs of its members
- parents do not demonstrate respect for each other's views on child-rearing practices
- inability to express/accept wide range of feelings
- inability to express/accept feelings of members
- family unable to meet security needs of its members
- inability of family members to relate to each other for mutual growth and maturation
- family uninvolved in community activities
- inability to accept/receive help appropriately
- rigidity in function and roles
- family not demonstrating respect for individuality and autonomy of its members
- family unable to adapt to change/deal with traumatic experience constructively
- family failing to accomplish current/past developmental tasks
- unhealthy family decision-making process
- failure to send and receive clear messages
- inappropriate boundary maintenance
- inappropriate/poorly communicated family rules, rituals, or symbols
- unexamined family myths
- inappropriate level and direction of energy

Related Factors
- situation transition and/or crises
- developmental transition and/or crisis

Examples of Specific Nursing Diagnoses

1. Altered family processes related to job loss and loss of major income.

   Altered family processes related to job loss and loss of major income as evidenced by client statement. "The stress is unbearable. We are all fighting and yelling at each other over things that 6 months ago we would have laughed off!" (PES format)

2. Altered family processes related to developmental transition (children entering adolescence).

   Altered family processes related to developmental transition (children entering adolescence) as evidenced by parent statements, "They never want to spend time at home. They test every rule. They refuse to go to church with us; it just isn't worth the battle to make them go. Our home life is really not happy at the present time." (PES format)

*Examples of Specific Outcomes**

1. Family members will verbalize their major worries related to loss of income and begin to develop a plan to resolve the worries within 1 week.

2. Family members will verbalize their anger and identify alternative outlets within 1 week.

3. Parents and teens will attend support group for families with adolescent members within 1 week.

4. Parents will discuss with nurse the developmental tasks of adolescence and compare to the behavior of their children before discharge.

5. Parents and adolescents will discuss with nurse the physiological changes of adolescence and their impact on behavior within 1 week.

Examples of Specific Nursing Interventions

Some of the interventions below are suited to a nurse working with a family in a community setting, others for a psychiatric setting, and some for the hospital. The nurse needs to select interventions and adapt them to individual client's needs.

---

*These outcomes focus on the family as client.

- See General Family and Growth/Development Nursing Interventions, page 352.
- Observe family interaction style and note especially who are the dominant members and who tends to withdraw from discussion.
- Invite family discussion by opening a conversation with, "So how are things going for your family?" This gives the family the opportunity to talk with the nurse or to answer at a level of a social pleasantry.
- Assist family members to assess their strengths and limitations considering both group skills and those of individual members. The nurse might encourage, "So Jennifer, what do you think are the things your mom does best?"
- Teach family members a problem-solving process that they can use as a group. It might be something like: name the problem, what caused it, brainstorm everything we can do about it, select solutions that we will all agree to try for a certain time period, then we will get together to see if it worked.
- Assist family to develop one or two house rules that everyone will agree to as well as consequences for breaking house rules. This might include church attendance, money management, guests in house, mealtimes, smoking.
- Develop a teaching plan for parents to learn normal adolescent growth and development (or the relevant developmental level). Invite discussion that relates observations of their children's behavior to the textbook picture.
- Provide experience in listening for family members. It might go something like this: "What I wish my mom/dad/family/sister/brother would understand about me is..." Each member may talk uninterrupted for a given time period (2 minutes) and then each family member repeats back to the speaker the message that was heard. The speaker agrees they got it right or disagrees, "No, that's not what I said. I said..."
- Encourage family to visit hospitalized member and to participate in care if they wish.
- Develop teaching plan for family members for home care after discharge.

- Assist family members to use coping strategies that were successful in the past.

   "Can you tell me about another difficult problem or situation in your past experience?"

   "What did you do about it?"

   "What was helpful to you then?"

   "Do you think you could try that now?"
- Provide access to financial counselor if family accepts offer.

Examples of Specific Evaluations for Outcome 1
1. Outcome not met. Family extremely worried about finances but refuses to discuss saying, "There is nothing we can do."
2. Outcome partially met. Family said they have talked about their problems as a group but has not been able to think of any plans.
3. Outcome met. Family made a list of worries and began a plan which included a request to see a financial counselor for help.

Key Index Words for Nursing Interventions
Look up these words in the index of fundamentals and medical-surgical nursing textbooks to find page references for additional nursing interventions and rationale for their selection:

- developmental steps/stages
- familial alcoholism
- family, single parent
- family systems theory
- family therapy
- growth and development

ALTERED GROWTH AND DEVELOPMENT

Definition
A state in which an individual demonstrates deviations in norms from own age-group.

Major Defining Characteristics
- delay or difficulty in performing skills (motor, social, or expressive) typical of age-group
- altered physical growth
- inability to perform self-care or self-control activities appropriate for age

Minor Defining Characteristics
- flat affect
- listlessness, decreased responses

Related Factors
- inadequate caretaking
- indifference
- inconsistent responsiveness, multiple caretakers
- separation from significant others
- environmental and stimulation deficiencies
- effects of physical disability
- prescribed dependence

Examples of Specific Nursing Diagnoses
1. Altered growth and development (right leg) related to hypoxia during the birth process.
   Altered growth and development (right leg) related to hypoxia during birth process as evidenced by unequal muscle development, foot abduction, and unequal leg length. (PES format)
2. Altered growth and development related to Down's syndrome.
   Altered growth and development related to Down's syndrome as evidenced by delayed intellectual and motor development: 4-year-old not toilet trained, unable to feed self, yes/no speech. (PES format)

Examples of Specific Outcomes
1. Client will demonstrate foot abduction exercises before discharge.
2. Parents will determine home exercise schedule for child before discharge.
3. Parental caregivers will verbalize and demonstrate appropriate sensory and motor stimulation activities to encourage continued development of child before discharge.
4. Parents will discuss how health care needs for their child may differ and develop an assessment plan assisted by the nurse before discharge.

Examples of Specific Nursing Interventions
- See General Family and Growth/Development Nursing Interventions, page 352.

- Assess and work through own feelings about working with clients with altered growth/development problems.
- Include client and parents in assessment interviews.
- Speak directly to client and maintain eye contact.
- Assess for client ability to perform ADLs (toileting, bathing, brushing teeth, hair care). Note modifications necessary and document for other staff to follow.
- Assure that client knows how to use call system for nurse.
- Assess normal routine for client and adapt hospital routine as much as possible: meals, snacks, bathing, bedtime routine.
- Encourage family members to visit ad lib.
- Provide family members with telephone numbers to reach a nurse 24 hours per day and assure them that they may call for information.
- Assess family need of respite services and provide information if requested.
- Offer to assist client to use phone to maintain contact with family/friends.
- Assist client/family to achieve/identify time achievable long-term and short-term goals.
- Provide feedback and reinforcement for progress toward goals as well as goal achievement.
- Teach client health care at level appropriate to ability, for example, handwashing, not to take medication unless given by caregiver, sleep needs, nutrition basics, what to do when you feel sick.
- Assess for hearing, vision, speech, and language problems which may be associated with nursing diagnosis.
- Assess for use of adaptive devices to enhance motor skills, for example, self-feeding is easier using special forks with handles molded to fit a hand.
- Identify community resources and provide written literature for the family. During the client's hospitalization they may not have the energy available to make use of these resources but it will be accessible at a later date.
- For adolescent clients, assess for knowledge about sex and sexuality, discuss with parents what information and instruction has been given, and offer to assist them in planning this education.
- Provide for appropriate sensory stimulation during

hospitalization when client is able to participate: consult with occupational therapist, get client out of bed, request parents to bring some activities from home that can be done in hospital.

- Assess parents/caregiver learning needs and motivation to learn.
- Assess client's existing home care routine and suggest any modifications to assist caregivers or meet client's needs.
- Demonstrate ability level sensory/motor stimulation and assess which activities client enjoys, selecting them for inclusion into a plan for home care.

Examples of Specific Evaluations for Outcome 1

1. Outcome not met. Parents refuse to have child do exercises because child complains of pain on movement. "She's been through too much to have her suffer any pain now."
2. Outcome partially met. Child does partial exercises with physical therapist but refuses therapy with parents.
3. Outcome met. Child demonstrates exercise routine assisted by parents.

Key Index Words for Nursing Interventions

Look up these words in the index of fundamentals and medical-surgical nursing textbooks to find page references for additional nursing interventions and rationale for their selection:

- Bender Visual-Motor Gestalt
- Denver Developmental Screening
- developmental tasks
- Draw-A-Person test
- performance skills

ALTERED PARENTING

Definition

A state in which a nurturing figure(s) experiences an inability to create an environment which promotes the optimum growth and development of another human being.

Defining Characteristics
- abandonment
- runaway
- verbalization of inability to control child
- incidence of physical and psychological trauma
- lack of parental attachment behaviors
- inappropriate visual, tactile, or auditory stimulation
- negative identification of infant/child characteristics
- negative attachment of meanings to infant/child characteristics
- constant verbalization of disappointment in gender or physical characteristics of infant/child
- verbalization of resentment towards infant/child
- verbalization of role inadequacy
- *inattention to infant/child needs
- verbal disgust at body functions of infant/child
- noncompliance with health appointments for self or infant/child
- *inappropriate caretaking behaviors (toilet training, sleep/rest, feeding)
- inappropriate or inconsistent discipline practices
- frequent accidents
- frequent illness
- growth and development lag in child
- *history of child abuse or abandonment by primary caretaker
- verbalization of caregiver desire to have a child call caregiver by first name versus traditional cultural tendencies
- child receives care from multiple caregivers without consideration for needs of the infant/child
- compulsive seeking of role approval from others

Related Factors
- lack of available role model
- ineffective role model
- physical and psychological abuse of nurturing figure
- lack of support between/from significant other(s)
- unmet social/emotional maturation needs of parenting figures

*Critical.

- interruption in bonding process (e.g., maternal, paternal, other)
- unrealistic expectations for self, infant, partner
- perceived threat to own physical or emotional survival
- mental and/or physical illness
- presence of stress (financial, legal, recent crisis, cultural move)
- lack of knowledge
- limited cognitive functioning
- lack of role identity
- lack of (or inappropriate) response of child to relationship
- multiple pregnancies

Examples of Specific Nursing Diagnoses
1. Altered parenting related to four pregnancies in 5 years.
   Altered parenting related to four pregnancies in 5 years as evidenced by frequent accidents of children, missed health care appointments, and mother's statement, "I just cannot be a good mother to four children all at the same time". (PES format)
2. Altered parenting related to lack of role model.
   Altered parenting related to lack of role model as evidenced by mother's statement: "I was raised by my sister who was 6 years older. My parents were never around". (PES format)

Examples of Specific Outcomes
1. Mother will express one positive statement of her ability as a mother in at least one area within 2 weeks.
2. Mother will keep appointment for immunization of infant within the next month.
3. Parents will attend parenting group within 2 weeks.
4. Parents will work with school to set action plan for their child within 2 weeks.

Examples of Specific Nursing Interventions
- See General Family and Growth/Development Nursing Interventions, page 352.
- Assess for safety of environment for child. Include physical assessment which notes unexplained bruises, scars, nutritional status, developmental lags. If indicated, report to authorities as required by law.

- Assess parent(s)/child interaction.
  - How do they speak to each other?
  - How is correction or discipline handled?
  - What is the overt stress level of each? Is eye contact maintained?
  - What kind of physical contact is used?
- Assess behavior of child: withdrawn, anxious, fearful, hyperactive, verbal, attention-seeking, response to discipline.
- Verbalize observations to parents; often parents are unaware of their actions.
- Assess readiness for change. Are parents satisfied with the way things are going or would they like to make some changes in the way they parent their children?
- Establish an environment where it is safe for a parent to talk about concerns without fear.
- Encourage parents to talk about their expectations of parenting. How does the reality compare to the expected.
- Assess parent's knowledge level of growth and development for their child's age-group. This is assessing their understanding of what is normal behavior and motor/intellectual skill for the particular age-group.
- Assess with parents their parenting assets. Write them out and give parents a copy to use as a basis for building new skills.
- Identify with parents what goals they would like to work on related to parenting, e.g., controlling my temper during discipline, setting rules for child, teaching child hygiene skills.
- Develop a teaching plan which incorporates both parent- and nurse-identified needs.
- Assist parents to develop parenting support systems such as extended family, community groups.
- Offer to contact financial counselor if this is needed and agreed to by family.
- Encourage attendance at parent effectiveness training classes and provide with schedules and contact persons.
- Assess for physical activity and recreational time. Assist parents to plan for meeting these needs.
- Teach parents about and assist them to meet the health needs of their child, for example, breast-feeding of infant, dental hygiene of preschool child, school-age immunizations, nutrition needs.

■ Establish schedule of meetings to evaluate progress on achieving mutually set parenting and health goals.

Examples of Specific Evaluations for Outcome 1

1. Outcome not met. Mother states, "I keep trying but I guess I'm just not cut out to be a mother. There is just too much to do!"
2. Outcome partially met. Mother states, "I'm trying. I tried reading a bedtime story to the kids every night but they wouldn't listen and bounced off the walls. Kids are supposed to like bedtime stories."
3. Outcome met. Mother states, "I made the kids breakfast every morning this week. They really liked that and I felt like I was helping them to do better at school."

Key Index Words for Nursing Interventions

Look up these words in the index of fundamentals and medical-surgical nursing textbooks to find page references for additional nursing interventions and rationale for their selection:

- abuse, physical
- abuse, psychological
- alcoholism
- blended families
- family systems theory
- family therapy
- parents/parenting
- single-parent family

HIGH RISK FOR ALTERED PARENTING

Definition

A state in which a nuturing figure(s) is at risk to experience an inability to create an environment which promotes the optimum growth and development of another human being.

Defining Risk Factors

- lack of parental attachment behaviors
- inappropriate visual, tactile, auditory stimulation
- negative identification of infant/child characteristics
- negative attachment of meanings to infant/child characteristics
- constant verbalization of disappointment in gender or physical characteristics of infant/child
- verbalization of resentment towards infant/child
- verbalization of role inadequacy

- *inattention to infant/child needs
- verbal disgust at body functions of infant/child
- noncompliance with health appointments for self or infant/child
- *inappropriate caretaking behaviors (toilet training, sleep/rest, feeding)
- inappropriate or inconsistent discipline practices
- frequent accidents
- frequent illness
- growth and development lag in child
- history of child abuse or abandonment by primary caretaker
- verbalization by caregiver of desire to have child call caregiver by first name versus traditional cultural tendencies
- child received care from multiple caregivers without consideration for needs of the infant/child
- compulsive seeking of role approval from others

Related Factors
- lack of available role model
- ineffective role model
- physical and psychological abuse of nurturing figure
- lack of support between/from significant other(s)
- unmet social/emotional maturation needs of parenting figures
- interruption in bonding process (e.g., maternal, paternal, other)
- unrealistic expectations for self, infant, partner
- perceived threat to own physical or emotional survival
- mental and/or physical illness
- presence of stress (financial, legal, recent crisis, cultural move)
- lack of knowledge
- limited cognitive functioning
- lack of role identity
- lack of (or inappropriate) response of child to relationship
- multiple pregnancies

*Critical.

Examples of Specific Nursing Diagnoses

1. High risk for altered parenting related to unwanted pregnancy and youth of mother.

   High risk for altered parenting related to unwanted pregnancy and youth of mother as evidenced by mother's statement, "I kept my pregnancy from my mother until it was too late for an abortion but she threw me out of the house when she found out. I don't want to be a mother." (PES format)

2. High risk for altered parenting related to inadequate income for family of four.

   High risk for altered parenting related to inadequate income for family of four as evidenced by father's statement, "I work two jobs, 60–70 hours per week, and we can't make it. Medical bills, food, clothes, rent, the car is falling apart and we would love to have a house but we can't save a nickel. We keep going deeper and deeper into debt. We fight a lot about money." (PES format)

Examples of Specific Outcomes

1. Client will participate in prenatal parenting classes at high school for the next 3 months.
2. Client will keep all scheduled prenatal clinic visits.
3. Parents will meet with financial counselor for assistance with budget planning within the next 2 weeks.

Examples of Specific Nursing Interventions

- See Specific Nursing Interventions for Altered Parenting, page 361.
- See General Family and Growth/Development Nursing Interventions, page 352.
- Assess for basic needs of parents and children, including health care needs of pregnant woman.
- Assess for the strengths of family unit, verbalize them to client, and use as basis for further teaching.
- Offer to contact financial counselor if this is indicated.
- Provide for transportation to health care appointments. This is a frequent cause of missed appointments.
- Assess for knowledge of pregnancy and health care need during this time.

- Aid in decision-making about future of unborn infant. Maintain a nonjudgmental attitude and present honestly all available options to client.
- Support the decision of client and work together on ways to make the decision succeed.
- Assist parents to prioritize demands on their time and energy expenditure.
- Identify community resources for parents to use in solving problems or in reducing stress.

Examples of Specific Evaluations for Outcome 1

1. Outcome not met. Client refuses to attend school, saying, "The kids waddle when they see me coming! I can't go back!"
2. Outcome partially met. Client has very erratic school attendance and states she is too tired to go to school.
3. Outcome met. Client refuses to attend academic classes but has perfect attendance at prenatal classes, "This is for my baby."

Key Index Words for Nursing Interventions

Look up these words in the index of fundamentals and medical-surgical nursing textbooks to find page references for additional nursing interventions and rationale for their selection:

- anxiety
- attachment
- bonding
- parenting

- physical safety
- psychological security
- role identity
- social support

CAREGIVER ROLE STRAIN

Definition

A caregiver's felt difficulty in performing the family caregiver role.

Defining Characteristics: Caregivers*

- do not have enough resources to provide the care needed
- find it hard to do specific caregiving activities

---

*Eighty percent of caregivers report one or more of defining characteristics.

- worry about such things as the care receiver's health and emotional state, having to put the receiver in an institution, and who will care for the care receiver if something should happen to the caregiver
- feel that caregiving interferes with other important roles in their lives
- feel loss because the care receiver is like a different person compared to the time before care began or, in the case of a child, that the care receiver was never the child the caregiver expected
- feel family conflict around issues of providing care
- feel stress or nervousness in their relationship with the care receiver
- feel depressed

Related Factors
Pathophysiological/Physiological
- illness severity of the care receiver
- addiction or codependency
- premature birth/congenital defect
- discharge of family member with significant home care needs
- caregiver health impairment
- unpredictable illness course or instability in the care receiver's health
- caregiver is female

Developmental
- caregiver is not developmentally ready for caregiver role, e.g., young adult needing to provide for a middle-aged parent
- development delay or retardation of the care receiver or caregiver

Psychosocial
- psychosocial or cognitive problems in the care receiver
- marginal family adaptation or dysfunction prior to the caregiving situation
- marginal caregiver's coping patterns
- past history of poor relationship between caregiver and care receiver
- caregiver is spouse
- care receiver exhibits deviant, bizarre behavior

Situational
- presence of abuse or violence
- presence of situational stressors which normally affect families such as significant loss, disaster or crisis, poverty or economic vulnerability, major life events, e.g., birth, hospitalization, leaving home, returning home, marriage, divorce, employment, retirement, death
- duration of caregiving required
- inadequate physical environment for providing care, e.g., housing, transportation, community services, equipment
- family/caregiver isolation
- lack of respite and recreation for caregiver
- inexperience with caregiving
- caregiver's competing role commitments
- complexity/amount of caring tasks

Examples of Specific Nursing Diagnoses
1. Caregiver role strain related to illness of caregiver.
   Caregiver role strain related to illness of caregiver as evidenced by reports of depression, weight loss, exhaustion, and sleeplessness of caregiver. (PES format)
2. Caregiver role strain related to caregiver lack of development readiness.
   Caregiver role strain related to caregiver lack of development readiness (28-year-old mother of two, ages 6 and 2, caring for own mother with Alzheimer's disease) as evidenced by crying, "I am not doing a good job at being a mother or taking care of my mother, and I'm so tired all the time." (PES format)

Examples of Specific Outcomes
1. Caregiver will report improved health status (uninterrupted sleep, no further weight loss, less severe depression) within 2 weeks.
2. Caregiver will meet with social worker for the purpose of identifying community resources and services available to assist in caregiving before discharge of care receiver.
3. Caregiver will report plans for one day or evening off per week prior to discharge of care receiver.

Examples of Specific Nursing Interventions

- See General Family and Growth/Development Nursing Interventions, page 352.
- Nurse assesses family in four areas: structure, communication, relationship to community, and health behaviors. Structure includes listing the members, where they live, and extended generations. Communication includes how they talk together and share information, feelings, and problems. Community includes what resources are available in the community. Is the family isolated or do they have a base of friends, neighbors, and church groups? Health practices include health beliefs and practices within the culture of the caregiver and care receiver.
- Offer time to meet with the caregiver privately since caregiver may be reluctant to talk in front of the care receiver.
- Assess strengths and limitations of caregiver.
- Assess other family members for potential contributions to the care of receiver.
- Facilitate family conference focusing on problem solving for care receiver. Identify resources within family group to assist the caregiver.
- Encourage the caregiver to say to other family members, "I need help!" Frequently caregivers are unable or reluctant to ask for needed help.
- Provide positive feedback/praise for the work the caregiver has done, acknowledge its importance, and accord it the respect it deserves.
- Solicit the caregiver's input into planning the nursing care of the care receiver in the hospital. The caregiver is an expert resource.
- Facilitate communication between caregiver and care receiver if necessary, giving voice to the needs of each person.
- Complete health assessment of caregiver.
- Assess receiver for potential to use assistive devices which may make caregiving easier: adaptive eating devices, lifts for moving the receiver, electric wheelchair, catheters or drainage devices.

- Assess receiver for adequacy of care. It is important to understand this is not a blame issue but the caregiver may not know how to provide some aspects of care.
- Assess receiver for self-care abilities which could be enhanced by training or assistive devices.
- Develop a teaching plan to provide knowledge and skill for the caregiver.
- Assess the caregiver for participation in recreational or diversional activities, "What do you do for fun?" If the answer is negative respond with, "What would you like to do?"
- Assist the caregiver to develop a plan which enables participation in regular recreation.
- Inventory all responsibilities of caregiver and identify those which could be delegated to others: home or lawn care, periods of child care, grocery shopping.
- Describe the care provided by a home health care aid and the insurance reimbursement that is available for the service.
- Introduce the consideration of agency/institution care if receiver's condition is progressively deteriorating. Caregiver may not be emotionally ready to implement the option at the time but may begin to consider it as a future choice.
- Plan conferences/consultations to involve the receiver as much as possible.
- Offer to coordinate interdisciplinary care planning conference of professionals: financial counselors, social workers, physicians, home health care workers, and members of other disciplines as indicated by the needs of the caregiver and care receiver.
- Identify support groups within the community and offer to facilitate contact for caregiver.

Examples of Specific Evaluations for Outcome 1

1. Outcome not met. Caregiver reports that receiver has been having bad nights and calls out to her two or three times each night, making sleep impossible.
2. Outcome partially met. Medication for the receiver is helping to allow caregiver as much as 4–5 hours of sleep without interruption, but caregiver continues to lose weight and feel depressed.

3. Outcome met. To help caregiver sleep, other family members have agreed to take turns sleeping at house. Caregiver reports gaining 2 lb and feeling less depressed.

Key Index Words for Nursing Interventions
Look up these words in the index of fundamentals and medical-surgical nursing textbooks to find page references for additional nursing interventions and rationale for their selection:

- discharge planning
- family assessment guide
- family social services
- home health care
- hospice care
- occupational therapy
- pain management
- rehabilitation therapy
- respite care

HIGH RISK FOR CAREGIVER ROLE STRAIN

Definition
A caregiver is vulnerable for felt difficulty in performing the family caregiver role.

Risk Factors
Pathophysiological
- illness severity of the care receiver
- addiction or codependency
- premature birth/congenital defect
- discharge of family member with significant home care needs
- caregiver health impairment
- unpredictable illness course or instability in the care receiver's health
- caregiver is female
- psychological or cognitive problems in the care receiver

Developmental
- caregiver is not developmentally ready for caregiver role, e.g., young adult needing to provide for a middle-aged parent
- developmental delay or retardation of the care receiver or caregiver

Psychosocial
- marginal family adaptation or dysfunction prior to the caregiving situation
- marginal caregiver coping patterns
- past history of poor relationship between caregiver and care receiver
- caregiver is spouse
- care receiver exhibits deviant, bizarre behavior

Situational
- presence of abuse or violence
- presence of situational stressors which normally affect families such as significant loss, disaster or crisis, poverty or economic vulnerability, major life events, e.g., birth, hospitalization, leaving home, returning home, marriage, divorce, employment, retirement, death
- duration of caregiving required
- inadequate physical environment for providing care, e.g., housing, transportation, community services, equipment
- family/caregiver isolation
- lack of respite and recreation for caregiver
- inexperience with caregiving
- caregiver's competing role commitments
- complexity/amount of caring tasks

Examples of Specific Nursing Diagnoses
1. High risk for caregiver role strain related to unpredictable illness course of spouse with multiple sclerosis.
   High risk for caregiver role strain related to unpredictable illness course of spouse with multiple sclerosis as evidenced by client statement, "It is so uncertain; we could have years of ups and downs or it could be steadily downhill!" (PES format)
2. High risk for caregiver role strain related to preexisting poor relationship between care receiver (mother) and caregiver (daughter).
   High risk for caregiver role strain related to preexisting poor relationship between care receiver (mother) and caregiver (daughter) as manifested by caregiver statement, "It is ironic that I should be in this role. My mother and I have never had a good relationship". (PES format)

Examples of Specific Outcomes

1. Caregiver will agree to participate in interdisciplinary care planning conference prior to discharge of client.
2. Caregiver will verbalize concerns about relationship with mother prior to discharge.
3. Caregiver will participate in problem solving to identify alternative care during periods of scheduled respite before client is discharged.

Examples of Specific Nursing Interventions

- See General Family and Growth/Development Nursing Interventions, page 352.
- Assist caregiver by providing a summary and schedule of the care presently required by client.
- Assist caregiver to identify what is a reasonable amount of care he/she is able to or desires to continue and what areas require assistance.
- Praise caregiver for past work.
- Offer to coordinate meeting of interdisciplinary team to assist in planning for future care. This should include social workers, financial counselors, physicians, nurses, representatives from home health care agencies.
- Discuss what recreational activities the caregiver enjoys and recent participation or lack of participation.
- Assist caregiver to identify opportunities for recreation and alternative respite caregivers.
- Assist client to develop an education plan for respite caregivers; consider such things as emergency assistance, toileting, safety of ambulation.
- Assess relationship between caregiver and care receiver during their interactions.
- Share observation (since caregiver has already reported a difficult relationship during the assessment phase) of relationship and ask if this is something the caregiver would like to improve. If the caregiver indicates this is something positive, the intervention can be as simple as teaching ways to respond to criticism, limit setting behaviors, expressing anger. It might include sessions with a counselor or clinical nurse specialist.

Examples of Specific Evaluations for Outcome 1

1. Outcome not met. Caregiver insists, "I can do it myself. No one has helped me so far."

2. Outcome partially met. Caregiver has agreed to meet with financial counselor to determine whether any assistance is available, "That is the only help I need."
3. Outcome met. Both caregiver and care receiver met with interdisciplinary team. Caregiver states, "It really helps to know that lots of alternatives are available. Now we can plan and make some choices."

Key Index Words for Nursing Interventions

Look up these words in the index of fundamentals and medical-surgical nursing textbooks to find page references for additional nursing interventions and rationale for their selection:

- dependence, independence, and interdependence
- discharge planning
- home health care
- hospice care
- mental health
- respite care
- support groups

FAMILY COPING: POTENTIAL FOR GROWTH

Definition

Effective managing of adaptive tasks by family member involved with the client's health challenge, who is now exhibiting desire and readiness for enhanced health and growth in regard to self and in relation to the client.

Defining Characteristics

- family member now attempting to describe growth impact of crisis on own values, priorities, goals, or relationships
- family member now moving in direction of health-promoting and enriching lifestyle which supports and monitors maturational processes
- client audits and negotiates treatment programs, and generally chooses experiences which optimize wellness
- individual expressing interest in making contact on a one-to-one basis or on a mutual-aid, group basis with another person who has experienced a similar situation

Related Factors
■ needs sufficiently gratified and adaptive tasks effectively addressed to enable goals of self-actualization to surface

Examples of Specific Nursing Diagnosis
1. Family coping: potential for growth related to effective coping with myocardial infarction.
   Family coping: potential for growth related to effective coping with myocardial infarction as evidenced by client statement, "We have all been talking about this as a family and decided that maybe this heart attack was the push we needed to make some changes in our diets and exercise patterns," (PES format)
2. Family coping: potential for growth related to coping with progressive illness of father (multiple sclerosis).
   Family coping: potential for growth related to coping with progressive illness of father (multiple sclerosis) as evidenced by daughter's statement, "I wish, of course, that he didn't have it, but I think it gave us a sense of family few others ever experience." (PES format)

Examples of Specific Outcomes
1. Family members will work as a group to develop and implement diet and exercise changes of their choosing before discharge.
2. Family members will be able to verbalize the impact of father's illness on life prior to client discharge.
3. Family members will identify coping strategies used when growing up in family of origin and relate them to the present situation before client discharge.
4. Family members will express to each other feelings of being supported during present crisis before discharge.

Examples of Specific Nursing Interventions
■ See General Family and Growth/Development Nursing Interventions, page 352.
■ Identify family members and relationships between members.
■ Support family coping skills by providing them privacy to interact and support each other.
■ Support family members participation in care of client.

- Provide information about community resources.
- Provide contacts with hospital system of caregivers.
- Engage in active listening.
  "That sounds like a healthy response...what kinds of changes are you thinking about?"
  "Your family sounds very important to you...what was it like growing up in your home?"
- Facilitate communication between family members.
  "Your sister has told me what a close family you were growing up. I guess that was a very special time for you all..."
- Provide health care information/teaching sessions as requested by the client and family.
- Assist client and family to verbalize previously successful coping strategies that may be appropriate in the present.
  "How did you cope with it when your father was diagnosed."
  "How did you handle that?"
  "What did you learn then that might be helpful now?"

Examples of Specific Evaluations for Outcome 1

1. Outcome not met. Family members unable to schedule joint session before discharge.
2. Outcome partially met. Family members met with dietician and were enthusiastic about learning new meal plans but will delay exercise program until father is given physician approval to join them.
3. Outcome met. Family is going as a group to Heart Smart classes which include diet and exercise content.

Key Index Words for Nursing Interventions

Look up these words in the index of fundamentals and medical-surgical nursing textbooks to find page references for additional nursing interventions and rationale for their selection:

- crisis intervention
- health: mental, physical
- health promotion
- health-seeking behaviors
- self-actualization

INEFFECTIVE FAMILY COPING: COMPROMISED

Definition

A usually supportive primary person (family member or close friend) is providing insufficient, ineffective, or compromised support, comfort, assistance, or encouragement which may be needed by the client to manage or master adaptive tasks related to own health challenge.

Subjective Defining Characteristics

- client expresses or confirms a concern or complaint about significant other's response to client's health problem
- significant person describes preoccupation with personal reaction (e.g., fear, anticipatory grief, guilt, anxiety) to client's illness, disability, or to other situational or developmental crises
- significant person describes or confirms an inadequate understanding of knowledge base which interferes with effective assistive or supportive behaviors

Objective Defining Characteristics

- significant person attempts assistive or supportive behaviors with less than satisfactory results
- significant person withdraws or enters into limited or temporary personal communication with client at the time of need
- significant person displays protective behavior disproportionate (too little or too much) to the client's abilities or need for autonomy

Related Factors

- inadequate or incorrect information or understanding by a primary person
- temporary preoccupation by a significant person who is trying to manage emotional conflicts and personal suffering and is unable to perceive or act effectively in regard to client's needs
- temporary family disorganization and role changes
- other situational or developmental crises or situations the significant person may be facing; in turn, little support provided by client for primary person
- prolonged disease or disability progression that exhausts supportive capacity of significant people

Examples of Specific Nursing Diagnosis
1. Ineffective family coping: compromised related to lack of support by spouse.
   Ineffective family coping: compromised related to lack of support by spouse as evidenced by client statement, "My husband just can't deal with my being sick. He hates hospitals and is afraid to even come in one, but I feel so alone and wish he could just be here with me." (PES format)
2. Ineffective family coping: compromised related to overprotective behavior of wife following husband's stroke.
   Ineffective family coping: compromised related to overprotective behavior of wife following husband's stroke as evidenced by wife's doing everything for client, brushing teeth, feeding, bathing, etc. (PES format)

Examples of Specific Outcomes
1. Client will make one statement that indicates client is feeling support of spouse prior to discharge.
2. Client's spouse will demonstrate ability to assist client with ADLs only when requested prior to discharge.
3. Client's spouse will verbalize individual stressors which interfere with ability to support client prior to discharge.
4. Client's spouse will verbalize support for client and identify ways to show support in own actions by discharge.

Examples of Specific Nursing Interventions
- See General Family and Growth/Development Nursing Interventions, page 352.
- Establish a therapeutic relationship with the family.
- Assess family interactions: who makes decisions, who talks to whom, dependency relationships, authority.
- Offer to schedule family meetings to assist family in coping with client's illness.
- Teach family members the skill of active listening and support them in practicing it in family meetings.
- Assess impact of client's illness on family member.
  "How has your wife's cancer affected you?"
  "What changes has it made in your life?"
  "What has it been like for you?"

- Encourage family to share meaning of illness with client and to express feelings to each other.
- Encourage family members to express their needs by teaching them to make statements which do not accuse the other person of a failure

    "I need…"

    "It is helpful to me when you…"

    "I feel…"

    "It felt good when you…"
- Encourage the client to ask for needed help.

    "Some people find it very difficult to ask for help. They feel that they should be able to handle things alone. I wonder if you are experiencing that?"

    "How do you think your family/spouse would respond if you were to ask for a visit, or whatever is needed?"
- Correct misperceptions or incorrect information that client or family members have. For example, "I thought everyone who had to have a mastectomy would die because I thought they used lumpectomy if there was hope. That just devastated me."
- Explain treatment/therapy plan and how family members can assist in promoting health of client. For example, "The exercise your husband gets by feeding himself will help him to maximize his recovery from the stroke by strengthening his muscles."
- Assist family members to identify strengths and limitations in coping with client illness.
- Assist family to develop a plan of home care after client is discharged. This could include both health care and recreation for all family members and should reflect priorities set by the family. For example, "Let's agree to clean house only once each week on Saturday mornings when everyone helps for an hour; always take half-hour walks each morning."
- Assess knowledge level of health care of family unit and plan teaching program to address needs.

Examples of Specific Evaluations for Outcome 1

1. Outcome not met. Client states spouse is unable to talk about client's cancer and client feels rejected.
2. Outcome partially met. Client states spouse has agreed

to attend meeting with physician prior to surgery and states that is a big step forward.
3. Outcome met. Client states, "I understand how hard it is for him to be here but we agree that we can face this together."

Key Index Words for Nursing Interventions

Look up these words in the index of fundamentals and medical-surgical nursing textbooks to find page references for additional nursing interventions and rationale for their selection:

- anxiety
- communication
- coping behavior
- fear
- health promotion

INEFFECTIVE FAMILY COPING: DISABLING

Definition

Behavior of significant person (family member or other primary person) that disables own capacities and the client's capacities to effectively address tasks essential to either person's adaptation to the health challenge.

Defining Characteristics

- neglectful care of the client in regard to basic human needs and/or illness treatment
- distortion of reality regarding client's health problem, including extreme denial about its existence or severity
- intolerance
- rejection
- abandonment
- desertion
- carrying out usual routines, disregarding client's needs
- psychosomaticism
- taking on illness signs of the client
- decisions and actions by the family which are detrimental to economic or social well-being
- agitation
- depression, aggression, hostility

- impaired restructuring of a meaningful life for self
- impaired individualization
- prolonged overconcern for client
- neglectful relationships with other family members
- client's development of helplessness, inactive dependence

Related Factors

- significant person with chronically unexpressed feelings of guilt, anxiety, hostility, despair, etc.
- dissonant discrepancy of coping styles for dealing with adaptive tasks by the significant person and client or among significant people
- highly ambivalent family relationships
- arbitrary handling of family's resistance to treatment, which tends to solidify defensiveness as it fails to deal adequately with underlying anxiety

Examples of Specific Nursing Diagnosis

1. Ineffective family coping: disabling related to chronic nature of cystic fibrosis.

Ineffective family coping: disabling related to chronic nature of cystic fibrosis as manifested by parent's statement, "I do the postural drainage and clapping routine when I think she needs it but not on a scheduled basis. I don't think it makes a difference." (PES format)

2. Ineffective family coping: disabling related to lack of understanding of mental illness and treatment.

Ineffective family coping: disabling related to lack of understanding of mental illness and treatment as evidenced by spouse's statement, "I get so mad at her. If she'd just get out of bed and try harder this could all be avoided." (PES format)

Examples of Specific Outcomes

1. Family members will participate in interdisciplinary conference to develop a plan of care for client before discharge.

2. Family members will verbalize understanding of home treatment routine and why it is necessary before discharge.

3. Spouse will make statement of understanding of signs and symptoms of depression, and how they affect client before discharge.

4. Spouse will identify three growth-promoting ways in which to help client during illness.

Examples of Specific Nursing Interventions

■ See Specific Nursing Interventions for Ineffective Family Coping: Compromised, Altered Family Processes and Caregiver Role Strain.

■ See General and Growth/Development Nursing Interventions, page 352.

■ Establish relationship with family members.

■ Assess what difficulties are being encountered in home care of the client in a supportive, nonthreatening, nonjudgmental conversation.

■ Encourage family members to express their feelings, however negative, and assist them in dealing with feelings.

■ Assure client, "Many people I have worked with tell me they feel...I wonder if you might be experiencing some of that too?"

■ Assure clients they are not bad or uncaring persons because they are having these feelings.

■ Provide teaching so each family member understands the client's illness and health care needs.

■ Assess for unmet physical and mental health care needs within the family that impair the ability of family members to cope with present situation.

■ Teach family some alternative coping skills: physical exercise, sharing workload, providing for respite care, relaxation techniques.

■ Offer client and family interdisciplinary care planning conference to assess and plan for home care.

■ Assess need for respite care and identify available resources for family.

■ Identify community resources and offer to make initial contact.

Examples of Specific Evaluations for Outcome 1

1. Outcome not met. Parent states, "After 4 years of taking care of this child I think I know what is best for her."

2. Outcome partially met. Parent states, "I know I should be doing all the drainage and clapping routine but I am just too tired."
3. Outcome met. Parents and teenage sibling worked out plan of care with nurse that provides for required care and considers family members' abilities.

Key Index Words for Nursing Interventions
Look up these words in the index of fundamentals and medical-surgical nursing textbooks to find page references for additional nursing interventions and rationale for their selection:

- anger/hostility
- anxiety
- defensive
- denial
- depression
- displacement
- mental health
- priority setting

PARENTAL ROLE CONFLICT

Definition
A state in which a parent experiences role confusion and conflict in response to crisis.

Major Defining Characteristics
- parent(s) expresses concerns/feelings of inadequacy to provide for child's physical and emotional needs during hospitalization or in the home
- demonstrated disruption in caretaking routines
- parent(s) expresses concerns about changes in parental role, family functioning, family communication, family heath

Minor Defining Characteristics
- expresses concern about perceived loss of control over decisions relating to their child
- reluctant to participate in usual caretaking activities even with encouragement and support
- verbalized, demonstrated feelings of guilt, anger, fear, anxiety, and/or frustrations about effect of child's illness on family process

Related Factors
- separation from child due to chronic illness
- intimidation with invasive or restrictive modalities (e.g., isolation, intubation) specialized care centers, policies
- home care of a child with special needs (e.g., apnea monitoring, postural drainage, hyperalimentation)
- change in marital status
- interruptions of family life due to home care regimen (treatments, caregivers, lack of respite)

Examples of Specific Nursing Diagnosis
1. Parental role conflict related to taking care of their dying child at home.
   Parental role conflict related to taking care of their dying child at home as evidenced by parent's statement, "Are we doing the right thing. She is in pain. Am I doing all that can be done. Would they be able to care for her better in the hospital? (PES format)
2. Parental role conflict related to meeting competing demands of needs of child in hospital, children at home, and job.
   Parental role conflict related to meeting competing demand of needs of child in hospital, children at home, and job as evidenced by parents' exhausted appearance and statement. "We're being pulled in all directions with taking care of all the kids, the job, being at the hospital for Jessica. And we have lots to learn about taking care of her at home in a cast." (PES format)

Examples of Specific Outcomes
1. Parent's will express confidence in their decision regarding home care of child within the week.
2. Parents will identify additional resources to use in coping with child's illness within the next week.
3. Parents will demonstrate care of child in cast before discharge.
4. Parents will develop plan for balancing needs of children and job within 24 hours assisted by nurse. Plan is to include adequate rest/nutrition for parents.

Examples of Specific Nursing Interventions
■ See General Family and Growth/Development Nursing Interventions, page 352.
■ Establish supportive therapeutic relationship with parents.
■ Encourage parents to do as much of their child's care as they wish without putting additional stress on them by establishing the expectation that they are to do all the care.
■ Encourage parents to practice care procedures assisted by a nurse so they can gain confidence in their ability.
■ Give parents support/feedback/evaluation of their caregiving skills.
■ Assure parents of the contribution they are making to their child's care and well-being.
■ Assist parents to make list of demands on them, prioritize demands, and develop a plan to meet them.
■ Identify knowledge and skills needed to care for child.
■ Develop teaching plan to meet parents' needs.
■ Provide parents with written care plan and instructions for procedures. This will give them something to refer to when they are at home.
■ Provide 24-hour telephone number for parents to call when they need help or have questions.
■ Identify supportive community resources.
■ Encourage parents to meet their own needs of respite and recreation.
■ Assure parents they may change their minds about the decision to do home care at any time and that decision will be accepted without question.
■ Assess need for home nursing assistance and secure referral.

Examples of Specific Evaluations for Outcome 2
1. Outcome not met. Parents have not had time to meet with nurse to develop scheduling plan and they continue to look progressively more exhausted.
2. Outcome partially met. Parents have begun a plan for balancing demands on their time but are unable to prioritize, insisting that everything needs to be done immediately.

3. Outcome met. Parents have developed a plan which enables them to get rest and meet needs of jobs and children. Both parents have agreed to try the plan for a 3-day period.

Key Index Words for Nursing Interventions

Look up these words in the index of fundamentals and medical-surgical nursing textbooks to find page references for additional nursing interventions and rationale for their selection:

- death and dying
- decision-making
- home care
- home care of the dying child

Chapter 19

Health Management Problems

FOCUSED ASSESSMENT GUIDE

Complete this focused assessment if a general nursing assessment indicates a possible problem. Then turn to page 388 of this text for the Data ⇒ Diagnosis Matching Guide for health management problems to help you select the best nursing diagnosis to match the client's data.

___ What kinds of things do you do at home to maintain your health: diet, exercise, hygiene, self-medication?
___ Do you have the equipment/supplies you need for your health problem or treatment?
___ What would you like to learn that might help you to improve your health status?
___ Who does the upkeep on your home/apartment: yard care/snow shoveling/raking?
___ Is getting help for home/apartment upkeep a problem for you?
___ How would you describe your financial status: stable, experiencing difficulty, crisis?
___ Are the things you are doing helping your health problem?
___ Is your health problem getting better, about the same, or rapidly worsening?
___ Have you been able to adapt your daily routine to include the care measures for your illness? What aspects of care are you having problems with?

___ Have you been able to follow the treatment plan for your condition?

___ Are there objective observations that indicate the client is not following the treatment regimen: lab tests, medication not taken, physical assessment?

DATA ⇒ DIAGNOSIS MATCHING GUIDE

Compare your client data from the Health Management Focused Assessment to these related health management nursing diagnoses and abbreviated descriptions. Select the nursing diagnosis which is the best match. Then turn to the page in this section with that specific diagnosis for help in planning care.

1. *Altered Health Maintenance: page 390*
   - definition: inability to do what is necessary to maintain health
   - data: lack of knowledge or interest in basic health practices; lack of resources (equipment/finance/other) for health care; impaired personal support system; expressed interest in improving health behavior

2. *Health-Seeking Behaviors (Specify): page 393*
   - definition: individual in good health seeks to improve health status
   - data: client asks for help in improving health or demonstrates readiness for higher level of wellness

3. *Impaired Home Maintenance Management: page 395*
   - definition: inability to maintain home in a safe manner
   - data: household members verbalize maintenance problems; verbalize debts or financial crises

4. *Ineffective Management of Therapeutic Regimen: page 398*
   - definition: way the client carries out the treatment program in daily lifestyle is not satisfactory for meeting health goals
   - data: daily living choices of client unlikely to achieve treatment goals; worsening of symptoms; statements of difficulty with or not following program

5. *Noncompliance (Specify): page 401*
   - definition: client's informed decision not to adhere to therapeutic recommendation
   - data: behavior, statements of client, or objective data that indicates failure to adhere to treatment plan

GENERAL OUTCOMES AND NURSING INTERVENTIONS

GENERAL HEALTH MANAGEMENT OUTCOMES

- Client will achieve the maximum level of health possible for the individual.
- Client will make informed choices among treatment regimens which promote recovery and health.
- Client will adhere to treatment regimen selected and agreed upon.
- Client will incorporate regimen into daily living activities.
- Client will maintain physical environment in manner that supports safety, health, and growth.
- Client will accept responsibility for own health.

GENERAL HEALTH MANAGEMENT NURSING INTERVENTIONS

- Assess the current health status of the client.
- Assess the meaning of health, illness, and specific treatments in the client's culture and value/belief system.
- Assess the client's readiness to change and ability to learn.
- Offer the client health teaching (in addition to illness teaching).
- Develop health teaching plans at the level of the client's knowledge and cognitive ability.
- Present care alternatives for client to select, give benefits and limitations of each.
- Accept the decision of the client.
- Adapt nursing and home care to reflect the cultural preferences of the client.
- Offer appropriate community resources and initiate the contact.

RELATED NURSING DIAGNOSIS

ALTERED HEALTH MAINTENANCE

Definition
Inability to identify, manage, and/or seek out help to maintain health.

Defining Characteristics
- demonstrated lack of knowledge regarding basic health practices
- demonstrated lack of adaptive behaviors to internal/external environmental changes
- reported or observed inability to take responsibility for meeting basic health practices in any or all functional pattern areas
- history of lack of health-seeking behavior
- expressed interest in improving health behaviors
- reported or observed lack of equipment, financial, and/or other resources
- reported or observed impairment of personal support systems

Related Factors
- lack of, or significant alteration in communication skills (writing, verbal, and/or gestural)
- lack of ability to make deliberate and thoughtful judgments
- perceptual/cognitive impairment; complete/partial lack of gross and/or fine motor skills
- ineffective individual coping
- dysfunctional grieving
- unachieved developmental tasks
- ineffective family coping
- disabling spiritual distress
- lack of material resources

Examples of Specific Nursing Diagnosis
1. Altered health maintenance related to smoking/lack of exercise.

   Altered health maintenance related to smoking/lack of

exercise as evidenced by, "I have smoked two or three packs a day for about 7 years. I'm hooked. I really should stop. And I get no exercise! A real candidate for a heart attack!" (PES format)

2. Altered health maintenance related to chronic alcoholism. Altered health maintenance related to chronic alcoholism as manifested by client reports of drinking about seven beers every night after work and a bit more on the weekend. "That's what men do in my family. Do you think that is too much?" (PES format)

Examples of Specific Outcomes

1. Client will make a decision to quit smoking and attend a Smoke Stopper program within 48 hours.
2. Client will identify factors contributing to smoking habit within 48 hours.
3. Client will contact community support groups related to goal of stopping smoking before discharge.
4. Client will plan exercise program assisted by nurse and approved by physician to include walking 15 minutes per day for the first 2 weeks.
5. Client will evaluate drinking pattern for impact on health status before discharge.

Examples of Specific Nursing Interventions

- See General Health Management Nursing Interventions, page 389.
- Assess client's perception of health status related to unhealthy behavior (smoking/drinking) and the feelings associated with health status: guilt, embarrassment, anger, satisfaction with level of health.
- Assess client readiness to change or reasons for reluctance to change, reasons for past failures.
- Offer support if client decides to attempt a change.
- Offer motivations for adapting healthy changes but accept that the decision is the client's and this is to be respected.
- Plan the change in steps the client can accept, e.g., is the goal to quit "cold turkey" or to cut down in small steps?
- Consult with physician if medication is required.
- Assess the client's level of knowledge of relationship of the behavior to health status: exercise/health/lung function/stress relief.

- Develop and implement a teaching plan to address health need.
- Consider cost of health promotion measure (smoke-stopping group or exercise program) and plan for resources to cover costs. This may involve meeting with a social worker or financial counselor. Some insurance may provide coverage.
- Secure physician approval prior to client beginning any exercise program.
- Encourage client to walk as a beginning exercise: no cost, no equipment, and has health benefits.
- Identify community supports for client and offer to initiate contact. Establish time/place of contact before discharge.
- Provide for evaluation of health care plan at predetermined intervals.

Examples of Specific Evaluations for Outcomes 1 and 4

1. Outcome not met. Client refused to participate in program to quit smoking, "I have to do it myself. Too busy to walk."
2. Outcome partially met. Client is eager to begin Smoke Stopper program but refuses to consider exercise because "I can't walk a flight of stairs without becoming winded."
3. Outcome met. Client has agreed to participate in the Fresh Start program sponsored by the American Cancer Society and will attend for the first time on 7/3 with MD approval. Client has started walking 1 mile per day.

Key Index Words for Nursing Interventions

Look up these words in the index of fundamentals and medical-surgical nursing textbooks to find page references for additional nursing interventions and rationale for the selection:

- addiction
- alcoholism
- altered nutrition
- diet/nutrition

- exercise
- lifestyle
- malnutrition
- smoking

HEALTH-SEEKING BEHAVIORS (SPECIFY)

Definition
A state in which an individual in stable health is actively seeking ways to alter personal habits and/or the environment in order to move to a higher level of health.*

Major Defining Characteristics
■ expressed or observed desire to seek a higher level of wellness

Minor Defining Characteristics
■ expressed or observed desire for increased control of health practice
■ expression of concern about current environmental conditions on health status
■ stated or observed unfamiliarity with wellness community resources
■ demonstrated or observed lack of knowledge in health-promoting behaviors

Examples of Specific Nursing Diagnosis
1. Health-seeking behavior: dietary planning for low fat diet for entire family related to concern about family's current eating habits.
   Health-seeking behavior: dietary planning for low fat diet for entire family related to concern about family's current eating habits as evidenced by mother's statement, "Lowering our fat intake is something we can do to decrease the risk of heart attacks, but I do not understand all the different fats and their uses." (PES format)
2. Health-seeking behavior: exercise plan to increase cardiovascular fitness related to approaching middle age.
   Health-seeking behavior: exercise plan to increase cardiovascular fitness related to approaching middle age as evidenced by client statement, "I think I'm in pretty good health but I'd like to be in better physical shape." (PES format)

---

*Stable health status is defined as achievement of age-appropriate illness prevention measures; client reported good or excellent health; signs and symptoms of disease, if present, are controlled.

Examples of Outcome Statements
1. Client will verbalize understanding of dietary fats and how to lower fat content in a family diet by discharge.
2. Client will bring 1 week of typical home menus and discuss with nurse modifications to lower fat intake.
3. Client will, with approval of MD, engage in physical activity designed to reach target heart rate, 20 minutes, 3 times per week within the next month.

Examples of Specific Nursing Interventions
- See General Health Management Nursing Interventions, page 389.
- Assess client's present lifestyle and culture as regards identified health practices.
- Assess client's knowledge level about identified health practices. The use of pre/post self-tests is helpful.
- Develop and implement teaching plan to meet client needs.
- Provide resources in a variety of formats: video/audio, books, pamphlets, discussion groups, lecture, programmed instruction.
- Secure physician/nurse practitioner approval for alterations in physical activity.
- Set measurable, realistic goals with client, increasing gradually.
- Obtain baseline data for client to compare to postprogram results. This might include such things as target heart rate and recovery period, cholesterol and HDL/LDH levels, average fat intake per week in grams, weight, as well as subjective responses to feeling of health.
- Support client in identified changes.
- Anticipate setbacks and problem-solve with client how to handle them constructively without abandoning program; identify sources of help for when this happens.
- Determine schedule of evaluation.
- Identify community resources and refer client as appropriate. Examples: American Cancer Society smoking cessation, American Heart CPR classes, Diabetes Association support groups.

Examples of Specific Evaluations for Outcome 1
1. Outcome not met. Client states, "That is all too complicated to learn."

2. Outcome partially met. Client attended four of the six Heart Smart sessions but states he is too busy to continue.
3. Outcome met. Client attended all the Heart Smart sessions with spouse and reports they really helped with understanding the fat issues in nutrition planning.

Key Index Words for Nursing Interventions

Look up these words in the index of fundamentals and medical-surgical nursing textbooks to find page references for additional nursing interventions and rationale for their selection:

- specific health change
- wellness
- teaching/learning process

IMPAIRED HOME MAINTENANCE MANAGEMENT

Definition
Inability to independently maintain a safe growth-promoting immediate environment.

Subjective Defining Characteristics
- *household members express difficulty in maintaining their home in a comfortable fashion
- *household requests assistance with home maintenance
- *household members describe outstanding debts or financial crises

Objective Defining Characteristics
- disorderly surroundings
- *unwashed or unavailable cooking equipment, clothes, or linen
- *accumulation of dirt, food wastes, or hygienic wastes
- offensive odors
- inappropriate household temperature
- *overtaxed family members (e.g., exhausted, anxious)
- lack of necessary equipment or aids
- presence of vermin or rodents
- *repeated hygienic disorders, infestations, infections

*Critical.

Related Factors
- individual/family member disease or injury
- insufficient family organization or planning
- insufficient finances
- unfamiliar with neighborhood resources
- impaired cognitive or emotional functioning
- lack of knowledge
- lack of role modeling
- inadequate support systems

Examples of Specific Nursing Diagnosis
1. Impaired home maintenance management related to inadequate financial resources.
   Impaired home maintenance management related to inadequate financial resources as evidenced by client statement, "I need a new furnace and a hot water heater but I can't afford it on a social security check." (PES format)
2. Impaired home maintenance management related to immobility and impaired eyesight.
   Impaired home maintenance related to immobility and impaired eyesight as evidenced by client's statement, "There's a lot that needs to be done but I'm afraid of falling on the ice so I don't take out garbage, shovel snow, or even take baths or showers very often." (PES format)

Examples of Specific Outcomes
1. Client will identify home maintenance that needs to be done and develop a plan with family members and nurse to complete repairs within 1 month.
2. Client will complete home safety assessment assisted by nurse to identify safety hazards to a person with impaired vision and mobility at next home visit.
3. Client will identify assistance needed to complete ADLs at home and develop plan for getting needed help assisted by nurse and social worker before discharge.

Examples of Specific Nursing Interventions
- See General Health Management Nursing Interventions, page 389.

- Assist client and family members to assess home for factors that are a threat to safety and health needs of the client. It is recommended to do a room by room walk-through. Make a determination if all the basic needs can be met in the environment. Note especially the bathroom facilities where the client will have to move from wheelchair (walker, canes, crutches) to toilet, bath, or shower. Can client easily use kitchen equipment?
- Assess client for ability to remain safely in the environment with self-care or assisted care.
- Identify equipment or assistive devices that would facilitate client's self-care and ability to remain in home.
- Identify simple modifications that can be made by moving or eliminating furniture or by rearranging equipment.
- List maintenance tasks that are required in order to maintain a safe environment.
- Identify what assistance is needed to complete maintenance tasks.
- Establish a realistic plan with client and family for both health care and home maintenance. Include priority setting as part of the planning process.
- Discuss financial needs with client and family and identify sources of assistance.
- Identify sources of community assistance: Meals-On-Wheels, home care aide, and housekeeping services; make initial referrals.
- Establish a periodic reevaluation schedule to determine effectiveness of plan and altered needs or condition of client.

Examples of Specific Evaluations for Outcome 1

1. Outcome not met. Family members decline to participate in planning session because they feel their parents belong in a nursing home and refuse to do anything that would encourage them to remain in their home.
2. Outcome partially met. Family has made a list of necessary repairs but need another meeting to continue to develop plan for accomplishing repairs.
3. Outcome met. Family has met twice with nurse and social worker and come up with a plan and timetable to accomplish necessary repairs. Social worker has assisted with securing financial aid.

Key Index Words for Nursing Interventions
Look up these words in the index of fundamentals and medical-surgical nursing textbooks to find page references for additional nursing interventions and rationale for their selection:

- Americans with Disabilities Act (ADA)
- aging process
- Department of Social Services (DSS)
- gerontology
- Medicare
- Medicaid
- poverty

INEFFECTIVE MANAGEMENT OF THERAPEUTIC REGIMEN

Definition
A pattern of regulating and integrating into daily living a program for treatment of illness and the sequelae of illness that is unsatisfactory for meeting specific health goals.

Major Defining Characteristics
- choices of daily living ineffective for meeting the goals of a treatment or prevention program

Minor Defining Characteristics
- acceleration (expected or unexpected) of illness symptoms
- client verbalizes desire to manage the treatment of illness and prevention of sequelae
- client verbalizes difficulty with regulation/integration of one or more prescribed regimens for treatment of illness and its effects or prevention of complications
- client verbalizes own inaction to reduce risk factors for progression of illness and sequelae

Related Factors
- complexity of health care system
- complexity of therapeutic regimen
- decisional conflicts
- excessive demands made on individual or family

- family conflict
- family patterns of health care
- inadequate number and types of cues to action
- knowledge deficits
- mistrust of regimen and/or of health care personnel
- perceived seriousness
- perceived susceptibility
- perceived barriers
- perceived benefits
- powerlessness
- social support deficits

Examples of Specific Nursing Diagnosis

1. Ineffective management of therapeutic regimen (congestive heart failure) related to lack of knowledge and economic difficulty.

   Ineffective management of therapeutic regimen (congestive heart failure) related to lack of knowledge and economic difficulty as evidenced by failure to take prescribed medication and to follow restricted sodium diet. (PES format)

2. Ineffective management of therapeutic regimen (follow-up on abnormal pap smear) related to excessive demands on individual and complexity of the health care system.

   Ineffective management of therapeutic regimen (follow-up on abnormal pap smear) related to excessive demands on individual and complexity of the health care system as manifested by failure to have repeat pap smears every 6 months and client statement, "I know I should do it but between my job, the house, and the kids it is hard to fit in. Plus it's a royal hassle getting an appointment. Never see the same person twice. Have to explain it all over again." (PES format)

Examples of Specific Outcomes

1. Client will verbalize understanding of medication/diet regimen for congestive heart failure within 48 hours.
2. Client will meet with hospital social worker within 24 hours to obtain funding for medications.
3. Client will agree to schedule follow-up monitoring for abnormal pap smear before discharge.

Examples of Specific Nursing Interventions
- See General Health Management Nursing Interventions, page 389.
- Assess client's understanding of illness, including causation of signs and symptoms: "What does it mean when your ankles get puffy or your shoes are too tight?"
- Assess client's understanding of treatment regimen and expected outcome of treatment.
    "What does the medicine do for you?"
    "Do you notice a difference when you take it/don't take it?"
    "Why did your doctor prescribe a low sodium diet?"
    "What does that do for your heart?"
    "What is your understanding of why it is necessary for you to have the repeat pap smears?"
- Provide realistic information about the consequences or potential risk associated with not following treatment regimen: "Remember how it was hard for you to breathe when you came to the emergency room. Well, the medication the doctor wants you to take will help to prevent that." This is not intended as a threat or scare tactic for the client but is information needed to make an informed decision.
- Identify problems client/family has experienced in adhering to treatment regimen.
    "Can you tell me some of the difficulties you have found in following the doctor's orders?"
    "What has gone well for you in taking care of your health problems?"
- Develop a teaching plan to provide information needed for health care or to remedy incorrect information.
- With client (and family) develop mutually agreed upon goals and a plan to achieve them. Include a predetermined time for evaluation.
- Brainstorm with client ways to avoid some of the hassle of the health care system, e.g., making next appointment before leaving the present appointment, knowing name of provider and requesting to be scheduled with the same provider, scheduling at least busy time and day.
- Identify additional resources available to client and make the initial contact: social work, clinic transportation, child care during appointments.

Examples of Specific Evaluations for Outcome 1

1. Outcome not met. Client refuses to learn about CHF or to plan for home care, "You just fix me up when I come back here."
2. Outcome partially met. Client understands therapeutic regimen for CHF but agrees to take medication only when "I start to have trouble breathing. Doesn't make sense to be taking medicine when I feel fine!"
3. Outcome met. Client has participated in teaching, has 1-month supply of medication, and verbalizes understanding of treatment regimen, "I will try to do this so I can stay out of the hospital."

Key Index Words for Nursing Interventions

Look up these words in the index of fundamentals and medical-surgical nursing textbooks to find page references for additional nursing interventions and rationale for their selection:

- adult learner
- social support
- specific disease/medication of the client
- teaching-learning process

NONCOMPLIANCE (SPECIFY)

Definition

A person's informed decision not to adhere to a therapeutic recommendation.

Defining Characteristics

- *behavior indicative of failure to adhere (by direct observation or by statements of client or significant others)
- objective tests (physiological measures, detection of markers)
- evidence of development of complications
- evidence of exacerbation of symptoms
- failure to keep appointments
- failure to progress

*Critical.

Related Factors
- client-provider relationships
- health beliefs, cultural influences, spiritual value
- client value system

Examples of Specific Nursing Diagnosis
1. Noncompliance with diet/foot care plan for diabetes related to health beliefs.
   Noncompliance with diet/foot care plan for diabetes related to health beliefs as evidenced by client statement, "They just discovered my diabetes so I must have lived with it for 43 years. Why should I do all that stuff now. Just give me the insulin and I'll be okay." (PES format)
2. Noncompliance with physical therapy routine following knee surgery related to negative perception of exercise.
   Noncompliance with physical therapy routine following knee surgery related to negative perception of exercise as evidenced by inability to increase weight load on knee, and by client statement, "Those exercises are just too boring." (PES format)

Examples of Specific Outcomes
1. Client will verbalize an understanding of the rationale for a diabetic diet and follow the diet for next 48 hours before discharge.
2. Client will verbalize the rationale for diabetic foot care and demonstrate correct self-care before discharge.
3. Client will verbalize understanding of importance of exercises and agree to physical therapy regimen before discharge.

Examples of Specific Nursing Interventions
- See General Health Management Nursing Interventions, page 389.
- Develop therapeutic relationship with client.
- Assess client's level of understanding of condition and treatment regimen.
- Develop a teaching plan to correct misinformation or provide additional information.
- Provide information for the client about the potential risks associated with not following the treatment plan. This is not used to scare or threaten the client, but is necessary for the client to make informed decisions.

- Assess client's perception of the treatment regimen. Are there cultural, economic, or other factors that make the plan unacceptable?
- Discuss with client modifications that might make the treatment plan more acceptable.
- Set small, frequently achievable, mutually agreed upon goals.
- Provide information for the client in various forms: videotapes, audiotapes, pamphlets, books, classes.
- Identify support groups within the community and provide contact information.
- Accept the informed decision of the adult client even if the nurse does not agree that it is in the best interest of the client's health.
- When/if the client faces illness/hospitalization caused by failure to follow the treatment regimen, it remains important to provide care in a nonjudgmental manner.

Examples of Specific Evaluations for Outcome 1
1. Outcome not met. Client refuses any discussion of diabetic diet and states, "I will try to watch it a bit but mealtime is pretty spontaneous at my house."
2. Outcome partially met. Client has followed the ADA diabetic diet for 48 hours but states, "On weekends I binge so this is impossible!"
3. Outcome met. Client has followed ADA diabetic diet for 48 hours and states, "I can handle this. I can still eat lots of my favorite foods."

Key Index Words for Nursing Interventions
Look up these words in the index of fundamentals and medical-surgical nursing textbooks to find page references for additional nursing interventions and rationale for their selection:

- addiction/addictive substances
- culture
- developmental level
- health promotion
- mutual goal setting
- nursing diagnosis: knowledge deficit
- readiness for learning
- teaching-learning process

Chapter 20

Roles/Relationship Problems

FOCUSED ASSESSMENT GUIDE

Complete this focused assessment if a general nursing assessment indicates a possible problem. Then turn to page 405 of this text for the Data ⇒ Diagnosis Matching Guide for roles/relationship problems to help you select the best nursing diagnosis to match the client's data.

SUBJECTIVE DATA

___ How do you spend your leisure time?
___ What activities do you enjoy doing with family and/or friends?
___ Approximately how much time each week, outside of your job, do you choose to spend with other people? Is that amount too much, too little, about right?
___ Who is the person you feel closest to?
___ To whom do you go for emotional support?
___ If you have a problem or if something great happens, who would you want to tell about it?
___ How do you think your friends/family/coworkers feel about you? How would they describe you?
___ What things are important to you? What drives you?
___ What are you responsible for in your life: job, care of children/parents, home care?

___ Has client been able to meet the responsibilities of roles identified above? If not, what has interfered with meeting those responsibilities?

OBJECTIVE DATA

___ Does physical appearance of client suggest identification with a subgroup not generally acceptable to dominant culture, e.g., pierced nose/lips, shaved head, strange hair color?

___ Has the client behaviors which are unacceptable to the dominant group in the culture, e.g., table manners, inability to play sport/game of peers, style of dress/hair?

___ Does the client appear sad, withdrawn, without eye contact?

___ Is there an angry tone in client's voice or nonverbal gestures?

DATA ⇒ DIAGNOSIS MATCHING GUIDE

Compare your client data from the Roles and Relationship Focused Assessment to these related roles and relationship nursing diagnoses and abbreviated descriptions. Select the nursing diagnosis which is the best match. Then turn to the page in this section with that specific diagnosis for help in planning care.

1. *Altered Role Performance: page 407*
   - definition: disruption in the way one perceives one's role performance
   - data: difficulties associated with role perception or performance

2. *Impaired Social Interaction: page 409*
   - definition: dissatisfying or dysfunctional ways of interacting
   - data: verbalized or observed discomfort in interacting with others, inability to communicate or receive sense of caring or belonging, family report change in client's interactions

3. Social Isolation: page 413
  ■ definition: being alone seen as imposed by others and experienced as negative or threatening
  ■ data: absence of significant others, expressed feeling of aloneness imposed by others, expressed feelings of rejection; physical appearance of sadness, uncommunicative, withdrawn or angry

GENERAL OUTCOMES AND NURSING INTERVENTIONS

GENERAL ROLES/RELATIONSHIP OUTCOMES

■ Client will establish satisfying relationships with family members or significant others.
■ Client will develop realistic role expectations for self.
■ Client will adapt to or modify roles with consideration of health problem.
■ Client will seek or accept assistance in meeting demands of role.
■ Client will identify barriers (personal, situational, other) to satisfying interpersonal interactions.
■ Client will establish amount of social interaction that is personally acceptable and satisfying.
■ Client will identify behaviors/conduct/aspects of appearance that client is willing to change to facilitate social acceptance.

GENERAL ROLES/RELATIONSHIP NURSING INTERVENTIONS

■ Establish therapeutic relationship which emphasizes the development of trust.
■ Recognize this area is very value-laden and unique to each culture; it is outside the practice of nursing to impose one's personal values or culture on the client.
■ Accept the client's perception as the beginning point for intervention.
■ Assess the client's comfort with the situation and willingness to consider change.

- Assess the duration and degree of the current problem. It may be more difficult to intervene effectively in long-standing problems, while clients in crisis are often more amenable to help.
- Include interventions which promote self-esteem.
- Identify appropriate community and health care system resources.

RELATED NURSING DIAGNOSES

ALTERED ROLE PERFORMANCE

Definition
Disruption in the way one perceives one's role performance.

Defining Characteristics
- change in self-perception of role
- denial of role
- change in other's perception of role
- conflict in roles
- changes in physical capacity to resume role
- lack of knowledge of role
- change in usual patterns of responsibility

Examples of Specific Nursing Diagnoses
1. Altered role performance related to unwanted pregnancy.
   Altered role performance related to pregnancy at age 15 years as evidenced by client statement, "I can never do anything with my friends because they don't want a baby along. And I'm always tired. And he cries all the time and I can't make him stop." (PES format)
2. Altered role performance related to chronic illness (multiple sclerosis).
   Altered role performance related to chronic illness (multiple sclerosis) as evidenced by client statement, "I work as a landscaper; that isn't something you can do from a wheelchair. How can I support this family?" (PES format)

Examples of Specific Outcomes
1. Client will verbalize own feelings about being a mother at next clinic visit.

2. Client will identify three parenting skills she would like to learn with help of nurse within 1 week.
3. Client and spouse will explore alternative roles within the family lifestyle prior to discharge.
4. Client will complete skills/interest assessment prior to discharge with the assistance of a vocational rehabilitation counselor.

Specific Nursing Interventions
- See General Roles and Relationship Nursing Interventions, page 406.
- Assess client's perception of impact of illness on role performance: mother/father, employee, husband/wife, student.
- Reflect, summarize, and restate client's perception in order to gain clarification of client's experience.
- Encourage and support the expression of feelings associated with the perception of client's experience.
- Support the client through the grief process: loss of normal adolescence, loss of career.
- Working with client and family (if client desires/permits) make realistic assessment of strength and limitations.
- Identify the aspects of the role which are altered or which client perceives as negative and positive.
- Provide openings for clients to discuss sexual concerns associated with the altered role: a paraplegic client with questions about ability to have intercourse, a single parent with concerns about dating relationships.
- With client, make problem list and work with client to prioritize direction of efforts.
- Develop a plan with client to work on top-priority problem/concern setting both long- and short-term goals.
- Identify usual coping strategies of client.
- Foster use of coping strategies that client has successfully used in dealing with past problems.
- Teach the client new coping strategies: relaxation, massage, biofeedback.
- Explore possibility with client of assuming new or altered roles.
- Promote self-esteem by recognition of client effort/achievement/progress.

- Provide referral to appropriate resources: vocational counselor, psychologist for interest testing, parenting classes.
- Provide referral to appropriate community support groups and offer to make the first contact: Parents Without Partners, Foster Grandparents, church groups, specific illness support groups.

Examples of Specific Evaluations for Outcome 3

1. Outcome not met. Client refuses to consider any alternatives to present family roles. Client states, "I am the head of the family. I will figure this out."
2. Outcome partially met. Client and spouse are beginning to consider other options but are unable to come up with any alternatives that they consider viable.
3. Outcome met. Client and spouse are considering spouse's return to work full-time while client attends accounting classes at the community college. Client states, "I have always been interested in accounting as a career and I could do that with an adapted computer even if my MS progresses."

Key Index Words for Nursing Interventions

Look up these words in the index of fundamentals and medical-surgical textbooks to find page references for additional nursing interventions and rationale for their selection:

- arrested development
- developmental tasks
- exacerbation/remission in chronic, progressive disease
- grief and loss
- paraplegia
- quadriplegia
- regression
- rehabilitation
- self-esteem
- vocational counseling

IMPAIRED SOCIAL INTERACTION

Definition

A state in which an individual participates in an insufficient or excessive quantity of social exchange or an ineffective quality of social exchange.

Major Defining Characteristics
- verbalized or observed discomfort in social situations
- verbalized or observed inability to receive or communicate a satisfying sense of belonging, caring, interest, or shared history
- observed use of unsuccessful social interaction behaviors
- dysfunctional interaction with peers, family, and/or others

Minor Defining Characteristics
- family report of change of style or pattern of interaction

Related Factors
- knowledge/skill deficit about ways to enhance mutuality
- communication barriers
- self-concept disturbance
- absence of available significant others or peers
- limited physical mobility
- therapeutic isolation
- sociocultural dissonance
- environmental barriers
- altered thought processes

Examples of Specific Nursing Diagnoses
1. Impaired social interaction related to peers' fear of contracting disease (AIDS).
   Impaired social interaction related to peers' fear of contracting disease (AIDS) as evidenced by client statement, "People I have been friends with all my life won't touch me or even shake hands with me." (PES format)
2. Impaired social interaction related to negative feelings about self associated with adolescent acne.
   Impaired social interaction related to negative feelings about self associated with adolescent acne as evidenced by client statement, "The kids don't want to go around with me because I look so gross." (PES format)

Examples of Specific Outcome Statements
1. Client will verbalize satisfactory amount/quality of social interaction with at least one peer prior to discharge.
2. Client will use telephone to maintain contact with old friend at least once during hospitalization.

3. Client will make positive statement about self and abilities prior to discharge.
4. Client will evaluate own interaction style, assisted by nurse, to determine if there is a social behavior client wishes to modify or change.

Examples of Specific Nursing Interventions

■ See General Roles and Relationship Nursing Interventions, page 406.
■ Assess the client's interaction style in conversation with nurse and note strength/limitations such as lack of eye contact, speech difficulties, lack of interest in discussion of events/persons in environment, withdrawal.
▪ Assess for physiological conditions which affect interaction: stroke, inability to speak dominant language, thought disorder, developmental disability, cultural barriers, medications, body odor, offensive breath, etc.
■ Assist the client to identify feelings associated with social interactions. What makes client or others uncomfortable?
■ Identify interventions that would make others more comfortable. For the AIDS client this might be meeting in a public place rather than the home, acknowledging the friend's fears directly though not confronting, "Some of my friends have told me they are afraid they might get AIDS from me. I wonder if you might be afraid too. I could tell you what I have learned about it."
■ Assist client to share with friends what their relationship means to client at a level that is appropriate, "We have been friends for years. I really want to maintain our friendship," or "It was great to have coffee with you and get filled in on what's happening at the office."
■ Encourage client to use telephone to maintain contact with friends.
■ Identify appropriate support/help group and offer to make initial contact for client.
■ If possible, intervene with family and friends to provide correct health care information.
■ Assist client to deal with health care problems that may interfere with satisfying interactions, e.g., medication and treatment regimen for acne, rest/activity balance for AIDS client, weight reduction plan for obese client who wants to participate in sports.

- Verbalize assessment of client's strengths and provide reinforcement for those behaviors.
- Verbalize limitation of client in interactions, give feedback on its effect on interaction, validate with client, and assist with behavior modification if client chooses, "I notice that when we talk, you keep looking around the room. That makes me feel that you are not interested or perhaps that you do not want to talk with me. Is that correct? I wonder if that is something other people feel also? Is that something you would want to work on with me?"
- Provide opportunities for client to practice new skill while in a safe, supportive environment.
- Assess the environment in which the client lives for opportunities for social interaction, for ways to meet people and make friends.
- List activities and/or interests the client enjoys as way to identify people having shared interest with client.
- Identify ways to place client in contact with peers having similar interests: school clubs, senior citizen center, church groups, volunteer activities, community service groups.
- Develop a plan with client to participate in new activity and evaluate at agreed date with nurse.

Examples of Specific Evaluations for Outcomes 1 and 2
1. Outcome not met. Client refuses to contact any school friends saying, "They know where I am. They should call me."
2. Outcome partially met. Client attempted to call a friend but was unable to reach her."
3. Outcome met. Client called school friend and talked for 45 minutes. Client states, "He really filled me in on what's happening. It felt good."

Key Index Words for Nursing Interventions
Look up these words in the index of fundamentals and medical-surgical textbooks to find page references for additional nursing interventions and rationale for their selection:

- acne vulgaris
- body image
- communication
- growth and development
- peer support
- relationship

■ group therapy ■ self-esteem

SOCIAL ISOLATION

Definition
Aloneness experienced by the individual and perceived as imposed by others and as a negative or threatening state.

Objective Defining Characteristics
■ *absence of supportive, significant others (family, friends, group)
■ sad dull affect
■ inappropriate or immature interests/activities for developmental age/stage
■ uncommunicative, withdrawn, no eye contact
■ preoccupation with own thoughts, repetitive meaningless actions
■ projects hostility in voice, behavior
■ seeks to be alone or exists in a subculture
■ evidence of physical/mental handicap or altered state of wellness
■ shows behavior unaccepted by dominant cultural group

Subjective Defining Characteristics
■ *expresses feelings of aloneness imposed by others
■ *expresses feelings of rejection
■ expresses feeling of difference from others
■ inadequacy in or absence of significant purpose in life
■ inability to meet expectations of others
■ insecurity in public
■ expresses values acceptable to the subculture group but unacceptable to dominant cultural group
■ expresses interests inappropriate to the developmental age/stage

Related Factors
■ factors contributing to the absence of satisfying personal relationships such as delay in accomplishing developmental tasks
■ immature interests

*Critical.

- alterations in physical appearance
- alterations in mental status
- unaccepted social values
- altered state of wellness
- inadequate personal resources
- inability to engage in satisfying personal relationships

Examples of Specific Nursing Diagnoses

1. Social isolation related to death of husband, living alone, and negative self-esteem.
   Social isolation related to death of husband, living alone, and negative self-esteem as evidenced by client statement, "I'm just another old woman alone. Not much good for anything. Who has time for me?" (PES format)
2. Social isolation related to lack of acceptance by peer group at school.
   Social isolation related to lack of acceptance by peer group at school as evidenced by client statement, "They don't ask me to come along or to help with anything. I always get left alone." (PES format)

Examples of Specific Outcomes

1. Client will verbalize one satisfying interaction with a friend within 24 hours.
2. Client will identify one activity at school to join within 1 week.
3. Client will identify one classmate to approach and invite to join in school activity within 2 weeks.

Examples of Specific Nursing Interventions

- See General Roles and Relationship Nursing Interventions, page 406.
- Encourage client to verbalize feelings of social isolation or aloneness.
- Reflect and summarize client's feelings for validation of nurse understanding of client perception.
- Assist client to distinguish between aloneness required by treatment regimen or necessary circumstances versus aloneness which is not necessary and not wanted.
- Assess causative factors which contribute to producing aloneness, either real or perceived.

- Assist visitors to understand requirements of treatment regimen (isolation precautions) so they are less fearful.
- Spend time with client when physical care is not required and sit down to appear unhurried and to indicate presence is a deliberate choice.
- Assist client to identify what types of interactions with people are desired.
- Assist client to identify peer group or group memberships of choice.
- Assist client to define personal strengths and limitations in interpersonal relationships.
- Discuss with client alternative ways of relating such as initiating an activity versus waiting to be asked.
- Support client in trying out new behaviors.
- Assist client in identifying personal and community resources which will aid in the development of satisfying relationships: recreation groups, volunteer needs, public transportation, money available to spend on recreation, free public entertainment.
- Assist client in developing a plan to achieve satisfying interactions aided by an interdisciplinary conference.
- Support client in assuming responsibility for initiating attempts at social interactions, e.g., phoning a friend when lonely, sharing cost of a joint meal, attending Book and Lunch brown bag at local library.

Examples of Specific Evaluations for Outcome 1

1. Outcome not met. Client states, "I am just the same as I ever was but now that I'm a widow no one wants to be around me."
2. Outcome partially met. Client states, "I know I tend to mope a lot when I should be getting out but my husband always was the one to take care of planning with friends."
3. Outcome met. Client states, "I've been sitting waiting for the world to come to me. I've a phone and I'm on a bus route. I'll make my own fun! I just called a friend to go to a movie."

Key Index Words for Nursing Interventions

Look up these words in the index of fundamentals and medical-surgical textbooks to find page references for additional nursing interventions and rationale for their selection:

- culture/subculture
  membership
- depression
- developmental stage
- grief and loss
- guilt

- isolation precautions
- protective isolation
- rejection
- self-esteem
- withdrawal

Chapter 21

Self-Esteem Problems

FOCUSED ASSESSMENT GUIDE

Complete this focused assessment if a general nursing assessment indicates a possible problem. Then turn to page 418 of this text for the Data ⇒ Diagnosis Matching Guide for self-esteem problems to help you select the best nursing diagnosis to match the client's data.

SUBJECTIVE DATA

___ How has this illness/surgery (name it) changed things for you?
   Check if present in response:
   ___ fear of rejection by significant others
   ___ negative feelings about body
   ___ emphasis on remaining strengths
   ___ helpless/hopeless/powerless
___ How have you been able to cope with this illness/surgery?
   Check if present in response:
   ___ negative self-evaluations
   ___ expression of shame/guilt
   ___ unable to cope
   ___ denial of problem, projection of blame
___ How long have you felt this way about yourself?
___ Does client seek excessive reassurance?
___ Since you have been sick, do you feel you cope with the stresses as well as most people, better than most people, or would you say you have great difficulty?

417

OBJECTIVE DATA

___ Does client refuse to look at or touch affected part of body?

___ Does client exhibit lack of eye contact?

___ Does client have a history of lack of success in jobs or courses at school

___ Is client indecisive, passive?

DATA ⇒ DIAGNOSIS MATCHING GUIDE

Compare your client data from the Self-Esteem Focused Assessment to these related self-esteem nursing diagnoses and abbreviated descriptions. Select the nursing diagnosis which is the best match. Then turn to the page in this section with that specific diagnosis for help in planning care.

1. *Body Image Disturbance: page 420*
   - definition: disruption in the way one perceives one's body image
   - data: verbal or nonverbal response about actual or perceived change in body

2. *Personal Identity Disturbance: page 423*
   - definition: inability to distinguish between self and nonself
   - data: to be developed by NANDA

3. *Self-Esteem Disturbance: page 423*
   - definition: negative evaluation of self or own capabilities
   - data: negative, "put down" statements about self, unable to accept compliment, oversensitive to criticism

4. *Chronic Low Self-Esteem: page 426*
   - definition: long-standing negative self-evaluation or capabilities
   - data: history of negative, "put down" statements about self, inability to deal with events; frequent lack of success in life events; passive, indecisive; excessively seeking reassurance

5. Situational Low Self-Esteem: page 429
- definition: negative self-evaluation in response to particular loss or situation from individual who previously had a positive-evaluation
- data: incident of negative self-evaluation related to specific event

GENERAL OUTCOMES AND NURSING INTERVENTIONS

GENERAL SELF-ESTEEM OUTCOMES

- Client will verbalize understanding of factors that contribute to negative self-evaluation: familial, situational, developmental.
- Client will accept responsibility for making changes in life to promote mental health and self-esteem.
- Client will verbalize a willingness to examine and change long-standing behavioral patterns that contribute to low self-esteem.
- Client will experience a positive sense of self-esteem.
- Client will identify realistic perception of strengths and limitations.
- Client will verbalize acceptance of body as altered by illness or surgery.
- Client will participate in self-care.

GENERAL SELF-ESTEEM NURSING INTERVENTIONS

- Identify and work through own feelings related to altered body of client.
- Support client in grieving body changes.
- Teach self-care required by body changes.
- With client, assess factors causing low self-esteem.
- Provide honest, realistic feedback of client's strengths and limitations.
- Assist identification of changes client is willing to make.
- Provide experiences that will result in positive self-evaluation.

- Provide feedback on client attempts to change negative evaluation behavior.
- Identify sources of referral for help and support after discharge.

RELATED NURSING DIAGNOSES

BODY IMAGE DISTURBANCE

Definition
Disruption in the way one perceives one's body image.

Defining Characteristics
A or B must be present to justify the diagnosis of body image disturbance: A = verbal response to actual or perceived change in structure and/or function; B = nonverbal response to actual and/or perceived change in structure and/or function. The following clinical manifestations may be used to validate the presence of A or B.

Objective Defining Characteristics
- missing body part
- actual change in structure and/or function
- not looking at body part
- not touching body part
- hiding or overexposing body part (intentional or unintentional)
- trauma to nonfunctioning part
- change in social involvement
- change in ability to estimate spatial relationship of body to environment

Subjective Defining Characteristics
- verbalization of change in lifestyle
- fear of rejection or of reaction by others
- focus on past strength, function, or appearance
- negative feelings about body
- feelings of helplessness, hopelessness, or powerlessness
- preoccupation with change or loss
- emphasis on remaining strengths and heightened achievement
- extensions of body boundary to incorporate environmental objects

- personalization of part or loss by name
- depersonalization of part or loss by impersonal pronouns
- refusal to verify actual change

Related Factors
- biophysical
- cognitive/perceptual
- psychosocial
- cultural or spiritual

Examples of Specific Nursing Diagnoses
1. Body image disturbance related to paraplegia.
   Body image disturbance related to paraplegia as evidenced by client statement, "I used to be the top forward on the basketball team. Thought maybe I could make the pros. Now look at me—an invalid!" (PES format)
2. Body image disturbance related to loss of breast.
   Body image disturbance related to loss of breast as evidenced by client refusal to look at surgical wound and statement, "Now I'm one of those lopsided people you see at the beach." (PES format)

Examples of Specific Outcomes
1. Client will verbalize the loss of use of legs and the associated feelings before discharge.
2. Client will verbalize the changes in his life related to paralysis by discharge.
3. Client will realistically assess own strengths and limitations by discharge from rehabilitation therapy.
4. Client will look at surgical wound and participate in self-care prior to discharge.

Examples of Specific Nursing Interventions
- See General Self-Esteem Nursing Interventions, page 419.
- Evaluate effect of changed body on the developmental stage of client and within client's culture.
- Recognize that anger and/or hostility expressed by client is part of the grieving process, not directed personally.
- Remain with client despite anger/hostile verbalizations and accept this as an indication that client is needing support.
- Assess interaction of client with family and/or significant others. If client is using maneuvers to distance self from

loved ones, support family during this period and encourage them to continue to support client.

- Support client/family members in the grief process.
- Assist family members to promote client's independence by encouraging self-care despite a natural tendency to "do for" the client.
- Verbalize for client what the surgical wound or changed body part looks like.
- Encourage client to view and touch the changed body part.
- Encourage client to participate in self-care, with progressive independence.
- Assist family to respond to client's changed body in healthy ways that promote growth such as modifying the home environment to maximize independence of the client.
- Encourage client to verbalize effects of changed body on lifestyle, plans, future.
- Encourage client to dress in street clothes (rather than hospital attire, if appropriate), use makeup (if usually does).
- Assist client to maintain contact (use of telephone) with friends during hospitalization.
- Assist client to identify alterations needed at home prior to discharge.
- Recognize that adaptation to change in body is a process that will not be complete at discharge from hospital so make appropriate referral to community health care providers including counseling or therapy if indicated.
- Coordinate interdisciplinary team meeting to assist client in planning posthospital care.
- Identify appropriate community support groups and offer to make the initial contact for the client.

Examples of Specific Evaluations for Outcome 2

1. Outcome not met. Client refuses to talk about loss of use of legs, "This is not permanent. I'll work hard and I'll be walking again in a year."
2. Outcome partially met. Client talks about paraplegia but refuses to acknowledge any lifestyle changes.
3. Outcome met. Client states, "This will change a lot of plans in my life and it will take some time and some help

to think through how to deal with it all. My family is right there for me though!"

Key Index Words for Nursing Interventions
Look up these words in the index of fundamentals and medical-surgical nursing textbooks to find page references for additional nursing interventions and rationale for their selection:

- anger/hostility
- developmental stage of client
- grief and loss
- growth and development
- nonverbal behavior
- paraplegia
- quadriplegia
- rehabilitation
- vocational counseling

PERSONAL IDENTITY DISTURBANCE

Definition
Inability to distinguish between self and nonself.

Defining Characteristics
To be developed by NANDA. This nursing diagnosis requires further development. The present authors refer students to a related nursing diagnosis, Altered Thought Processes.

SELF-ESTEEM DISTURBANCE

Definition
Negative self-evaluation/feelings about self or self-capabilities, which may be directly or indirectly expressed.

Defining Characteristics
- self-negating verbalizations
- expression of shame/guilt
- evaluates self as unable to deal with events
- rationalizes away/rejects positive feedback and exaggerates negative feedback about self
- hesitant to try new things/situations
- denial of problems obvious to others
- projection of blame/responsibility for problems
- rationalizing personal failures
- hypersensitive to being slighted or criticism
- grandiosity

Examples of Specific Nursing Diagnoses

1. Self-esteem disturbance related to inability to cope with stressful academics and social life of college.

   Self-esteem disturbance related to inability to cope with stressful academics and social life of college as evidenced by failing grades, unsatisfying social interactions and client statement, "Everyone else can handle this and even enjoy it but I can't! Guess I just don't have what it takes." (PES format)

2. Self-esteem disturbance related to chronic illness (congestive heart failure) and treatment regimen.

   Self-esteem disturbance related to chronic illness (congestive heart failure) and treatment regimen as evidenced by client statement, "I'm incapable of doing anything. I can't handle the demands of my job or do anything for my family." (PES format)

Examples of Specific Outcomes

1. Client will make positive statement of ability to succeed in college within 1 week.
2. Client will be able to accept compliment without adding self-negative response by discharge.
3. Client will make positive statement of self-regard prior to discharge.

Examples of Specific Nursing Interventions

- Match interventions to related factors causing self-esteem disturbance.
- See General Self-Esteem Nursing Interventions, page 419.
- Nursing interventions focus on the therapeutic use of self. Begin by considering own sense of self-esteem and how it affects own ability to work with clients.
- Consider impact of client's culture on self-esteem (e.g., are men supposed to be dominant and in control?)
- Convey unconditional positive regard by listening with understanding and responding nonjudgmentally.
- Express interest in client by active listening.
- Assess history of self-esteem disturbance. Are there identifiable precipitating factors causing or contributing to the problem?

- Assess potential for suicide or other destructive behavior. "Have you ever thought about harming yourself? Do you have a plan?" If answer is yes, report to physician.
- Use of nontask-oriented touch to convey caring such as touching the shoulder of a client who begins to cry.
- Offer self-affirming messages.
     "You are not alone. Many clients I have worked with feel this way."
     "You are going through some very difficult times."
     "I like your honesty in acknowledging your feelings."
     "You handled that well."
- Offer the hospitalized client the opportunity to control aspects of environment to increase sense of competence.
     "How would you like this done?"
     "When would you like your treatment?"
- Discuss past strategies for coping with stress that client has used and assist client to evaluate their effectiveness.
- Assist client to write a list of personal strengths and limitations.
- Ask whether client wishes to change any aspects of the listing. Use this as a beginning plan to assist the client in behavioral changes.
- Identify one specific current stressor the client is experiencing. List coping strategies which have been unsuccessful and work with client on new strategies to use.
- Assist client to select alternative coping strategies and develop a plan to implement a new strategy. For example, plan for learning a study skill to decrease exam stress, plan to schedule evening with a friend, plan to prioritize the demands of job and limit work to 40 hours per week.
- Set a time for evaluation of plan with client and modify as necessary.
- Teach alternative coping strategies to meet the need of specific situation: delegation, time management, physical exercise, decision-making process.
- Identify sources of interpersonal support: family members/significant others, health professionals, peers, colleagues.
- Assist client to "repeople" environment with persons who are supportive and positive (as opposed to individuals who "drag you down").

Examples of Specific Evaluations for Outcome 1
1. Outcome not met. Client states, "I'll probably be just another college dropout."
2. Outcome partially met. Client states, "I did do well in English but that's an easy course anyone can do well in."
3. Outcome met. Client states, "It was a tough adjustment going from high school to college but I think I can make it now. There's an academic support center on campus and I've an appointment for some extra help."

Key Index Words for Nursing Interventions
Look up these words in the index of fundamentals and medical-surgical nursing textbooks to find page references for additional nursing interventions and rationale for their selection. For diagnoses related to self-esteem it is also helpful to consult psychiatric nursing textbooks.

- culture
- depression
- lethality assessment
- nonverbal communication
- self-esteem
- suicide
- withdrawal

CHRONIC LOW SELF-ESTEEM

Definition
Long-standing negative self-evaluation/feelings about self or self capabilities.

Major Defining Characteristics
Long-standing or chronic
- self-negating verbalization
- expressions of shame/guilt
- evaluates self as unable to deal with events
- rationalizes away/rejects positive feedback and exaggerates negative feedback about self
- hesitant to try new things/situations

Minor Defining Characteristics
- frequent lack of success in work or other life events
- overly conforming, dependent on other's opinions
- lack of eye contact
- nonassertive/passive
- indecisive
- excessively seeks reassurance

Examples of Specific Nursing Diagnoses

1. Chronic low self-esteem related to history of comparison to achievements of older sibling.

   Chronic low self-esteem related to history of comparison to achievements of older sibling as evidenced by client statement, "Nothing I do is ever good enough. I could never equal anything my brother did so I quit trying." (PES format)

2. Chronic low self-esteem related to birth deformity of right foot.

   Chronic low self-esteem related to birth deformity of right foot as evidenced by client's statement, "All my life people have avoided me because I can't keep up with my bad leg. I can't face new situations or new people." (PES format)

Examples of Specific Outcomes

1. Client will verbalize own understanding of causative factors associated with chronic low self-esteem prior to discharge.
2. Client will identify and record in writing one successful accomplishment each day prior to discharge.
3. Client will make contract to stop self-negating verbalizing prior to discharge.

Examples of Specific Nursing Interventions

- Match interventions to related factors causing self-esteem disturbance.
- See General Self-Esteem Nursing Interventions, page 419, and Specific Nursing Interventions for Self-Esteem Disturbance.
- Focus on the therapeutic use of self. Begin by considering own sense of self-esteem and how it affects own ability to work with clients.
- Because this self-esteem problem is long-standing, it is probably quite resistant to change and progress will be in small steps. However, the client who is suffering a great deal of psychological pain may be ready for help and able to make rapid progress.
- Assess client's readiness to change and learn new behavior patterns: "It sounds like you've been feeling badly about yourself for some time. I wonder if you would like to work on changing how you feel about yourself?"

■ Assist client to identify factors causing low self-esteem: "I notice that you seem to have a hard time saying anything good about yourself or accepting compliments. I wonder why that is? Could you tell me how that came to be?"
■ Verbalize specific positive feedback to client.

> "I notice you did XXX very well."
>
> "That was especially thoughtful of you to do XXX."
>
> "You were very patient over something that usually irritates me."

■ Engage the client in a contract not to verbalize self-negations (as this tends to make them "real") but to focus on "I" statements: "I feel...when that happens." The goal here is to recognize the feeling without giving power to the negative verbalization. It is also important that the client does not use statements like "You make me feel...when you do that." The "you" statements give the power of control over one's feelings to another person.
■ Assist client to make a written list of own strengths.
■ Assist client to identify potential strengths to develop: "If I could respond to stress any way I want, I think I would like to..."
■ Develop a plan to teach client identified coping skills.
■ Encourage use of a journal in which client records one successful accomplishment that day. Review journal weekly to verbalize progress. Later the journal habit can be expanded to include other entries.
■ Provide opportunity for client to rehearse positive behavior by role playing with nurses or other clients. Discuss the feelings encountered during the role play and explore alternative ways of handling the situation.
■ Involve family/significant others in supporting the process of self-change for client.
■ Observe family/significant other interaction; provide feedback and seek validation: "I notice when client is speaking, there are frequent interruptions. I wonder if this is how you usually communicate?"
■ Assist client to share feelings with family/significant others.

> "Can you tell your mother how it feels when you are talking and she interrupts you?"

"Can you tell your father how you feel when he says, 'When Tom was your age he...'"
■ Reinforce client efforts at expression of direct communication.
■ Acknowledge family/significant other's willingness to participate and communication efforts as well as the difficulty of the efforts: "It is difficult to talk about some of these things and I appreciate the great effort you are making to be here and to work on communication."
■ Identify other sources of support or continued therapy for client posthospitalization.

Examples of Specific Evaluations for Outcome 1

1. Outcome not met. Client refuses to discuss feelings and states, "It's just the way I am."
2. Outcome partially met. Client able to discuss feelings of low self-esteem but states, "Nothing caused it. It's just in the genes."
3. Outcome met. Client talked about factors associated with his low self-esteem and commented, "Wow, I certainly listened to other people a lot and gave them a lot of power, didn't I?"

Key Index Words for Nursing Interventions

Look up these words in the index of fundamentals and medical-surgical nursing textbooks to find page references for additional nursing interventions and rationale for their selection. For diagnoses related to self-esteem it is also helpful to consult psychiatric nursing textbooks.

■ family coping
■ family communication patterns
■ family functioning
■ family systems theory
■ family therapy

See also:
  Self-Esteem Disturbance

SITUATIONAL LOW SELF-ESTEEM

Definition

Negative self-evaluation/feelings about self which develop in response to a loss or change in an individual who previously had a positive self-evaluation.

Major Defining Characteristics
- episodic occurrence of negative self-appraisal in response to life events in a person with a previous positive self-evaluation
- verbalization of negative feelings about the self (helplessness, uselessness)

Minor Defining Characteristics
- self-negating verbalizations
- expressions of shame/guilt
- evaluates self as unable to handle situations
- difficulty making decisions

Examples of Specific Nursing Diagnoses
1. Situational low self-esteem related to loss of job.
   Situational low self-esteem related to loss of job as evidenced by client statement, "I always thought people liked me and that I was doing a good job and now I find out I really wasn't any good." (PES format)
2. Situational low self-esteem related to recent divorce.
   Situational low self-esteem related to recent divorce as evidenced by client statement, "I feel like such a failure. I couldn't even keep a marriage together and everyone tells me he seemed to be the nicest man in the world. It had to be my fault." (PES format)

Examples of Specific Outcomes
1. Client will assess factors contributing to own termination from job within 48 hours.
2. Client will develop a plan, assisted by a nurse, to pursue a new job within 1 week.
3. Client will complete written list of strengths and achievements in all areas of life: family, social, work, community within 1 week.
4. Client will agree to counseling with the goals of getting rid of feelings of blame or guilt from the divorce within 1 week.

Examples of Specific Nursing Interventions
- See General Self-Esteem Nursing Interventions, page 419.
- Focus on the therapeutic use of self. Begin by considering own sense of self-esteem and how it affects own ability to work with clients.

- See Specific Nursing Interventions for Self-Esteem Disturbance and Chronic Low Self-Esteem.
- The interventions for this nursing diagnosis focus on the immediate situation causing the low self-esteem. Because the nursing diagnosis is of shorter duration and the person had a previously healthy sense of self-esteem, maximize the capabilities and independence of the client in seeking solutions.
- Assist client to assess factors causing the low self-esteem in a written format.
- Identify person client trusts who will work with client to enhance self-esteem and who will be the one person to whom negative feelings will be verbalized. This approach helps to contain the negativism of the situation and leave other spheres of functioning intact.
- Assist client to identify alterable factors.
- Having identified the factors within client's control, assist the client to make a plan to begin to resolve the causative factors.
- Assist client by providing resources or information.
- Work with client to identify all areas of life in which client functions: community services groups, a career, recreation, church, family, etc. Then, within each of these spheres encourage client to write down own contributions over the years, successes, and friends made. It may be helpful to compile this list in a chronological order. This list is then reviewed as a strategy for coping with negative feelings.
- Encourage the client to maintain social relationships and circle of friends.

Examples of Specific Evaluations for Outcome 1

1. Outcome not met. Client refuses to talk about situation.
2. Outcome partially met. Client talks about loss of job but can only identify unsatisfactory performance.
3. Outcome met. Client indicates several factors contributing to own low self-esteem, "It's not only the loss of this job. I could see that coming with the merger and the decreased sales volumes. But I don't have a good education, I don't have the new computer skills I need to get another job. And I'm afraid I will have to begin at a lower salary this time."

Key Index Words for Nursing Interventions
Look up these words in the index of fundamentals and medical-surgical nursing textbooks to find page references for additional nursing interventions and rationale for their selection. For diagnoses related to self-esteem it is also helpful to consult nursing textbooks.

- coping skills
- crisis intervention
- problem-solving process
- self-esteem
- time-limited therapy

Chapter 22

Violence Problems

FOCUSED ASSESSMENT GUIDE

Complete this focused assessment if a general nursing assessment indicates a possible problem. Then turn to page 434 of this text for the Data $\Rightarrow$ Diagnosis Matching Guide for Violence problems to help you select the best nursing diagnosis to match the client's data.

SUBJECTIVE ASSESSMENT

___ Have you ever been so depressed you felt that life wasn't worth living?

___ Have you ever thought about harming yourself?

___ Have you ever thought about committing suicide?

___ Do you think about harming yourself or committing suicide now?

___ Have you a plan? What is your plan?

___ Have you ever cut/scratched/hurt yourself on purpose?

___ Have you ever been accused of a crime? What was the crime? When did this occur? What were the circumstances?

___ Have you ever hit anyone in anger? Who? When? Under what circumstances?

___ Do members of your family settle arguments by physically fighting?

___ Have you ever experienced a major trauma like a car crash, fire, earthquake, life-threatening illness, or injury?

___ Do you ever have nightmares or flashbacks about it?

___ Who are the persons you feel close to, go to for support?

____ Have you a will? Have you recently made a new will? Have you changed an insurance policy? Have you recently given away a prized possession?

____ Has the client reported a rape?

____ Has the client/spouse/boyfriend reported sudden change in sexual behavior?

____ Have you any fears that started recently and suddenly?

OBJECTIVE ASSESSMENT

____ Is the client making threats, clenching fists?

____ Is the client pacing, restless, agitated, crying?

____ Is the client throwing objects, smashing furniture?

____ Has the client been drinking, using drugs?

DATA ⇒ DIAGNOSIS MATCHING GUIDE

Compare your client data from the Violence Focused Assessment to these nursing diagnoses and abbreviated descriptions related to violence. Select the nursing diagnosis which is the best match. Then turn to the page in this section with that specific diagnosis for help in planning care.

1. High Risk for Self-Mutilation: page 436
- definition: individual is at high risk to injure (not kill) self producing tissue damage and tension relief
- risk factors: females age 16–25 years with borderline personality disorder; psychotic clients; battered children; inability to cope with tension; feelings of depression, rejection

2. High Risk for Violence: Self-Directed or Directed at Others: page 439
- definition: individual experiences behaviors that can harm self or others
- risk factors: clenched fists, angry speech, increased motor activity; prior incidents of violence; possession of weapons; suspicious of others; substance abuse

3. Post-trauma Response: page 443
- definition: sustained painful response to overwhelming traumatic event

- data: reexperiences the event in nightmares, dreams, flashbacks; verbalizes survival guilt; altered lifestyle in negative direction; irritable; explosive

4. *Rape-Trauma Syndrome: page 446*
   - definition: the trauma syndrome that occurs as a result of rape
   - data:
     acute phase: anger, fear, and multiple physical symptoms
     long-term: change in lifestyle, nightmares, seeking support

5. *Rape-Trauma Syndrome Compound Reaction: page 450*
   - definition: the trauma syndrome that occurs as a result of rape added to preexisting psychiatric or physical illness or substance abuse
   - data: as in rape plus reactive symptoms of previous illness or substance abuse

6. *Rape-Trauma Syndrome Silent Reaction: page 452*
   - definition: the trauma that occurs as a result of rape but without the verbalization of the rape
   - data: abrupt changes in relationships with men; changes in sexual behavior; onset of phobic reactions

GENERAL OUTCOMES AND NURSING INTERVENTIONS

GENERAL VIOLENCE OUTCOMES

- Client will acknowledge traumatic event and effect on life
- Client will not harm self or others.
- Client will learn appropriate ways of dealing with anger.
- Client will identify sources of help in dealing with emotional pain and anxiety.
- Client will participate in therapy specific to the identified problems.
- Client will seek medical treatment for problems associated with the violence.
- Client will establish interpersonal relationships which foster mental health.

GENERAL VIOLENCE NURSING INTERVENTIONS

These interventions require expertise and specialized nursing care. Often care providers who have skills beyond those of an entry-level nurse are consulted. The novice nurse has two considerations in providing nursing care. First, the nurse keeps communication open, provides support, and affirms client self-esteem. Secondly, the nurse seeks the consultation of a skilled clinician or refers to the appropriate professional.

- Establish trusting, interpersonal, therapeutic relationship with client.
- Reaffirm client sense of self-esteem and worthiness.
- Provide safe environment where client is unable to harm self, other clients or staff.
- Provide psychologically secure environment for clients who have been victims of violence.
- Provide contact with sources of legal assistance as appropriate.
- Seek consultations with other health care professionals.
- Identify need for long-term therapy and provide referrals.
- Identify and provide contact with sources of community support.

RELATED NURSING DIAGNOSES

HIGH RISK FOR SELF-MUTILATION

Definition
A state in which an individual is at high risk to perform an act upon the self to injure, not to kill, which produces tissue damage and tension relief.

Risk Factors
Groups at risk:

- clients with borderline personality disorder, especially females aged 16–25 years
- clients in psychotic state—frequently males in young adulthood
- emotionally disturbed and/or battered children
- mentally retarded and autistic children
- clients with a history of self-injury

- history of physical, emotional, or sexual abuse
- inability to cope with increased psychological/physiological tension in a healthy manner
- feelings of depression, rejection, self-hatred, separation, anxiety, guilt, and depersonalization
- fluctuating emotions
- command hallucinations (e.g., voices tell client to do something)
- need for sensory stimuli
- parental emotional deprivation
- dysfunctional family

Examples of Specific Nursing Diagnoses
1. High risk for self-mutilation related to history of childhood sexual abuse.
2. High risk for self-mutilation related to mental retardation.
3. High risk for self-mutilation related to lack of impulse control.
4. High risk for self-mutilation related to past episodes of harmful behavior.

Examples of Specific Outcomes
1. Client will remain safe from physical harm throughout hospitalization.
2. Client will verbalize understanding of own self-mutilating behaviors prior to discharge.
3. Client will verbalize feeling state immediately preceding episode of self-mutilation before discharge.
4. Client will learn and use alternative activities to provide tension release prior to discharge.

Examples of Specific Nursing Interventions
These clients require highly specialized nursing care. A clinical nurse specialist or psychiatric nurse is often consulted even if the client is in the hospital with a medical or surgical condition. The staff nurse assesses the client and thoroughly documents all observed behaviors as a starting point of intervention.

- See General Violence Nursing Interventions, page 436.
- Provide a safe environment for client. Every environment

contains some objects which may be potentially dangerous to client. Do a room check to assure there are no weapons, glass objects, ropes, razor blades, silverware, shoelaces, or other objects that could be harmful to the client.

- The client may need to be temporarily placed in restraints to prevent self-harm. Review hospital rules for the application of restraints: who may authorize them, frequency of checks, required documentation.
- Administer medication as ordered.
- Assure that visitors do not bring anything to the client without having it first checked by a nurse. Visitors may be unaware of the potential risk of objects they bring to a client.
- Establish trusting therapeutic relationship with client. This may be done in very small steps and may be very difficult.
- Make careful physical assessment and medication history as physical conditions and medications could cause symptoms of mental illness.
- Observe client every 15 minutes (at least) or require client to be in area where intense observation is possible; it may be necessary to place client on suicide precautions which require constant observation.
- Introduce No Harm contract to client; both nurse and client sign.
- Assist client to verbalize feelings and to identify situations/events/persons which precede self-harm episodes.
- Teach client alternative tension-reducing strategies; provide opportunities to practice them within safe hospital environment.
- Provide for physical activity as release for tension. Identify activities the client likes and plan for inclusion into routine.
- Ask whether client ever hears voices or sees things that other people cannot; ask whether client is hearing/seeing them now and if so, talk with client to try to redirect cognitive involvement.
- Provide for psychiatric consult if client is not admitted to a psychiatric unit.
- Provide for discharge planning which includes continued therapy and medication.

Examples of Specific Evaluations for Outcome 1
1. Outcome not met. Client scratched lower legs until bloody while in bed.
2. Outcome partially met. Client had one attempted episode of self-harm in past 24 hours and nurse intervened.
3. Outcome met. Client has no episodes of self-harm and asked nurse for help when feeling desire to harm self.

Key Index Words for Nursing Interventions
Look up these words in the index of fundamentals and medical-surgical nursing textbooks to find page references for additional nursing interventions and rationale for their selection. For this diagnosis it will also be helpful to consult textbooks of psychiatric nursing.

- antisocial personality disorder
- borderline personality disorder
- dementia
- delusion
- hallucination
- illusion
- mood disorder
- No Harm contract
- psychological abuse
- sexual abuse
- suicide

HIGH RISK FOR VIOLENCE: SELF-DIRECTED OR DIRECTED AT OTHERS

Definition
A state in which an individual experiences behaviors that can be physically harmful either to the self or others.

Defining Characteristics
Presence of risk factors such as:

- body language: clenched fists, tense facial expression, rigid posture, tautness indicating effort at control
- hostile, threatening verbalization: boasting to or prior abuse of others
- increased motor activity
- pacing, excitement, irritability, and agitation
- overt and aggressive acts: goal-directed destruction of objects in environment
- possession of destructive means: guns, knives, or other weapons

- rage
- self-destructive behavior, active aggressive suicidal acts
- suspicion of others
- paranoid ideation, delusions, and hallucinations
- substance abuse/withdrawal

Other Possible Characteristics
- increased anxiety level
- fear of self or others
- inability to verbalize feelings
- repetition of verbalizations: continued complaints, requests, or demands
- anger
- provocative behavior (argumentative, dissatisfied, over-reactive, hypersensitive)
- vulnerable self-esteem
- depression (specifically active, aggressive, suicidal acts)

Related Factors
- antisocial behavior
- battered women
- catatonic excitement
- child abuse
- manic excitement
- organic brain syndrome
- panic states
- rage reactions
- suicidal behavior
- temporal lobe epilepsy
- toxic reactions to medication

Examples of Specific Nursing Diagnoses
1. High risk for self-directed violence related to psychotic state.

   High risk for self-directed violence related to psychotic state accompanied by delusions and hallucinations, "The voices are telling me what to do." (PES format)
2. High risk for violence directed at others related to lack of impulse control and attention deficit hyperactivity disorder.

   High risk for violence directed at others related to lack of impulse control and attention deficit hyperactivity disorder as manifested by sudden outbursts of rage, throwing furniture, knowledge of karate. (PES format)

Examples of Specific Outcomes

1. Client will not injure self or others throughout hospitalization.
2. Client will sign contract not to harm self within 48 hours.
3. Client will recognize situations or factors which signal approaching outbursts or loss of control within 1 week.
4. Client will take medication as prescribed and begin a daily log evaluating the effect of the medication within 48 hours.

Examples of Specific Nursing Interventions

These clients often require highly specialized nursing care. A clinical nurse specialist or psychiatric nurse is often consulted even if the client is in the hospital with a medical or surgical condition. The staff nurse assesses the client and thoroughly documents all observed behaviors as a starting point of intervention.

- See General Violence Nursing Interventions, page 436.
- First assure client's safety. The client may need to be temporarily placed in restraints, in a seclusion room, or medicated in order to decrease the risk of violence. Review hospital rules for the application of restraints: who may authorize them, frequency of checks, required documentation.
- Provide a safe environment for the client: do a room check to assure there are no weapons, glass objects, ropes, razor blades, silverware, shoelaces, or other objects that could be used to harm self/others.
- Assure that visitors do not bring anything to the client without having it first checked by a nurse. Visitors may be unaware of the potential risk of objects they bring to a client.
- Establish trusting therapeutic relationship with client. This needs to be done in very small steps and may be very difficult.
- Complete a physical assessment and medication history since both physical conditions and medications could cause symptoms of mental illness.

- Medicate client as ordered and assure client actually takes medication. It may be necessary to check the client's mouth to assure oral medication has been swallowed.
- Secure scheduled order for medication rather than prn in effort to prevent destructive behavior.
- Observe client every 15 minutes (at least) or require client to be in area where intense observation is possible; it may be necessary to place client on suicide precautions which require constant observation.
- Introduce No Suicide contract (or No Harm contract) to client; both nurse and client sign.
- Assist client to verbalize feelings and to identify situations/events/persons which precipitate violent feelings.
- Teach client alternative coping strategies and offer opportunities to practice them within safe hospital environment.
- If client is becoming increasingly agitated, decrease stimuli within the situation, talk in short sentences, low voice, slow speech, do not touch client, attempt to redirect client attention.
- If physical intervention or restraint is necessary follow procedure of hospital and assure there are adequate numbers of trained staff. This intervention requires practiced teamwork and must be directed by a leader who acts decisively and calmly.
- After physical intervention and the client is again in control, work with client to identify alternative behaviors and ways of handling violent feelings.
- Ask whether client ever hears voices or sees things that other people cannot; ask whether client is hearing/seeing them now and if so, talk with client to try to redirect cognitive involvement.
- Provide for psychiatric consult if client is not on a psychiatric unit.
- Provide for discharge planning which includes continued therapy and medication.

Examples of Specific Evaluations for Outcome 1
1. Outcome not met. Client attempted to scratch wrist with broken plastic cup.

2. Outcome partially met. Client safe on unit but talking about hurting self after discharge.
3. Outcome met. Client remained safe throughout hospitalization and did not harm others.

Key Index Words for Nursing Interventions
Look up these words in the index of fundamentals and medical-surgical nursing textbooks to find page references for additional nursing interventions and rationale for their selection. For this diagnosis it will also be helpful to consult textbooks of psychiatric nursing.

- crisis intervention
- delusion
- hallucination
- illusion
- impaired reality testing
- lethality assessment
- manic behavior
- mood disorder
- physical management
- schizophrenia
- seclusion and restraint
- suicide
- suicide precautions

POST-TRAUMA RESPONSE

Definition
The state of an individual experiencing a sustained painful response to an overwhelming traumatic event(s).

Major Defining Characteristics
- reexperience of traumatic event which may be identified in cognitive, affective, and/or sensory motor activities (flashbacks, intrusive thoughts, repetitive dreams or nightmares, excessive verbalization of traumatic events, verbalization of survival guilt or guilt about behavior required for survival)

Minor Defining Characteristics
- psychic/emotional numbness (impaired interpretation of reality, confusion, dissociation or amnesia, vagueness about traumatic event, or constricted affect)
- altered lifestyle (self-destructiveness, such as substance abuse, suicide attempt, or other acting-out behavior, difficulty with interpersonal relationship, development of phobia regarding trauma, poor impulse control/irritability, and explosiveness)

Related Factors
- disasters, wars, epidemics, rape, assault, torture, catastrophic illness, or accident

Examples of Specific Nursing Diagnoses
1. Post-trauma response related to military duty in the Persian Gulf War.
   Post-trauma response related to military duty in the Persian Gulf War as evidenced by inability to sleep and recurrent nightmares. (PES format)
2. Post-trauma response related to house fire in which child died.
   Post-trauma response related to house fire in which child died as evidenced by weight loss, irritability, depression, inability to sleep, and client statement, "Why couldn't it have been me? Why do I have to go on living?" (PES format)

Examples of Specific Outcomes
1. Client will be able to discuss the traumatic event with the support of the nurse prior to discharge.
2. Client will verbalize the feelings associated with the traumatic event before discharge.
3. Client will be able to identify situations, persons, or events which trigger the emotions associated with the trauma and in role play develop alternative responses to cope with the anxiety prior to discharge.
4. Client will practice sleep hygiene plan and be able to sleep uninterrupted for at least 6 hours per day within 1 month.

Examples of Specific Nursing Interventions
These clients often require highly specialized nursing care. A clinical nurse specialist or psychiatric nurse may be consulted even if the client is in the hospital with a medical or surgical condition. The staff nurse assesses the client and thoroughly documents all observed behaviors as a starting point of intervention.

- See General Violence Nursing Interventions, page 436.
- Assess for risk of suicide; if so, provide a safe environment for the client, removing all objects client might use for

self-harm. (see Specific Nursing Interventions for High Risk for Violence: Self-Directed).

- Begin suicide precautions if indicated or 15-minute checks for first 24 hours of hospitalization.
- Assess for health conditions that may be contributing to the traumatic stress: chronic pain, disfigurement from the event, stress ulcers, blindness, deafness, sexually transmitted disease (in the case of rape).
- Assure that basic physical human needs are met and client feels safe before proceeding to psychosocial interventions: food, clothing, shelter, warmth. Meet same needs for client's family so client is able to focus on resolving the traumatic stress.
- Assess for substance abuse: alcohol and drugs.
- Make appropriate referral if substance abuse is indicated.
- In daylight, encourage client to verbalize traumatic event; support client in a warm, comforting style, accepting the entire scope of emotions the client describes.
- Assist client to "name" own emotions as the event is relived.
- Support client in expression of anger associated with the event.
- Assist/support client in grieving, if relevant.
- Assess the degree of anxiety client is experiencing and teach alternative coping strategies (see Specific Nursing Interventions for Anxiety).
- Involve family members and significant other in the treatment plan.
- Plan for physical exercise to promote sleep, decrease anxiety, and as a possible outlet for anger.
- Medicate as ordered: hypnotics, antidepressants, anti-anxiety medications.
- Plan with client for a sleep hygiene routine to promote sleep (see Specific Nursing Interventions for Sleep Pattern Disturbance).
- Identify community support group for persons with similar experiences.
- Anticipate a recurrence of emotions associated with the event on the anniversary of the event or at holiday times when a deceased member would ordinarily be present. Assist client to plan coping strategies for these times.

Examples of Specific Evaluations for Outcome 1

1. Outcome not met. Client declines to discuss the event stating, "It hurts too much."
2. Outcome partially met. Client describes the traumatic event but recounts it chronologically and without any emotion.
3. Outcome met. Client describes military duty in the Gulf War and sobs while telling of a wounded 20-year-old friend crying for help when the client was unable to get to him.

Key Index Words for Nursing Interventions

Look up these words in the index of fundamentals and medical-surgical nursing textbooks to find page references for additional nursing interventions and rationale for their selection. For this diagnosis it will also be helpful to consult textbooks of psychiatric nursing.

- anxiety
- depression
- guilt
- physical or sexual abuse
- post-trauma response

- psychological abuse
- rape
- substance abuse
- suicide

RAPE-TRAUMA SYNDROME

Definition

Forced, violent sexual penetration against the victim's will and consent. The trauma syndrome that develops from this attack or attempted attack includes an acute phase of disorganization of the victim's lifestyle and a long-term process of reorganization of lifestyle.*

Defining Characteristics

Acute Phase

- emotional reactions (anger, embarrassment, fear of physical violence and death, humiliation, revenge, and self-blame)

---

*This syndrome includes the following three subcomponents: rape-trauma, compound reaction, and silent reaction. In this text, each appears as a separate nursing diagnosis.

- multiple physical symptoms (gastrointestinal irritability, genitourinary discomfort, muscle tension, and sleep pattern disturbance)

Long-Term Phase
- changes in lifestyle (changes in residence)
- dealing with repetitive nightmares and phobias
- seeking family support
- seeking social network support

Examples of Specific Nursing Diagnoses
1. Rape-trauma syndrome (long term phase) related to lack of familial support.
   Rape-trauma syndrome (long-term phase) related to lack of familial support as evidenced by client statement, "I need to tell my family but it is so humiliating..." (PES format)
2. Rape-trauma syndrome (acute phase) related to date rape.
   Rape-trauma syndrome (acute phase) related to date rape as evidenced by emotional reactions, sleep pattern disturbance and by client statement, "I had known John for 2 years before we starting dating. I didn't think he was like this." (PES format)

Examples of Specific Outcomes
1. Client will verbalize understanding of rape as a violent crime and own part as faultless victim within 1 week.
2. Client will maintain physical health with no sexually transmitted disease or genitourinary infections within 3 months.
3. Client will identify persons in own environment that would be supportive and share own experience with them in the next 2 weeks.
4. Client will resume usual lifestyle within 1 week.
5. Client will agree to attend support group for victims of rape within 1 week.

Examples of Specific Nursing Interventions
These clients often first present at the emergency room (ER) where they may or may not be accompanied by a police officer. The ER nurse needs to be well trained to provide the specialized care required by this client. A clinical nurse specialist or psychiatric nurse may be consulted if additional

intervention is indicated.

- See General Violence Nursing Interventions, page 436.
- On presentation at ER triage, show client to a room immediately as this is a medical and psychological emergency.
- Establish a trust relationship with the client, talking slowly and soothingly.
- Explain each examination procedure to client and indicate that you will be with her through each step of the process. Most clients find this a very difficult time and psychological support and maintaining the privacy of the client is crucial.
- Do a head-to-toe physical assessment noting any evidence of trauma: bruises, rectal tears, hematoma, fractures.
- Document if client has bathed prior to the examination.
- Do a mental status examination using both objective and subjective data: ability to follow directions, response to questions, evidence of depression, suicidal ideation, confusion, self-blame, availability of family/other interpersonal support for client.
- Assess individual response to the trauma, not making any assumptions about how the victim should behave.
- Assess current coping strategies and evaluate for health impact: denial, anger, hysterics, intellectualization, substance abuse.
- Ask the client if there is anyone she would like the nurse to call to be with her.
- Offer to call rape counselor who will remain with the client.
- Reinforce that the client is a victim of a crime.
- Maintain chain of custody of evidence (nail clippings, vaginal smears, clothing, etc); obtain samples, seal and witness the collection, and never let it out of sight until turned over to police officer. It is not sufficient to lock evidence in a safe; it must be held on person without interruption until it is turned over to police.
- Teach client about sexually transmitted diseases and possibility of pregnancy, and pregnancy prevention, and the follow-up required. Many victims will be unable to attend to teaching at this time so it is important to provide them with written instructions for follow-up.

- Assure client has a safe place to return to after treatment. If the client indicates this is a problem, consult a social worker for assistance.
- During the long-term phase, assist client to work through anger and feelings of guilt/responsibility.
- Assist the client to reestablish healthy relationships with men.
- Refer to mental health specialist (psychiatrist, psychologist, clinical nurse specialist, psychiatric social worker) for additional therapy.
- Offer to put in contact with community support group and survivors of rape.
- Assist client to develop a sleep hygiene/physical exercise program to promote rest.
- Discuss strategies to prevent rape.

Examples of Specific Evaluations for Outcome 1

1. Outcome not met. Client states, "I should not have walked home alone. It was my fault."
2. Outcome partially met. Client states, "In my head I know that I'm not at fault, but I could have prevented it."
3. Outcome met. Client states, "I have a right to walk at night and I'm going to press criminal charges."

Key Index Words for Nursing Interventions

Look up these words in the index of fundamentals and medical-surgical nursing textbooks to find page references for additional nursing interventions and rationale for their selection. For this diagnosis it will also be helpful to consult textbooks of psychiatric nursing.

- depression
- pregnancy prevention
- rape
- self-esteem
- sexually transmitted disease (STD)
- suicide
- violence
- pregnancy prevention

RAPE-TRAUMA SYNDROME: COMPOUND REACTION

Definition
Forced, violent sexual penetration against the victim's will and consent. The trauma syndrome that develops from this attack or attempted attack includes an acute phase of disorganization of the victim's lifestyle and a long-term process of reorganization of lifestyle.*

Defining Characteristics
Acute Phase
- emotional reactions (anger, embarrassment, fear of physical violence and death, humiliation, revenge, and self-blame)
- multiple physical symptoms (gastrointestinal irritability, genitrourinary discomfort, muscle tension, and sleep pattern disturbance)
- reactivated symptoms of previous conditions (e.g., physical illness, psychiatric illness)
- reliance on alcohol and/or drugs

Long-Term Phase
- changes in lifestyle (changes in residence)
- dealing with repetitive nightmares and phobias
- seeking family support
- seeking social network support

Examples of Specific Nursing Diagnoses
1. Rape-trauma syndrome: compound reaction related to previous recent rape.
   Rape-trauma syndrome: compound reaction related to recent rape as evidenced by recurrence of previous alcohol problem. (PES format)
2. Rape-trauma syndrome: compound reaction related to recent rape.
   Rape-trauma syndrome: compound reaction related to recent rape with recurrence of previously unresolved depression as evidenced by remaining in home, not going

---

*This syndrome includes the following three subcomponents: rape-trauma, compound reaction, and silent reaction. In this text, each appears as a separate nursing diagnosis.

to job, withdrawing from friends and family, complaining, "I just can't do anything. I have no energy." (PES format)

Examples of Specific Outcomes

1. Client will join/rejoin Alcoholics Anonymous while hospitalized and plan continued participation before discharge.
2. Client will remain safe from physical injury throughout hospitalization.
3. Client will identify three alternative strategies for coping with anxiety and practice them during hospitalization.
4. Client will verbalize positive self-esteem prior to discharge.

Examples of Specific Nursing Interventions

Clients with this diagnosis are often seen some time after the rape has occurred. Unsuccessful attempts to deal with the anxiety associated with the rape have resulted in substance abuse or recurrence of previously resolved mental or physical illness.

- See Specific Nursing Interventions for Rape Trauma Syndrome.
- See General Violence Nursing Interventions, page 436.
- Assess for potential of self-harm.
- Provide a safe environment for client: remove dangerous objects and provide for psychological security by providing consistency of caregivers and a planned therapeutic routine.
- Identify sources of community support and offer to initiate the first contact with the identified group.
- Assist client to verbalize unresolved feelings.
- Assist client to recognize the relationship between recurrence of substance abuse/mental illness/physical illness and the rape.
- Support client to develop understanding of own part as victim of a violent crime and therefore not to blame.
- Assist family/significant others to understand client's feelings and to offer support.
- Assist client to identify situations that may trigger feelings of anxiety related to the rape and to deal with those issues within therapy sessions.
- Refer for substance abuse treatment evaluation.

Examples of Specific Evaluations for Outcome 1
1. Outcome not met. Client denies substance abuse problem.
2. Outcome partially met. Client acknowledges a connection between the rape and substance abuse but refuses to attend AA meetings stating, "I did that once and look at all the good it did me."
3. Outcome met. Client has rejoined AA and states, "I think I can make it one day at a time. They never give up on you."

Key Index Words for Nursing Interventions
Look up these words in the index of fundamentals and medical-surgical nursing textbooks to find page references for additional nursing interventions and rationale for their selection. For this diagnosis it will also be helpful to consult textbooks of psychiatric nursing.

- anxiety
- defense mechanisms
- depression
- phobias
- pregnancy prevention
- rape
- self-esteem
- sexually transmitted disease (STD)
- substance abuse
- suicide
- violence

RAPE-TRAUMA SYNDROME: SILENT REACTION

Definition
Forced, violent sexual penetration against the victim's will and consent. The trauma syndrome that develops from this attack or attempted attack includes an acute phase of disorganization of the victim's lifestyle and a long-term process of reorganization of lifestyle.*

Defining Characteristics
- abrupt changes in relationships
- increase in nightmares
- increased anxiety during interview (e.g., blocking of

*This syndrome includes the following three subcomponents: rape-trauma, compound reaction, and silent reaction. In this text, each appears as a separate nursing diagnosis.

associations, long periods of silence, minor stuttering, and physical distress)
■ pronounced changes in sexual behavior
■ no verbalization of the occurrence of rape
■ sudden onset of phobic reactions

Examples of Specific Nursing Diagnoses
1. Rape-trauma syndrome: silent reaction related to blaming self for the rape.
   Rape-trauma syndrome: silent reaction related to blaming self for the rape as evidenced by abrupt breakup with fiancé, and increased anxiety, and statement, "I can't even tell him what happened. How can I marry him?" (PES format)
2. Rape-trauma syndrome: silent reaction related to lack of knowledge of how to obtain help.
   Rape-trauma syndrome: silent reaction related to lack of knowledge of how to obtain help as evidenced by client statement, "I knew I needed help but I didn't know what to do." (PES format)

Examples of Specific Outcomes
1. Client will verbalize understanding that she was the victim of a violent crime and tell fiancé about the crime prior to discharge.
2. Client will verbalize positive sense of self-esteem prior to discharge.
3. Client will maintain/regain physical health within 1 month.
4. Client will join community support group for survivors of rape within 2 weeks.

Examples of Specific Nursing Interventions
These clients are usually seen some time after the rape has occurred. It is important that they are not made to feel guilty for not reporting the rape promptly. When they are seen, they may be experiencing the failure of coping mechanisms for dealing with the anxiety generated by the rape. These clients require caring support and assessment for Compound Rape-Trauma Reaction, in addition to the interventions for Rape-Trauma Syndrome. Please see the nursing diagnoses: Rape-Trauma Syndrome and Rape Trauma Syndrome: Compound Reaction for nursing interventions.

Examples of Specific Evaluations for Outcome 1
1. Outcome not met. Client states, "I can't talk to him about this, it's too humiliating."
2. Outcome partially met. Client states, "I really want to tell him but I have to think about what to say. It really is a horrible crime."
3. Outcome met. Client states, "I told my fiancé about it and he was wonderful. He said he loves me more than ever and will help me to heal and survive this crime."

Key Index Words for Nursing Interventions
Look up these words in the index of fundamentals and medical-surgical nursing textbooks to find page references for additional nursing interventions and rationale for their selection. For this diagnosis it will also be helpful to consult textbooks of psychiatric nursing.

- anxiety
- defense mechanisms
- depression
- pregnancy prevention
- self-esteem
- sexually transmitted disease (STD)
- substance abuse
- suicide
- violence

References and Bibliography

Ackley, B., Ladewig, G. (1993). *Nursing Diagnosis Handbook: A Guide to Planning Care*. St. Louis: Mosby.

Acute Pain Management Guideline Panel (February, 1992). *Acute Pain Management: Operative or Medical Procedures and Trauma. Clinical Practice Guidelines.* AHCPR Pub. No. 92-0032, Rockville, MD: Agency for Health Care Policy and Research, Public Health Serivce, U.S. Department of Health and Human Services.

Acute Pain Management Guideline Panel (February, 1992). *Acute Pain Management in Adults: Operative Procedures. Quick Reference Guide for Clinicians.* AHCPR Pub. No. 92-0019, Rockville, MD: Agency for Health Care Policy and Research, Public Health Service, U.S. Department of Health and Human Services.

Acute Pain Management Guideline Panel (February, 1992). *Acute Pain Management in Infants, Children and Adolescents: Operative and Medical Procedures. Quick Reference Guide for Clinicians.* AHCPR Pub. No. 92-0020, Rockville, MD: Agency for Health Care Policy and Research, Public Health Service, U.S. Department of Health and Human Services.

Agency for Health Care Policy and Research (April, 1993). *Depression in Primary Care: Clinical Practice Guidelines.* Rockville, MD: Agency for Health Care Policy and Research, Public Health Service, U.S. Department of Health and Human Services.

Agency for Health Care Policy and Research (April, 1993). *Depression is a Treatable Illness: A Patient's Guide.*

455

Rockville, MD: Agency for Health Care Policy and Research, Public Health Service, U.S. Department of Health and Human Services.

Agency for Health Care Policy and Research (May, 1992). *Pressure Ulcers in Adults: Prediction and Prevention. Clinical Practice Guidelines.* Rockville, MD: Agency for Health Care Policy and Research, Public Health Service, U.S. Department of Health and Human Services.

American Pain Society (1992). *Principles of Analgesic Use in the Treatment of Acute Pain and Cancer Pain* (3rd ed.) Skokie, IL: American Pain Society.

American Nurses Association (1991). *Standards of Clinical Nursing Practice.* Washington: American Nurses Association, NP-79 20M 12/91.

American Nurses Association (1980). *A Social Policy Statement.* Washington: American Nurses Association.

Carpenito, L. (1993). *Nursing Diagnosis: Application to Clinical Practice* (5th ed.). Philadelphia: J.B. Lippincott.

Carroll-Johnson, R., Paquette, M. (eds.) (1994). *Classification of Nursing Diagnoses: Proceedings of the Tenth Conference.* North American Nursing Diagnosis Association. Philadelphia: J.B. Lippincott.

Craven, R., Hirnle, C. (1992). *Fundamentals of Nursing: Human Health and Function.* Philadelphia: J.B. Lippincott Company.

Food Guide Pyramid (August 1992). Home and Garden Bulletin, No. 252. U.S. Department of Agriculture.

Guyton, A. (1991). *Textbook of Medical Physiology* (8th ed.). Philadephia: W.B. Saunders Co.

Herr, K., Mobily, P. (June, 1992). Interventions related to pain. *Nursing Clinics of North America* **27**(2):347–371.

Jacox, A., Carr, D.B., Payne, R., et al. (March, 1994). *Management of Cancer Pain. Clinical Practice Guideline No. 9.* AHCPR Pub. No. 94-0592, Rockville, MD: Agency for Health Care Policy and Research, U.S. Department of Health and Human Services, Public Health Service.

Jacox, A., Carr, D.B., Payne, R., et al. (March, 1994). *Management of Cancer Pain: Adults. Quick Reference Guide for Clinicians.* No. 9. AHCPR Pub. No. 94-0593, Rockville, MD: Agency for Health Care Policy and

Research, U.S. Department of Health and Human Services, Public Health Service.

Kozier, B., Erb, G., Olivieri, R. (1991). *Fundamentals of Nursing: Concepts, Process and Practice* (4th ed.). Redwood City, CA: Addison-Wesley Nursing.

Long, B.C., Phipps, W.J., Cassmeyer, V.L. (1993). *Medical-Surgery Nursing: A Nursing Process Approach.* (3rd ed.). St. Louis: C.V. Mosby.

Lyke, E.M. (1992). *Assessing for Nursing Diagnosis.* Philadelphia: J.B. Lippincott.

McCaffery, M. (Winter, 1993). *Confidence in Cancer Pain Management.* Los Angeles, CA 90045: Margo McCaffery.

McCaffery, M., Beebe, A. (1989). *Pain: Clinical Manual for Nursing Practice.* St. Louis: C.V. Mosby.

McFarland, G., McFarlane, E. (1993). *Nursing Diagnosis & Intervention.* (2nd ed.). St Louis: C.V. Mosby.

McKenna, M. (Winter, 1991). Patient discharge outcome audits: improving quality and reducing cost. *Definition* **6**(1):1,3.

Metheny, N. (1992). *Fluid and Electrolyte Balance* (2nd ed.). Philadelphia: J.B. Lippincott.

Murray, M., Atkinson, L. (1994). *Understanding the Nursing Process: The Next Generation* (5th ed.). New York: McGraw-Hill.

NANDA (1992). *NANDA Nursing Diagnosis; Definitions and Classification 1992–1993.* Philadelphia: North American Nursing Diagnosis Association.

Olds, S., London, M., Ladewig, P. (1992). *Maternal-Newborn Nursing: A Family Centered Approach* (4th ed.). Redwood City, CA: Addison-Wesley Nursing.

O'Toole, M. (ed.) (1992). *Miller-Keane Encyclopedia & Dictionary of Medical, Nursing, & Allied Health* (5th ed.). Philadelphia: W.B. Saunders.

Smeltzer, S., Bare, B. (1992). *Brunner and Suddarth's Textbook of Medical-Surgical Nursing.* (7th ed.), Philadelphia: J.B. Lippincott.

Taylor, C., Lillis, C., LeMone, P. (1993). *Fundamentals of Nursing.* (2nd ed.). Philadelphia: J.B. Lippincott.

Thompson, J.M., Mcfarland, G.K., Hirsch, J.E., Tucker, S.M. (1993). *Mosby's Clinical Nursing.* St. Louis: C.V. Mosby.

Urinary Incontinence Guideline Panel (March, 1992). *Urinary Incontinence in Adults: Clinical Practice Guidelines.* AHCPR Pub. No. 92:0038. Rockville, MD: Agency for Health Care Policy and Research, Public Health Services, U.S. Department of Health and Human Services.

Vitas Healthcare Corporation (1992). *Pain Management Formulary.* Miami: Vitas Healthcare Corporation of Florida.

Wilson, H.S., Kneisl, C.R. (1992). *Psychiatric Nursing.* (4th ed.). Redwood City, CA: Addison-Wesley.

Woodyard, L., Sheetz, J. (October, 1993). Critical pathway patient outcomes: The missing standard. *Journal of Nursing Care Quality* **8**(1):51–57.

Zander, K. (1992). Critical pathways. In: Melum, M., and Sinioris, M. (eds.) *Total Quality Management,* Ch. 9. Chicago: American Hospital Association.

Zander, K. (Fall, 1988). Why managed care works. *Definition* **3**(4):1–3.

Zander, K. (September, 1988). Nursing case management; Resolving the DRG paradox. *Nursing Clinics of North America* **23**(3):503–520.

Zander, K. (May–June, 1992). Focusing on patient outcomes: case management in the 90's. *Dimensions of Critical Care Nursing* **11**(3):127–129.

Zander, K. (Fall, 1992). Quantifying, managing and improving quality, Part III: Using variance concurrently. *The New Definition* **7**(4):1–4.

APPENDIX

Case Management/Clinical Pathway Examples*

*All examples are from the Battle Creek Health System, Battle Creek, MI, and are reproduced with permission.

Battle Creek Health System
300 North Avenue
Battle Creek, MI 49016

DRG 089
Expected LOS 6–8 Days

Date Initiated ___/___/___ Time _____

PATIENT DATA

COMPLICATED PNEUMONIA

	Initial	ADMISSON / SURGERY 0 – 24 hrs	DAY 1 24 – 48 hrs Date	DAY 2 48-72 hrs Date	DAY 3 Date	DAY 4 Date	DAY 5 Date
Unit		Medical					
Tests	___ ___ ___ ___	CBC c̄ diff. ___ Blood C&S x2 MDG / Chem I ___ CXR UA ___ ABG or Pulse O Sputum C&S ___ PPD		___ CBC c̄ diff ___ Chem I ___ Consider CXR 48° p̄ Adm		___ CBC c̄ diff ___ CXR (early AM c̄ report prior to discharge)	
Meds	___ ___ ___	IV / Helplock IV Antibiotics ----------- as indicated <aminophylline> < steroids> IV -----------	___ If PO intake adeq -----------	Theodur ↑ Prednisone ↑	Begin PO antibiotic 24° prior to DC	
Consults	___ ___ ___	Pharmacist Resp Care to eval for approp tx Physical Therapy evaluation			___ Consider Pulmonologist if not improving		
Diet	___	Dietary Consult or DAT -----------			NPO if bronch		
Treatments	___ ___ ___	VS q 4° / 8° --------------- I & O ---------------- O2 -----------------		DC O2 per order ↑	↑	↑	↑

				Review isolation needs
	Assess lung sounds q 4° / 8° ⟶			
	C&DB q 4° ⟶			
	Assess need for respiratory isolation			
	Respiratory tx			
Activity	Bedrest / ↑ HDB BRP Act as tolerated	↑ Chair Amb in Room as tol	Amb c̄ assist BID or >	Amb as tol
Teaching	C&DB ⟶ Medications / procedures ⟶ Review clinical path c̄ patient or significant other			
Discharge Planning	Medical Social Work referral Current Living Environment_____	Assessment	Identify discharge plan	Case conference if indicated

*Nursing initials q shift

Clinical Path / Care Plans **DO NOT** represent a standard of care—they are guidelines for consideration which may be modified according to the individual patient's needs

INITIALS			
	Signature		Signature
	Signature		Signature
	Signature		Signature

CLINICAL PATHWAY / PATIENT CARE PLAN

om #N-7003   7/94   Page 1 of 4

Battle Creek Health System
300 North Avenue
Battle Creek, MI 49016

PATIENT DATA

	DAY 6 Date____	DAY 7 Date____	DAY 8 Date____	DAY 9 Date____	DAY 10 Date____	DAY 11 Date____	DAY 12 Date____	DAY 13 Date____
Unit	Medical							
Tests								
Meds								
Consults								
Diet	___DAT							
Treatments Procedures	___VS q 4⁸ / 8⁸ ___I&O ___Assess Lung sounds ___C&DB							

Activity	Amb as tol							
Teaching	C&DB Medications Prevision Signs /symptoms Early intervention							
Discharge Planning								

Clinical Path / Care Plans **DO NOT** represent a standard of care—they are guidelines for consideration which may be modified according to the individual patient's needs

INITIALS

INITIALS	Signature		INITIALS	Signature
	Signature			Signature
	Signature			Signature

xm #N-7003 7/94   Page 2 of 4

CLINICAL PATHWAY / PATIENT CARE PLAN

Battle Creek Health System
300 North Avenue
Battle Creek, MI 49016

PATIENT DATA

DRG 089 COMPLICATED PNEUMONIA

PROBLEMS IDENTIFIED *(Date & initial)*

_____ 1. Altered respiratory function

_____ 2. Altered nutritional status

_____ 3. Altered activity

_____ 4. Alteration in fluid volume

_____ 5. Lack of knowledge

_____ 6.

_____ 7.

OUTCOMES *(Date & initial)*

_____ 1. Improved ventilation & oxygenation WNL for pt

_____ 2. Tolerates diet unl for pt.

_____ 3. Activity as tolerated WNL for pt

_____ 4. Demonstrates fluid balance

_____ 5. Verbalizes understanding of medication, disease process & tx

_____ 6.

_____ 7.

COMMENTS / PATIENT COMPLICATION OR COMORBIDITIES

PATIENT EDUCATION

(Date & initial to indicate the following has been reviewed with the pt/significant other and they verbalize understanding)

___ 1. Patients instructed in the importance of:

    a. Keeping HOB up and frequent movement while in bed

    b. Increasing activity

    c. Oral hygiene

    d. Using purse lip breathing during periods of SOB

Clinical Path / Care Plans **DO NOT** represent a standard of care—they are guidelines for consideration which may be modified according to the individual patient's needs

INITIALS		INITIALS	
	Signature		Signature
	Signature		Signature
	Signature		Signature

CLINICAL PATHWAY / PATIENT CARE PLAN

orm #N-7003   7/94   **Page 3 of 4**

BATTLE CREEK HEALTH SYSTEM
300 NORTH AVENUE – BATTLE CREEK, MI 49016

Patient Name _____   DRG 127 DX Congestive Heart Failure

Nurse Coordinator _____   Date Activated _____

Physician _____

STAMP HERE

	adm	Day 1	Day 2	Day 3	Day 4	Day 5 – 6
UNIT	Critical Care vs Med–Surg	If in Critical Care consider transfer to Med–Surg				DC
TESTS	CXR EKG ABG/Pulse Ox CBC Chem I	Chem I Pulse Ox if > 90% consider DC O2 then repeat Pulse Ox p̄ 15min on room air - - - - →	Chem I	Repeat CXR	Chem I	
NURSING/ ACTIVITY/ TREATMENTS	VS q̄ 4° I/O VS q̄ 2° if PCU Daily weights - - - → O2 per order - - - → Foley per order→ Telemetry per order - - - - → ↑ HOB	VS q̄ 8° I/O - - - - - - - - → Consider DC per order Consider DC	Refer to Pulse Ox DC per order			

ACTIVITY	BR c̄ BRP Encourage rest during 1st hour p̄ meals Provide rest periods between activities Freq position chgs	↑ Activity, as tolerates			
MEDS	Diuretics IV/Heplock ------>	Consider Oral Meds	Oral Meds D/C Heplock		
DIET	Low Na limit fluids per order				
DISCHARGE PLANNING	Referral to Social Services	Psychosocial Assessment	Validate needs for home care (notify VNS)	Finalize home care plan	DC
TEACHING	Make appropriate referrals Discuss care plan c̄ pt & SO	Begin CHF Educ Dietary teaching for Sodium/K+ and/or fluid restrict		Reinforce diet and home care instructions	
CONSULTS	Referrals to Dietary/Card Hlth				
PROGRESS CORRESPONDS TO CLINICAL PATH	Date & Sign Daily				

*Indicates variance, see reverse side.

Discharge Date _____ Total LOS _____ M/S _____ PCU _____ ICU _____

mdr(drg127)   CLINICAL PATH/PATIENT CARE PLAN

FORM # N-2018 (1 of 4) 5/92

NN-9-30

* Key:
1. Patient

Admission Date: _____
Discharge Date & Time: _____
Actual LOS: _____

DATE	VARIATION	* CAUSE	KEY	ACTION TAKEN	SIGNATURE

VARIANCE REPORT FORM DRG 127

FORM # N2018 (2 of 4)

BATTLE CREEK HEALTH SYSTEM
300 NORTH AVENUE – BATTLE CREEK, MI 49016

CONGESTIVE HEART FAILURE – DRG 127

stamp here

DATE OR REVIEW/INITIAL:

PATIENT PROBLEM	Day 1	Day 2	Day 3	4	5	6	7
		OUTCOMES					
1. ↓ CO/Fluid volume excess		VS WNL for patient ↓ Dyspnea & angina ↑ U.O. and ↓ weight Maintain UO > 1000cc/24 hours - - - - - - - →		Dysrhythmia absent/ controlled Free of skin breakdown Free of S & Sx of failure Documented weight loss > 5#			
Date Initiated							
Date Resolved							
2. Activity intolerance			Activity ↕: ↑ HR > 10 BPM ↑ dysrhythmia S & Sx of CHF	Activity level/ADLS maintained/regained			
Date Initiated							
Date Resolved							
3. Impaired gas exchange		Pulse ox/ABGs WNL for patient		Lungs clear to auscultation O2 disconnected			

Date Initiated			
Date Resolved			
4. Knowledge Deficit. (After instruction pt. and/or SO will state importance of O2)	Report: Palpitations, ↑ SOB, Chest Pain	Verbalizes under-standing of disease process medications treatments and condition	Demonstrate ability to take pulse
Date Initiated			
Date Resolved			
5.			
Date Initiated			
Date Resolved			

Signature _____

Signature _____

❷

PATIENT CARE PLAN

* Date & Initial

c:\123r31\DRG\127PCP

FORM # N-2018 (1/93)
   .3 of 4

DRG 127 – Congestive Heart Failure

stamp here

DESCRIPTION	DATE INITIATED*	DATE DISCONTINUED*

1. Assess
  A. Lung sounds for rales q _____ °
  B. Tissue perfusion, edema, JVD q _____ °
  C. Call UO < _____		

2. Daily weight		
3. Assess response to activity/ADLs daily		
4. Turn q 2° while on BR		
5. C & DB vs IS q _____ °		
6. Skin care q _____ ° Reduce pressure on boney prominces ↑ edematous extremities		
7. Other		

	DATE OF INSTRUCTION*	RETURN DEMONSTRATION VERBALIZES INSTRUCTION DATE & INITIAL*

8. Education
   A. Avoid activity which causes shortness of breath and/or fatigue
   B. Weigh yourself daily and keep records
   C. Avoid exposure to communicable disease (ie, colds, flu)
   D. Arrange for rest periods during day between activities
   E. Do not sit with legs crossed
      Keep feet elevated when sitting for long periods of time
   F. Notify physician if
      1. Shortness of breath, fatigue, chest pain and/or pressure
         with normal activity or at rest
      2. Increased swelling, especially of feet, ankles, hands
         and/or abdomen
      3. Weight gain of 2 – 3 lbs for two or more consecutive days
      4. Increased coughing and/or production of sputum
      5. Decrease urinary output
      6. Nail bed and/or lips are blue or purple in color
      7. Rapid heart rate and/or palpitations

Signature

*Include your initials after date. ©

c:\123\31\DRG\127SNI   **STANDARD NURSING INTERVENTIONS**

FORM # N–2018 (1/93)

BATTLE CREEK HEALTH SYSTEM
300 NORTH AVENUE
BATTLE CREEK, MI 49016

Patient Name _____   DRG 209 DX Total Joint (Knee or Hip)

Nurse Coordinator _____

Date Activated _____   Physician _____

	PAT	adm SURG	HD1 PO 1	HD2 PO 2	HD3 PO 3	HD4 PO 4	HD5 PO 5
UNIT		SDS/OPS	Ortho				
TESTS	CBC diff EKG UA MDG Sed Rate Pro time PTT T&C 2u CXR (lat CS if RA)	PAT results on chart	Protime qd if on Coumadin →→→→→ H & H Chem I	H & H	H & H		
NURSING TREATMENTS		Ted hose as ordered →→→ Foley prn →→→ Hemovac →→→		D/C D/C	chg drsg		
ACTIVITY		PT evaluation & TX	Stand at bedside	Walker amb sit as tol in Total Hip Chair	act as tol →→→→→→→→→→		

stamp here

NN-9-30

MEDS	IV -----→ Ancef Gm 1 q 8° x 24–48° Coumadin or aspirin Protocol	D/C & Heplock x 24° ---------→ D/C ----------↑ Consider oral pain meds		
DIET	clr liq post op	dat ---------		
DISCHARGE PLANNING	Information packet sent 6 weeks prior Telephone interview	Social Services re-evaluation	Finalize transfer plans	SWMRH transfer or DC
TEACHING		Rev & reinforce PT precautions--------		
CONSULT	Anesthesia SWMRH PT evaluation OT evaluation	Dr Chamberlin	OT evaluation & TX ----------	
PROGRESS CORRES- PONDS TO CLINICAL PATH	Date & Initial Daily			

*indicates variance, see reverse side.

Discharge Date _____ Total LOS _____

mdr(DRG 209)

	M/S	PCU	ICU
	CLINICAL PATH – PATIENT CARE PLAN		

FORM # N-2001   (5/92)

* Key:
1. Patient

Admission Date: _____
Discharge Date & Time: _____
Actual LOS: _____

DATE	VARIATION	* CAUSE	KEY	ACTION TAKEN	SIGNATURE

VARIANCE REPORT FORM DRG 209

BATTLE CREEK HEALTH SYSTEM
300 NORTH AVENUE
BATTLE CREEK, MI 49016

stamp here

TOTAL JOINT/FRACTURED HIP – DRG 209/210

DATE OF REVIEW/INITIAL _____

PATIENT PROBLEM	Day 1	Day 2	Day 3	Day 4–7
		OUTCOMES		
1. Alteration in skin integrity				Evidence of wound healing No sign of infection Patient free of skin breakdown
Date Initiated				
Date Resolved				
2. Potential for impaired gas exchange		Lungs clear to auscultation		
Date Initiated				
Date Resolved				
3. Fluid volume deficit	Moist mucous membrane	H & H WNL Chem I WNL		Vital signs are WNL
Date Initiated				
Date Resolved				
4. Alteration in comfort			Verbalizes decreased pain with activity Relief of discomfort with oral meds	
Date Initiated				

PATIENT CARE PLAN

	Date Resolved
5. Knowledge deficit	Verbalizes under-standing of positioning & precautions / Weight bearing limitation
Date Initiated	
Date Resolved	
6. Alteration in elimination bowel/bladder	Voiding without difficulty. Bowel movement prior to discharge
Date Initiated	
Date Resolved	
7. Impaired tissue perfusion	Palpable pulses without c/o numbness in affected extremity Skin warm/dry
Date Initiated	
Date Resolved	
8. Impaired mobility	Maximize Mobility Potential
Date Initiated	
Date Resolved	

Signature

Date & Initial

123|31|DRG|209|pcp

FORM # N-2001 (12/92)

BATTLE CREEK HEALTH SYSTEM
300 NORTH AVENUE
BATTLE CREEK, MI 49016

STANDARD NURSING INTERVENTIONS
DRGs 209 and 210

stamp here

DESCRIPTION	DATE INITIATED/INITIALS	DATE DISCONTINUED/INITIALS
1 Cough and deep breathe q 2 hours		
2 Turn q 2 – 3 hours		
3 Assess skin condition q shift A Order pressure reduction mattress PRN B Consult Enterostomal Therapy Nurse PRN		
4 Encourage fluids		
5 Check pedal pulses q shift		
6 Elevate legs PRN for pressure relief		

	DATE OF INSTRUCTION	RETURN DEMONSTRATION/ VERBALIZES INSTRUCTION DATE/INITIAL
7 Education		

A Use of Incentive Spirometer

B Explain
  1—TED Hose
  2—Ice
  3—Pain management
  4—Constavac/Drains
  5—Positioning and Abduction Pillow
  6—Hip precautions
  7—Ankle exercises (Dorsi/Plantar Flexion)

C Remove TED stockings at least once daily

D Sleep with abduction pillow between legs (Joint Replacement pts)

E Elevate legs slightly while sitting

F Report the following
  1—Pain, redness, warmth
  2—Swelling, redness, drainage from incision
  3—Unexplained fever greater than 101

Signature

Key:
Include your initials after date.

c:123r31\drg\209sni

STANDARD NURSING INTERVENTIONS

Alphabetized Listing of Nursing Diagnoses

Index

ISBN 0-07-105466-9

9 780071 054669